The Social Policy of the AKP toward the Kurds

Culture, Society and Political Economy in Turkey

Isabel David and Kumru Toktamiş
General Editors

Vol. 1

İlker Cörüt

The Social Policy of the AKP toward the Kurds

Healthcare Provision in Hakkâri
(2003–2014)

PETER LANG
Lausanne • Berlin • Bruxelles • Chennai • New York • Oxford

Library of Congress Cataloging-in-Publication Control Number: 2022047545

Bibliographic information published by the **Deutsche Nationalbibliothek**.
The German National Library lists this publication in the German
National Bibliography; detailed bibliographic data is available
on the Internet at http://dnb.d-nb.de.

Cover design by Peter Lang Group AG

ISSN 2832-1367 (print)
ISSN 2832-1359 (online)
ISBN 978-1-4331-9576-1 (hardcover)
ISBN 978-1-4331-9578-5 (ebook pdf)
ISBN 978-1-4331-9579-2 (epub)
DOI 10.3726/b19533

© 2023 İlker Cörüt
Peter Lang Group AG, Lausanne
Published by Peter Lang Publishing Inc., New York, USA
info@peterlang.com - www.peterlang.com

All rights reserved.
All parts of this publication are protected by copyright.
Any utilization outside the strict limits of the copyright law, without the permission of the
publisher, is forbidden and liable to prosecution.
This applies in particular to reproductions, translations, microfilming, and storage and
processing in electronic retrieval systems.

This publication has been peer reviewed.

To my father, Abdullah Cörüt

Table of Contents

List of Figures	xi
List of Tables	xiii
Preface	xv
Acknowledgements	xxiii
List of Abbreviations	xxvii

1	Introduction	1
	1.1 Research Objective	5
	1.2 Theoretical Framework	6
	1.3 Fieldwork: Field and Methodology	17
	1.4 Overview	36
2	The Kurdish Question, Sovereign Violence, and Hakkâri	43
	2.1 Historical Background of the Kurdish Question	43
	2.2 Sovereign Violence and State Incapacity	46
	2.3 Dehumanization: Sovereign Violence and the Official Discourse on Kurds	55
	2.4 Sovereign Violence in Hakkâri	58
	2.5 Privatization of Sovereignty in Hakkâri	73
	2.6 Conclusion	77

3 Indirect State Racism, Healthcare Provision, and Hakkâri — 83
　3.1 Indirect State Racism — 85
　3.2 Indirect State Racism toward Hakkâri: Not an Ethnic Phenomenon? — 88
　3.3 Poverty of Healthcare Provision as Indirect State Racism toward Hakkâri — 94
　3.4 Conclusion — 124

4 Turkish Nationalism, the Kurdish Question, and Hakkâri: Discourses and Practices, 2003–2014 — 131
　4.1 The AKP: From Conservative Democracy to Authoritarian Conservatism — 132
　4.2 The AKP and the Kurdish Question — 134
　4.3 The AKP's Turkish Nationalism — 137
　4.4 The AKP's Turkish Nationalism and Hakkâri — 151
　4.5 The Limits of the AKP's Turkish Nationalism in Hakkâri — 163
　4.6 Conclusion — 167

5 The Persistence of Patient Dissatisfaction as a Mass Phenomenon — 173
　5.1 Dissatisfaction with Healthcare Provision in Hakkâri: A Mass Phenomenon — 176
　5.2 An Analysis of Dissatisfaction with Healthcare Provision in Hakkâri — 183
　5.3 Conclusion: Dissatisfaction as Citizenship versus Turkishness — 221

6 The Compulsory Public Service of Doctors (CPSD) in Hakkâri — 229
　6.1 CPSD, the Production of National Space, and the Kurdish Question — 230
　6.2 Unitary Theory of Space as a Key to Understanding Doctors in Hakkâri — 233
　6.3 Production of Space as Endurance: Nothing to Be Discovered, but a Bundle of Problems to Be Passively Managed — 234
　6.4 The Production of Hakkâri as Endurance as the Outcome of a Trialectical Relationship — 236
　6.5 Essentialist and Discriminatory Discourses and Practices of the Doctors — 257
　6.6 An Exception: Nursing and Midwifery Professionals — 269
　6.7 Conclusion — 273

7 Discussion   279
  7.1 Patient Dissatisfaction and Essentialist Discourses as Limits of Turkish State-Nationalism   280
  7.2 The Issue of the Rationality of Ethnopolitical Challenges: Gains and Losses   285

Appendix   295
Bibliography   301
Index   317

List of Figures

Figure 1a.	Regional Location of Hakkâri.	19
Figure 1b.	The Province and Main Settlements of Hakkâri.	19
Figure 2.	Rural and Urban Population in Hakkâri (1965–2000).	22
Figure 3.	Kicking Garbage or Cursing His Fate? A Man Wanders the Hakkâri City Neighborhood of Keklikpınar, Formed by Village Evacuees.	23
Figure 4.	Showing the Effects of Tear Gas (Hakkâri City).	34
Figure 5.	A Shanty Hut Filled with Smuggled Fuel (Şemdinli).	63
Figure 6a.	Public Expenditure Per Capita (Education, Public Works, Health, Agriculture) between 1946 and 1960.	91
Figure 6b.	Public Investment Per Capita between 1963 and 1981.	91
Figure 6c.	Public Investment Per Capita between 1982 and 2002.	92
Figure 7a.	The Ratio of 0-4 Age Group Mortalities to All Mortalities (Hakkari and Nationwide, Urban Settlements).	118
Figure 7b.	The Ratio of 0-1 Age Group Mortalities to All Mortalities (Hakkari and Nationwide, Urban Settlements).	118
Figure 8.	The Ratio of Mortalities from Pneumonia, Enteritis and Other Diarrheal Diseases, and Perinatal Mortalities Combined to All Mortalities in Hakkâri, 1975–2005 (Urban Settlements).	120

List of Figures

Figure 9.	From "How Happy is the One Who Calls Himself a Turk" to "Peace at Home, Peace in the World."	144
Figure 10a.	Old Central Health Post in Şemdinli (opposite the Şemdinli Public Hospital).	156
Figure 10b.	New Central Health Post in Şemdinli.	157
Figure 11a.	Responses to the Statement on Hakkâri Public Hospital: "I'm Fairly Satisfied with the Healthcare Provision at Hakkâri Public Hospital."	182
Figure 11b.	Responses to the Statement on Hakkâri Public Hospital: "I Do not Have Any Significant Complaints About Hakkâri Public Hospital."	183
Figure 12.	The Level of Satisfaction of Hakkârians with Healthcare Provision.	183
Figure 13.	Responses to the Statement "I Trust the Diagnosis Made by the Doctors in Hakkâri Public Hospital."	188
Figure 14.	Responses to the Statement "I Always Trust the Results of Tests and X-Ray, Ultrasound and MR Imaging."	189
Figure 15.	Responses to the Statement "I am Fairly Satisfied with the Healthcare Provision of Hakkâri Public Hospital."	190
Figure 16.	Hakkâri Public Hospital Wall Panel: "The Philanthropists Making Donations to Our Hospital."	193
Figure 17.	Responses to the Statement "Some of the Behavior and Actions of the Doctors and Nurses at Hakkâri Public Hospital Sometimes Lead Me to Think that I am not Paid Satisfactory Attention because I am Kurdish."	204
Figure 18.	Responses to the Statement "Doctors in Hakkâri Public Hospital Approach Patients Whose Turkish is Better in a Markedly Better Way."	205
Figure 19.	Children Watching Clashes between Demonstrators and the Police.	251
Figure 20.	Yüksekova Central Health Post-2.	271

List of Tables

Table 1.	Healthcare Provision in Hakkâri, 2002 and 2010	3
Table 2.	Population of Hakkâri Districts and Province in 1891 by Religious Belonging	21
Table 3.	Illiteracy Rate in Southeastern Anatolia Region and Hakkâri, 1950–1990 (%)	47
Table 4.	Proportion of Kurdish Population in Kurdish Provinces, 1935–1990 (%)	48
Table 5.	Provincial Proportions of Villages with Electricity, Telephone, and Road and of Rural Population in Kurdish Provinces at the end of 1983 (%)	49
Table 6.	Number of Banned Uplands and Meadows in Hakkâri	73
Table 7.	Health Workforce in Hakkâri (Numbers of State Professionals Employed, Five-Yearly), 1955–2005	95
Table 8.	Performance of Hakkâri Health Center, 1956–1967	110
Table 9.	Performance of Hakkâri Public Hospital, 1968–1980	111
Table 10.	Performance of Hakkâri Public Hospital, 1981–2002	112
Table 11.	TT Vaccination Coverage for Hakkâri and Turkey (%), 1996–1999	122

Table 12.	Measles Vaccination Coverage for Hakkâri and Turkey (%), 1997–2002	123
Table 13.	Progressive Rates of Increase in Nominal Public Investment in the Kurdish Provinces and the Rest of the Country in 2003–13 (index: 2003=100)	139
Table 14.	PKK Guerillas Killed Yearly in Military Operations, 2003–2016	148
Table 15.	Progressive Rates of Increase in Nominal Public Investment in Hakkâri, Kurdish Provinces, and the Rest of the Country (index: 2003=100), 2003–2013	152
Table 16.	Surgical Operations Performed in Hakkâri Public Hospital (by category), between 1995 and 2013	153
Table 17.	Performance of Hakkâri Public Hospital, 1995–2013	155
Table 18.	Maternal and Child Health Services in Hakkâri, 1996–2014	158
Table 19.	Immunization Rates in Hakkâri and Turkey, 1996–2012	159
Table 20.	Hakkârian PKK Guerillas Killed, 2003–2014	160
Table 21.	Gender and Age Composition of the Sample and Hakkâri City (%)	179
Table 22.	Educational Background of the Sample and Hakkâri City (%)	180
Table 23.	The Level of Out-Patient Satisfaction with Hakkâri Public Hospital, March 2013	186

Preface

This research focuses on the period 2003–14, which was exceptional in the history of the Turkish Republic for its radical shift in the official, government stance adopted toward Kurds and the "Kurdish problem" (*Kürt sorunu*). What made this radical shift possible was the election and coming to power of an Islamist-oriented party, the Justice and Development Party (Adalet ve Kalkınma Partisi, AKP), which opened the gates to a new era in Turkish politics, reshaping its norms and institutions and the composition of leading cadres.

The pre-AKP period of the Republic—or "Kemalist Turkey"—had been characterized by a normative allegiance to bourgeois-secular civilization, privileged place of the military as the guardian of the political system, and intolerance for Kurdish ethnic claims. Thus, other than during partial exceptions in the early and late 1990s prompted by the European Union (EU) membership process, Turkish governments had never really had a Kurdish policy. Rather, they had addressed the Kurdish problem as an issue of public order, security, and state sovereignty.

Recently, the post-2014 period of the AKP has seen a return and replication of Kemalist norms in another reduction of Turkey's Kurdish issue to counterinsurgency, now with a highly developed military and surveillance capacity. From the point of view of the AKP today, the ethnic and social rights of Kurds have been restored—by the AKP governments—so there is no longer any Kurdish question worth mentioning.

The 2003–14 period is thus specified here by the AKP's governance and approach to the Kurdish issue. It includes and extends the AKP's early "golden period" to the time when it entered into and then backed away from its "Kurdish Opening," diluted and renamed a "Democratic Opening." Despite all the policy fluctuations, the hopes and tragedies and missed opportunities—from the original foregrounding of civil rights in the EU-accession process to the Roboski massacre and siege of Kobanê (when Ankara favored the attacking Islamic State over the PKK-linked Kurdish resistance), and through it all the ground-breaking, mostly secret negotiations with Kurdistan Workers' Party (Partiya Karkerên Kurdistanê, PKK) representatives in Oslo culminating in the "Peace" or "Solution Process" (Çözüm Süreci) and open talks with jailed PKK leader Abdullah Öcalan—this period represented a real divergence from the past (as well as from what came after, the post-2014 violence).

Between 2003 and 2014, that is, for first time in the history of the Republic, the Turkish government developed an approach to the Kurdish issue that went beyond oppression and nonengagement, state security considerations, and the dirty war of counterterrorism. Although there were continuing tensions, distrust, and military operations during these years—including lethal PKK attacks in Hakkâri in 2007 and a massive response from the Turkish military in 2008 with an incursion into Iraq to attack PKK bases there—the period overall was one of relative peace and progress. The PKK announced ceasefires and the government began to recognize Kurdish language and cultural rights and seemed to have public opinion more or less on its side, favoring the steps necessary for a resolution (or at least the party's electoral support was strong enough for it to take a calculated political risk).

During this period, the AKP addressed Kurds as equal members of the nation (*millet*), essentially a Muslim one, whose ethnic and social rights had been systematically violated by the secular Kemalist elites alienated from the (Muslim) nation as a whole. The political calculus of the AKP approach was evident. The more the violated ethnic and social rights of Kurds were restored, the smaller would be the grounds for the exploitation of Kurds by the PKK and the more peaceful the state-Kurd relations, the AKP reasoned.

In other words, the overall Kurdish policy of the AKP in 2003–14 was part of a wider agenda of refashioning the nation on an anti-Kemalist, anti-elitist, and essentially pro-Muslim basis. This reconstruction of the nation and state was built on the populist claim to be ending the varying levels of social and cultural exclusion that the religious masses, Kurds, informal employees, and poorly educated rural masses had been subject to as subaltern groups of the Republic.

Although liberatory in many respects, the AKP's Kurdish policy between 2003 and 2014 had many limitations. These account for how the government could so easily slide from a reformist stance (e.g., negotiating with the PKK over an amnesty for its fighters) into a complete counter-insurgency strategy, finally, thus, to make a full circle (with methods recalling the horrifying tactics of the 1990s as that era's village evacuation was now replaced by the military destruction of city centers).

In fact, the AKP's challenge to Kemalist Turkey bore the character of a "passive revolution."[1] It was a passive revolution both because it contained the subaltern opposition to social exclusion and reconciled this with structures of capitalism and also because it sought to satisfy Kurdish demands in order to weaken the Kurdish national movement and consciousness yet without any major concession on the constitutive principles of the Turkish nation-state. To put it in Ranajit Guha's Gramscian terms, the AKP's Kurdish policy between 2003 and 2014 reflected a shift rather than removal of Turkish "dominance" over Kurds, from one without "hegemony" to one with it; in fact, the change in state policy was rather more (just) a shift in its balance or makeup, from coercion outweighing persuasion to persuasion outweighing coercion.[2]

This policy did not work. The AKP failed to establish Turkish hegemony over Kurds and could not suppress the Kurdish national movement. On the contrary, the Kurdish movement reached the peak of its power, with its legal, political representation, the People's Democratic Party (Halkların Demokratik Partisi, HDP) even capturing enough votes nationwide to pass the old 10 percent threshold maintained to keep Kurdish parties out of the parliament in Ankara. Why was this? How was it that even the barely functioning Hakkâri Public Hospital, which for decades had served little better than a large health post, could be upgraded to a fairly well staffed, modern facility as part of a national policy to remove inequities in health provisioning, and yet this seemed not to be appreciated by the local population and did not translate into the expected levels of votes?

This book looks for an explanation of the failure of the Kurdish policy of the AKP by considering the limits of its social policy in instituting a compliant, cooperative, submissive Kurdish subjectivity. To do this, it focuses on the persistence of patient dissatisfaction in Hakkâri, a small Kurdish province in the southeast corner of Turkey, as an example or case study of a widespread phenomenon during the period despite the very considerable improvements to healthcare provision achieved in these years.

I look for the answer in social policy for two reasons. First, social policy was crucial to the AKP's Kurdish strategy; it was effectively instrumentalized by the AKP government to win over the Kurds. In the first decade of AKP rule, one can observe a striking expression of the change in the "organic composition of power"[3] of the state over Kurds. The relative weight of coercive and persuasive elements in the composition of state policy tools in the Kurdish region was shifted away from security measures and militarization and toward the deployment of a social policy, specifically in response to the Kurdish issue. Since the coercive elements had been employed in the securitization approach applied by the Kemalist state forces—the army, primarily—this was actually an entirely logical type of "democratizing" move for the new government. And indeed, the region had suffered from a lack of relevant social programs in Kemalist Turkey, as is evident in the statistics for public investment and social assistance presented in this work.

A second reason to look for the reason for the failure of the AKP social policy approach to win Kurdish "hearts and minds"—one that is mostly overlooked in Turkish and Kurdish studies—concerns the fact that processes of redistribution are intertwined with *recognition*.[4] What occurs during a redistribution of resources involves a realignment of recognition. The relative positions of groups involved are altered, and new hierarchies are built, fortified, or challenged. In other words, an analysis of Turkish hegemonic attempts to incorporate Kurds into the Turkish national body and of Kurdish ethnopolitical resistance to being co-opted in a moment of redistribution needs to go well beyond an analysis of high politics. It must also pay close attention to how subjectivities are instituted and relative positions are taken in everyday processes that are not immediately political. In this respect, I should also acknowledge that one of my basic motivations in this research was my own critical distance from the dominant tendency in discussions in Turkish and Kurdish studies limiting the issue of the recognition of Kurdishness to that of cultural and political rights.

The main focus of this book, patient dissatisfaction in Hakkâri, was also not chosen without reason. My sense was that the nature of the social policy in the Kurdish strategy under the AKP, which comprised much more than a mere distribution of resources and directly pertained to the issues of recognition, subjectivities, and the (re)negotiation of the relative positions of the sides involved, could not be better revealed than through a research study in Hakkâri. This has been among the poorest and most stigmatized and marginalized of the Kurdish provinces throughout the history of the Republic; if social policy were only an issue of resource distribution, the AKP government would have been expected to weaken the Kurdish movement and emerge as the leading political power there, given that the 2003–14 period saw armed combat and deadly incidents at their lowest levels overall since the first clashes between the PKK and the state in the province in the early 1980s.

It would not be an overstatement to argue that Hakkârians could now access a more or less adequate health service in Hakkâri for the first time ever, and this was directly due to the central government policies and investments introduced from 2003. And yet, the electoral base of the AKP in Hakkâri never did expand beyond a third of the electorate, and Hakkâri remained a bastion of the Kurdish national movement throughout the period.

The empirical findings of this study show a widespread persistence of patient dissatisfaction in Hakkâri even after a decade of material improvements that effected a complete major upgrade of the healthcare system. Interpreting this, we need to say that the issue for patients was more a matter of perspective and political subjectivity than of biomedical dissatisfaction. It was a daily symptom of an ethnopolitical resistance to being interpellated by the AKP as citizens-in-the-making who would compare past and present, realize the progress, and thus appreciate the current quality of healthcare provision by tolerating any shortcomings as a minor price to pay for relative material comfort.

This book thus reveals two factors that prevented Hakkârians from subscribing to the AKP transition narrative. One was the history of state-citizen relations in Hakkâri—that is, the firmly established conviction on the part of Hakkârians that their lives counted for little in the eyes of the Turkish state. The other was a strong, egalitarian insistence on the "here and now," which reflects an anticolonial intolerance of any promissory talk of something "in the making" that will fully manifest "later, not now."

It was when I came to finishing the dissertation on which this book is based, in the middle of 2015, that the negotiation process between the PKK and the AKP finally ended. Thereafter, the Turkish state launched a full-fledged assault on the PKK and affiliated NGOs and political parties. This was quite different from the violent interruptions that had occurred between the different rounds of negotiations, for it signaled a strategic move by the AKP indicating and acknowledging that the party's Kurdish policy had failed to weaken the hegemony of the Kurdish movement.

But the ending of the negotiations was more than just a pragmatic calculation; it testified to the limits of the AKP reformism. In terms of the Kurdish question, the reformism had involved ensuring the disarmament of the PKK, on the one hand, and recognition of the language and cultural rights of Kurds, on the other. Importantly, the rights recognition was performed on an individual basis and never extended to any negotiation over the collective demand of a nation claiming the right to self-determination. Thus, by 2015, the Kurdish question as framed and understood by the AKP was answered. The PKK, meanwhile, was buoyed by the gains made both electorally in Turkey via the HDP and in northern Syria (Rojava), where the autonomous political system advocated by its leader, Abdullah Öcalan, was established (through constantly shifting compromises on the ground between the (mainly) Kurdish militia and leadership, Assad regime/Russia, and the United States).

It was, therefore, very clear to both sides that the gap between their expectations was unbridgeable and negotiations no longer sustainable. The AKP replaced its earlier Kurdish policy with a fully-fledged counterterrorism policy in the summer of 2015. The resulting destruction (of cities) and oppression (of Kurdish-identity politics) has arguably been as intense as any before, during the Kemalist period. While the cultural rights granted during the reform process have not been withdrawn, and the state continues to provide social services and social assistance as before, the problematic giving shape to the way it rules Kurds has changed sharply.

The findings of this research may be considered as offering fresh insights into two areas in particular. First, by examining the shift and then shift back in the governmental approach to the Kurdish issue, the profound change and yet deeper continuities between the pre-AKP and AKP periods are revealed. Second, the research also shows the nature of the unbridgeable gap between the Turkish state addressing the Kurd as an object, as the projective entity of a (Turkish) nationalist fantasy, and Kurds' expectation of and struggle for recognition as subjects in their own right, as (a) people with "a separate and equivalent center of self."[5] This means a true peace process is not possible without a complete breakdown of the Turkish nationalist fantasy that has no room for an independent Kurdish subjectivity.

Notes

1 Cihan Tuğal, *Passive Revolution: Absorbing the Islamic Challenge to Capitalism* (Stanford, CA: Stanford University Press, 2009).
2 Ranajit Guha, *Dominance without Hegemony: History and Power in Colonial India* (Cambridge, MA: Harvard University Press, 1997), 1–99.
3 Ibid., 22–23.

4 See Axel Honneth's arguments in his philosophical exchange with Nancy Fraser, in Nancy Fraser and Axel Honneth, *Redistribution or Recognition?: A Political-Philosophical Exchange* (London and New York: Verso, 2003).
5 Jessica Benjamin, "An Outline of Intersubjectivity: The Development of Recognition," Supplement, *Psychoanalytic Psychology* 7 (1990): 35.

Acknowledgments

This book is an outcome of a great deal of labor expended in various research sites, from archives and libraries in Ankara and Istanbul to the health posts, family health centers, hospitals, and local neighborhoods of Hakkâri. The happiness in finally being able to complete this research with this book is immense. I hope that it will meet its intended reader, provide input for further similar research projects, and contribute to our understanding of the present inability to bring a peaceful resolution to "the Kurdish issue."

Many people have contributed to this book in its different phases of making. During my postgraduate education, starting at the Atatürk Institute for Modern Turkish History at Boğaziçi University in Istanbul and ended at the Sociology and Social Anthropology Department of Central European University in Budapest, where I submitted the dissertation that built the basis of this book, I benefited from the presence and intellectual work of some very distinguished professors. Among these, Nazan Üstündağ, with her uniquely critical mind, expertise on the Kurdish issue and uncompromising political stance, provided me with critical standards against which I always felt compelled to measure the arguments developed in this book. Ayşe Çağlar, my doctoral thesis supervisor, was available whenever I needed her support and contribution. With her sound academic professionalism and experience, she always provided timely suggestions and helpful warnings.

Elsewhere, in the Netherlands, Joost Jongerden hosted me at Wageningen University, generously shared his insightful comments and questions on my initial research findings based on his command of the field and encouraged me to contribute with a piece on Hakkâri to the book he was editing at the time on the Kurdish issue. I would also like to thank Prem Kumar Rajaram and John Clarke for their invaluable input into the research during its different phases.

I am grateful to Jürgen Mackert, who enabled me to conduct my postdoctoral research at the Centre for Citizenship, Social Pluralism and Religious Diversity at the University of Potsdam. Had he not shown his strong solidarity at a time when I needed it most, this book simply would not have been possible.

I would like to thank friends and colleagues from the University of Hakkâri, Yaşar Akdağ, Mustafa Rüstemoğlu, Sebahattin Şen, and İhsan Seddar Kaynar, with whom I had pleasant, stress-relieving, and thought-inspiring hours discussing Hakkâri, politics, and Kurds while sipping our delicious smuggled tea. Their companionship and solidarity made my fieldwork easier and more productive and joyful. I would like to express my special thanks to Yaşar Akdağ for his invaluable contribution to my fieldwork. He helped me overcome many of the practical challenges of researching at a site where building relationships and winning the trust of people is not easy. Thank you, *mamoste*.

Among many Hakkârian friends, I must mention Ömer Özcan, who provided me with the first local contacts through which I stepped into the field. Leyla Kurt contributed as an excellent research assistant, and İrfan Sarı, Yusuf Demir, Abdurrahman Keskin, İlkay Şimşek, İsmail Akbulut, Serdar Akbulut, and Nazım Elmas generously shared their experiences and helped me collect more data and reach further contacts.

I need to acknowledge my gratitude to the American University of Central Asia (AUCA), in Bishkek, Kyrgyzstan, and its Sociology Department, where I worked between 2017 and 2020. Thank you, Galina Gorborukova and Mehrigul Ablezova, for giving me the opportunity to continue my academic research at a time when I was excluded from the Turkish universities due to my critical stance toward authoritarian, one-man rule in Turkey. My special thanks go to Clyde R. Forsberg, with whom I shared my desk during my AUCA years. Unfortunately, he was defeated by corona-related complications. Clyde, your true friendship, unique sense of humor, and very strong solidarity will be always remembered.

I need to thank also Isabel David and Kumru F. Toktamış, the editors of *Culture, Society and Political Economy in Turkey*, a new series by Peter Lang Publishing. They carefully read the whole manuscript and helped me quickly proceed toward publishing in the most practical way possible with their very useful advice. I also am grateful to Andy Hilton, the copy editor of the book, whose corrections and remarks made major improvements to the expression style of the book.

Thanks are due, too, to the publisher of the journal *Nations and Nationalism* for allowing me to include in this book, especially in Chapters 4 and 5, the revised sections of a previously published article entitled "Ethno-political Subordination and Patient Dissatisfaction: The Kurdish case in Hakkâri during the AKP period in Turkey, 2003–2013" (*Nations and Nationalism* 26, no. 3, pp. 553–75). I am also thankful to Routledge for allowing me to include, especially in Chapter 6, revised sections of "An Ethnographic Account of Compulsory Public Service by Doctors in Hakkari: The Limits of the AKP Assimilation Strategy and the Production of Space" (in Zeynep Gambetti and Joost Jongerden, eds., *The Kurdish Issue in Turkey: A Spatial Perspective* [London: Routledge, 2015], 105–35).

I could not have continued my academic research without a loving and supportive family. My brother Soner not only helped me find some of the documents I used in the research—he has also always been there as my *birader*. I have had great support from my parents-in-law, Ertan and Nilgün Yazıcı, during both the research and writing periods of this book. We shared the same apartment for a few years, during the most critical part of my research. This book testifies to their unlimited trust, understanding, and support.

My most special thanks are for my wife and daughter. They have been at the center of my life over the last 12 years, which also correspond to the story of making of this book. I am not sure if I can fully express my gratitude to Gözde Yazıcı Cörüt, my *Gozo*. Every single line, page, and argument of this book are embedded in her love, self-sacrificing support, and patience. Thank you for everything, Gozo! And with her unique presence, joy, and love, making me feel likes the luckiest of dads, Sümela Cörüt, my *Sümoto*, has helped to boost me with the energy and dynamism I needed to bring this project to a conclusion. I should thank her also for being able to adapt to the countries that we moved through over the years.

Finally, the contribution of my parents, Esin and Abdullah Cörüt, to this work has been multidimensional. They provided me with strong support at each stage of my education process, taught me to aim always high, and never failed to show their endless confidence that I could achieve those goals. The value of the unconditional, unlimited support and love they have given me was immeasurable. My father, my *Cörüdo*, recently passed away. I dedicate this book to his memory. He was always proud of me. If only he could hold this book in his hands, if only I could see the gleam of happiness and the look of pride then that would appear in his eyes . . .

List of Abbreviations

AKP	Justice and Development Party (Adalet ve Kalkınma Partisi)
AP	Justice Party (Adalet Partisi)
Bağ-Kur	Social Security Institution of Craftsmen, Tradesmen, and Other Self-Employed Workers (Esnaf ve Sanatkârlar ve Diğer Bağımsız Çalışanlar Sosyal Sigortalar Kurumu)
BBP	Great Union Party (Büyük Birlik Partisi)
BDP	Peace and Democracy Party (Barış ve Demokrasi Partisi)
CHP	Republican People's Party (Cumhuriyet Halk Partisi)
CPSD	Compulsory Public Service of Doctors
CUP	Committee of Union and Progress (İttihat ve Terakki Cemiyeti)
DİE	State Statistical Institute (Devlet İstatistik Enstitüsü)
DP	Democratic Party (Demokrat Parti)
DPT	State Planning Organization (Devlet Planlama Teşkilatı)
DTP	Democratic Society Party (Demokratik Toplum Partisi)
Eğitim-Sen	Education and Science Workers' Union (Eğitim ve Bilim Emekçileri Sendikası)
FP	Virtue Party (Fazilet Partisi)
GP	General Practitioner
GSS	General Health Insurance Scheme (Genel Sağlık Sigortası)

HDP	Peoples' Democratic Party (Halkların Demokratik Partisi)
IMF	International Monetary Fund
İHD	Human Rights Association (İnsan Hakları Derneği)
JİTEM	Gendarmerie Intelligence and Counterterrorism Organization (Jandarma İstihbarat ve Terörle Mücadele Teşkilatı)
KCK	Association of Communities in Kurdistan (Koma Civakên Kurdistan)
Mazlumder	Association of Human Rights and Solidarity for Oppressed People (İnsan Hakları ve Mazlumlar için Dayanışma Derneği)
MHP	Nationalist Action Party (Milliyetçi Hareket Partisi)
MHSA	Ministry of Health and Social Assistance (Sağlık ve Sosyal Yardım Bakanlığı)
MİT	National Intelligence Agency (Milli İstihbarat Teşkilatı)
MoH	Ministry of Health (Sağlık Bakanlığı)
PKK	Kurdistan Workers' Party (Partiya Karkerên Kurdistanê)
SES	Health and Social Services Laborers' Union (Sağlık ve Sosyal Hizmet Emekçileri Sendikası)
SGK	Social Security Institution (Sosyal Güvenlik Kurumu)
SSK	Social Insurance Institution (Sosyal Sigortalar Kurumu)
TSK	Turkish Armed Forces (Türk Silahlı Kuvvetleri)
TTB	Turkish Medical Association (Türk Tabipleri Birliği)
TUS	Medical Specialty Exam (Tıpta Uzmanlık Sınavı)
TÜİK	Turkish Statistical Institute (Türkiye İstatistik Kurumu)
TÜSİAD	Turkish Industry and Business Association (Türk Sanayicileri ve İş Adamları Derneği)
UNDP	United Nations Development Programme

1

Introduction

This research looks at the Kurdish policy of the governing conservative AKP during the period between 2003 and 2014. Analyzing the discourses, subjectivities, and practices around a particular aspect of the party's social policy, it focuses on healthcare provider involvement and patient responses to the improvement of healthcare provision in Hakkâri, a small, homogenously Kurdish province in Turkey's southeast. The healthcare providers comprise health institutions, general practitioners (GPs), medical specialists (surgeons, cardiologists, etc.), nurses, midwives, and other health professionals, while the healthcare provision, in addition to the health workforce, ranges from the material, such as medical infrastructure, to areas like administration and preventive medicine.

The improvement of healthcare provision in Hakkâri is approached as part of a comprehensive Kurdish policy aimed at a resolution or at least addressing and containment of Turkey's "Kurdish problem," in particular its expression in the unrest and violent resistance instigated by the PKK since 1984. This research should thus be regarded as an example of anthropology of policy in that it uses healthcare provision as "a lens for exploring" the workings of a political system and thus puts into practice the suggestion that "examination of particular policies can provide unique avenues for analyzing wider issues of governance, including various ways [used] ... to manufacture consent."[1] As an anthropology of policy, that is, it seeks to shed light on the nature, application, and functioning of Turkish state-nationalism in respect to Kurds and the Kurdish-dominated region ("the Southeast") through a critical analysis of the role of social policy in the assimilation of Kurds into Turkishness and thence control of social space.

Even though the assimilation of Kurds into Turkishness is an old story, which dates back to the early days of the foundation of the Turkish state in 1923, the employment of social policy as an instrument of Turkish assimilationism was something new and should be regarded as distinctive of the AKP's period in office. Despite many fluctuations and the profound challenges faced, internal to the party as well as in the political and other spheres more generally, the AKP can be said to have had a coherent Kurdish policy between 2003 and 2014. This was characterized by a major change of approach with a shift in the relative weight of persuasive as against coercive elements in the instrumental composition of policy tools deployed.

In the period following its accession to office and subsequent years—approximately its first decade in government—the AKP addressed the Kurdish issue by, on the one hand, relaxing the security approach, which included covert negotiations with the PKK, and on the other, committing to a fully-fledged assimilation policy. Thus, it moved Ankara somewhat away from coercive and constraining instruments of sovereignty—at least insofar as these did not constitute the only or predominant approach. Indeed, the move toward productive and life-affirming technologies was a major adjustment to the nation-state's typical repertoire of violent governance. The AKP placed an emphasis on the biopolitical care of Kurds, which it framed as a "politics of service." This was situated at the heart of its Kurdish policy and asserted against what the government dubbed the "useless" and "ideological" kind of "politics of identity" associated with Turkish nationalists (Kemalists and Turkist far-right movements) and Kurdish nationalists (PKK).

This adroit positioning was not as centrist as it appeared, however. First, the opposition of the politics of identity with the politics of service was performed in a partial way that involved Islamic references to the divisive role of ethnic and tribal belongings. The AKP thus delivered the message to Kurds that ethnic identity was not worth fighting for. Second, and contrary to its claim to be forging a middle ground between Turkish and Kurdish nationalisms that excluded the old extremes, the AKP reserved collective cultural and political rights for Turks only, made no concession on the major principles of the Republic of Turkey, and rather enacted a reformism limited to curbing certain of its more extreme aspects, such as the power of the military. Recognizing Kurdish rights on an individual basis, therefore—with a special emphasis on Islam—the new regime sought to diminish ethnicity with respect to religion as the primary self-identification (but still under the old mantle of Turkish national and state-centrist power).

The improvement of healthcare provision in Hakkâri during 2003–14 may be one of the most striking expressions of the AKP's reliance on its politics of service in the Kurdish issue. It was only after the introduction of the 2005 law on compulsory public service for doctors (CPSD), and construction and opening of two new, modern public hospitals at the end of 2008—one in the provincial capital, Hakkâri city, the other in the largest district (county) of the province, Yüksekova—that the inhabitants of Hakkâri were able to access a more or less adequate health service in their local area. Before the CPSD law and the new hospitals, patients would either make the four-hour journey to Van or, in more serious cases, take the even longer route to Ankara or Istanbul, or else cross the border for the hospitals in Orumieh, in Iran.

The striking improvement to healthcare provision in Hakkâri during the early period of AKP rule was not limited to the enactment of the CPSD law, purchase of new equipment, and construction of modern hospitals. As Table 1 confirms, healthcare provision in Hakkâri as a whole considerably improved during this time.

This remarkable improvement signified a notable shift in Hakkâri politics toward productive technologies of power centered on raising the quality of life. It may have been the most striking change but was by no means the only one. After 2004, means-tested conditional cash transfers requiring pregnant women to attend regular check-ups during the prepartum period and parents to ensure school attendance and regular check-ups of their children became an

Table 1. Healthcare Provision in Hakkâri, 2002 and 2010

Provision	2002	2010
No. medical specialists	11	91
No. GPs	11	89
No. emergency medical stations	2	9
No. ambulances	2	24
No. transfers by air ambulance*	0	63
Vaccination rate (BCG)	49	94

Source: Presentation to Provincial Director of Health.
* Van region air ambulance (operational from December 2009).

important source of income for thousands of families in Hakkâri, as in other, mainly Kurdish-populated provinces.[2] Also, with the enactment of The Law on Compensation for Losses Resulting from Terrorism and the Fight against Terrorism in 2004, thousands of Hakkâri-resident victims of the village evacuations of the counter-insurgency strategy of the 1990s were allocated an average of fifteen-twenty thousand lira (equivalent at that time to around 7–10k USD). Among other signs of development in the province, one may also mention the opening of a public university in 2008 and the construction of an airport in Yüksekova (initiated in 2010, opened in 2015).

The change in the form and rationality of state violence during this period further confirmed the new orientation, placing its main emphasis on service and development rather than sovereignty. Until the late 1990s, the effort of the Turkish state to manufacture a Turkish national body corresponded in Hakkâri, as in the Kurdish region generally, with overwhelmingly violent policies enacted through extraordinary forms of rule intended to constitute Turkish sovereignty in the region. These ranged from the Law for the Restoration of Order (1925–27), through the establishment of the First General Inspectorate (1927–47),[3] to martial law (1979–87) and emergency rule (1987–2002). State violence persisted in 2003–14, but now aimed at forcing Hakkârians to make the government-framed choice between the identity politics of the Kurdish movement and the politics of service of the AKP. When the AKP came to power in November 2002, there had already been a remarkable decrease in counter-insurgency tactics directly targeting Kurdish activists, including the assassinations and systematic torture perpetrated by the special units of army and police. This was mainly due to a unilateral ceasefire declared by the PKK in 1999 that lasted until 2004 and the annulment of the state of emergency in the Kurdish provinces in 2002 as part of the democratization reforms enacted in the EU membership process that had begun in 1999.[4] The AKP built on this environment. The primary form of violent policies enacted under the AKP government in the 2003–14 period was rather the arrest of political opponents. The large scope for initiative left to special courts and anti-terror teams by the Anti-Terror Law led to thousands of Hakkârians being arrested, accused of affiliation with the PKK or the Association of Communities in Kurdistan (Koma Civakên Kurdistan, KCK).

Considered from a comparative perspective, this new setting of the encounter of the Turkish state and Kurds exemplifies a not atypical multiethnic setting in which the state-nationalism, facing the limits of coercion, uses social policy for the containment of ethnic movements. In these settings,

A state struggling against powerful nationalist movements can choose to launch new social programmes to gain, regain, or preserve the loyalty of a population being targeted by nationalist leaders seeking to increase political autonomy or achieve independence. In the short term, the objective may be to "buy" the loyalty of these citizens by offering them more generous social benefits . . . but from this perspective a perhaps more significant objective is to foster a sense of identification with the state and the nation it projects.[5]

In the UK, for instance, where some of the most heated debates on the issue occurred as a consequence of the growing Scottish nationalism, "the development of the post-war welfare state . . . created a sense of belonging related to the concrete, institutionalized forms of economic solidarity and redistribution rooted in the notion of British social citizenship."[6] This "helps to explain why Scottish nationalism, at least in its home rule or independence-seeking manifestations, remained weak until the 1980s"[7] and subsequently grew stronger. The development of Quebec nationalism in Canada and Flemish nationalism in Belgium and the responses given by the states to these sub-state nationalisms also had much to do with the use of social policy instruments.[8]

It can be stated, then, that the precise topic addressed by this research concerns whether healthcare provision did in fact serve as an instrument of state-nationalism for the AKP and support the containment of ethnopolitical unrest among Hakkârian Kurds. In addition to exemplifying the anthropology of policy by using healthcare provision as a lens for exploring the larger mechanism behind it, this research should also be seen as a work of critical social policy and nationalism studies as it focuses on attempts at nation-building and the institution of a compliant, cooperative, submissive Kurdish subjectivity incorporated into the Turkish state.

The remainder of this chapter establishes the main concerns of the book with a presentation of the research objective and theoretical framework. This is followed by a consideration of the research field, broadly, the province of Hakkâri, and the mode of investigation, or methodology, and concluded with a preview of the different chapters.

1.1 Research Objective

Somewhat surprisingly, even strikingly, perhaps, the change in the relative weight of coercive and persuasive elements in the instrumental composition of the Turkish policy tools toward Hakkâri and Kurds did *not* result in a steady and meaningful increase of support for the AKP in the province. On the contrary, it was the pro-Kurdish party—the Democratic Society Party, later Peace and Democracy Party (Demokratik Toplum Partisi, DTP and Barış ve Demokrasi Partisi, BDP)—that was backed by the majority of Hakkârians, as the history of election results reveals. While the AKP share of the total vote of Hakkâri in general elections held in 2002, 2007, and 2011 rose from 6 to 33 and then fell to 16 percent, respectively, the Kurdish party (DTP/BDP) vote-share increased from 45 through 56–80 percent.[9] The DTP/BDP confirmed its overwhelming electoral superiority over the AKP in Hakkâri in local elections held in 2009 and 2014. In 2014, six of the eight mayors in Hakkâri were members of the BDP. The AKP, on the other hand, was so marginalized by 2009 that it even had difficulty in finding a place to rent in the city.[10]

The main question that I seek to answer in this contribution, therefore, concerns the failure of the Kurdish policy in Hakkâri. Why was it not successful? The answer to this question should shed some light on the limits of the instrumentalization of social policy as a tool of the Turkish assimilation strategy and thus contribute to the academic body of knowledge at two levels. At the local level, which is of particular concern to scholars of Kurdish and Turkish studies, the dominance of coercive elements in Turkish nationalist policy toward the Kurds until the end of 1990s has meant that nonviolent, everyday processes have not been placed at the center of Kurdish studies.[11] Therefore, our knowledge about the subjectivities, shortcomings, achievements, and discourses generated by the use of social policy and life-affirming instruments in the management of the Kurdish issue is largely lacking. This book aims to contribute to filling this lacuna. At the wider, global level, which is of particular concern to scholars focusing on the relationship between ethnopolitics and social policy, this research shows how the deployment of social policy for the containment of ethnopolitical challenge is a more complicated issue than it may appear at first sight. Relying on less violence and more social policy does not automatically entail the decline of ethnopolitical challenge.

1.2 Theoretical Framework

The origin of the theoretical questions addressed in this research dates back to 2007, when, as a member of the organization committee of the graduate conference, *History, Politics, Turkey: Social Questions and Critical Approaches*, I assumed responsibility for classifying the papers into the conference sessions. During this work, I realized two interesting and interrelated issues. One had to do with my difficulty in grouping the presentations. While I found many papers difficult to group into our designed sessions as they fit more than one session, I had little difficulty in grouping the papers into the session on Turkish nationalism, for there was a common conception, which I shared, that Turkish nationalism refers to a very specific phenomenon: a particular extremist ideology and movement and labeled thus, "Turkish nationalism." The other issue pertained to the papers on the Kurdish question, all of which focused on aspects of political and ideological resistance to the extremist policies of the Turkish nation-state. Actually, once Turkish nationalism is identified with extremism, it is unsurprising that scholars of Kurdish studies should place political and ideological resistance to that at the center of their studies.

The question that emerged from this classifying task concerned how it was possible that while we are living under the strict control of the nation-states, yet we still manage to identify nationalism with extremist movements and ideologies and yet not with the very "network of apparatuses and daily practices" of the nation-states through which we are instituted "as *homo nationalis* from cradle to grave."[12]

As Michael Billig shows in his famous work *Banal Nationalism,* this deficiency was not confined to a group of graduate students:

> In both popular and academic writing, nationalism is associated with those who struggle to create new states or with extreme right-wing politics. According to customary usage, George Bush is not a nationalist but separatists in Quebec or Brittany are; so are the leaders of extreme right-wing parties such as the Front National in France; and so, too, are the Serbian guerrillas, killing in the cause of extending the homeland's borders.[13]

Parallel to my readings on everyday nationalism, I saw that the answer to my question was there in the question itself. It is precisely *because* we are living under the strict control and hegemony of nation-states that we tend to identify nationalism with extremist movements and ideologies. We are all, in varying degrees, *homo nationalis,* unable to realize the "network of apparatuses and daily practices" that institute us thus. Nationalism has become such a normalized phenomenon that it has become naturalized, an ontological constant. This is seen also in the preference of Benedict Anderson for grouping nationalism with kinship and religion rather than with ideologies like fascism and liberalism.[14] In other words:

in the established nations, there is a continual "flagging", or reminding, of nationhood ... In so many little ways, the citizenry are daily reminded of their national place in a world of nations. However, this reminding is so familiar, so continual, that it is not consciously registered as reminding. The metonymic image of banal nationalism is not a flag which is being consciously waved with fervent passion; it is the flag hanging unnoticed on the public building.[15]

1.2.1 The Literature on Everyday Nationalism: Suggestions and Limits

The scholars of everyday nationalism, though varying in their focal points and sites of expertise, together represent "a movement away from the 'grand narratives' of ethnicity and nationalism with their concentration on elite projects to a systematic study of the role of popular beliefs, sentiments, and practices."[16] Their point of departure is not complicated: "The nation ... is not simply the product of macro-structural forces; it is simultaneously the practical accomplishment of ordinary people engaging in routine activities."[17]

This understanding of nationalism has entailed a shift in research topics and updating of methodologies to render them more compatible with new research topics. As Anthony D. Smith emphasizes, alongside the emergence of new research topics covering everyday phenomena, such as consumption practices, rituals, everyday speech, and habits, standard ethnographic methods, like surveys, in-depth interviews, focus groups, and participant observation of everyday life, have acquired a great importance in the literature on everyday nationalism.[18] For instance, Jon E. Fox and Cynthia Miller-Idriss propose that research topics of everyday nationalism studies should be "the discursive construction of the nation through routine talk in interaction, ... nationhood as it is implicated in the decisions ordinary people make, ... the production of national sensibilities through the ritual enactment of symbols, ... [and] the constitution and expression of national difference through everyday consumption habits."[19]

This research recognizes the insights enabled by the perspective of everyday nationalism, but it also provides a critique of a tendency in everyday nationalism studies to underestimate the role played by states in the everyday production of nation. This tendency, which we can follow in the research topics proposed by Fox and Miller-Idriss, is, I argue, based on an implicit assumption that the contribution of the state to nation-building is limited to the construction of the basic structural and institutional bases of a nation. In this understanding of nation-building through the state, which is in fact in a clear conflict with the spirit of everyday nationalism studies, "nation-building through the state is, more often than not, analyzed only as a process specific to the eighteenth and nineteenth centuries, that is, it is considered to have come to a stop sometime in the twentieth century."[20]

Yet, we know that "the process of nation-building is not merely a phenomenon associated with the period of state formation. It is also evident ... in well-established states seeking to maintain their legitimacy and territorial integrity in the face of internal or external challenges."[21] In the words of Daniel Béland and André Lecours, "states continuously engage in nation-building through routine and seemingly innocuous practices such as distributing social benefits and delivering social services."[22] The newly flourishing anthropology of policy enables a better understanding of the fact that nations are not just formed and finished in a once-and-for-ever moment of foundation and establishment. The state is involved in the everyday production of nation via policy-making and implementation processes, through which the state also reproduces itself.[23] The anthropology of policy shows that state discourses and governmental programs not only produce material effects but also impose identities and operate as mechanisms of interpellation on a daily basis:

> Like the modern state (to which its growth can be linked), policy now impinges on all areas of life so that it is virtually impossible to ignore or escape its influence. More than this, policy increasingly shapes the way individuals construct themselves as subjects. Through policy, the individual is categorized and given such statuses and roles as "subject", "citizen", "professional", "national", "criminal" and "deviant". From the cradle to the grave, people are classified, shaped and ordered according to policies ...[24]

Subject-formation taking place through policies employed by nation-states, especially in multiethnic contexts, is necessarily informed by the agenda of nation-building. In multiethnic contexts, the nation-states are largely driven by state-nationalism, "the nationalism of the aspiring nation state" which "aims to render the boundaries of the nation and governance unit congruent by transforming a multinational state into a national one."[25]

To sum up, my formulation of the research topic, objective, and methodology of the research is guided by the insights provided by the literature on everyday nationalism, as well as its shortcomings. The basic argument of the literature on everyday nationalism that nationalism exists in the very materiality of our ordinary lives provided the theoretical grounds of my concern about the identification of nationalism with extremism in Turkish and Kurdish studies.

The emphasis placed on ethnographic methods also aided development of the research subject. Yet, the literature on everyday nationalism does less to suggest the type of theoretical framework necessary to make ethnographic sense of the role of the state in everyday nationalism. In the following sections, I attempt to formulate the basic concepts of a methodology that may be useful in making sense of the operation of state-nationalism through ordinary nation-state practices in which nationalism does not take the shape of imposing visible signifiers of national identity.

1.2.2 The Analytic of Nation of State-Nationalism: Being and Becoming of Nation

Taking and adapting its title from Dipesh Chakrabarty's "Histories and the Analytic of Capital", this section addresses the analytic of nation of state-nationalism.[26] The being and becoming of nation are overviewed from the perspectives of time, homogeneous and heterogeneous, and resistance and assimilation.

1.2.2.1 Being of Nation, or Nation in Homogeneous and Empty Time

The distinction Dipesh Chakrabarty makes between the "being" and "becoming of capital" is fundamental to the framework provided here. Chakrabarty develops these concepts in the second chapter of his work *Provincializing Europe*, subtitled *The Two Histories of Capital*, in which he focuses on the complicated relationships of difference, exchange, and commodity. Chakrabarty starts his analysis by underlining the conflict between difference and exchange, which is embedded in the very structure of commodity:

> Fundamental to Marx's discussion of capital is the idea of the commodity, and fundamental to the conception of the commodity is the question of difference ... commodity exchange is about exchanging things that are different in their histories, material properties, and use-value. Yet the commodity form, intrinsically, is supposed to make differences—however material they may be in their historical appearance-immaterial for the purpose of exchange.[27]

In order to make the products of incommensurable concrete labors exchangeable with one another, the labors need to be reduced to abstract labor, where this is measurable by a common standard. This common standard is the homogeneous empty time of the clock, which has an objective existence indifferent to and independent of the human subject. Therefore, what is at stake in the reduction is the separation of the laborer from the laboring process. This is a violent practice in that capitalists utilize disciplinary mechanisms to prevent the diverse times and histories embedded in the laborer and their effort from interrupting the uniformity and regularity imposed during the laboring process. In Chakrabarty's words, "to organize life under the sign of capital is to act as if labor could indeed be abstracted from all the social tissues in which it is always embedded and which make any particular labor ... concrete."[28]

With the phrase "being of capital," Chakrabarty refers to the ideal case in which this abstraction is fully achieved. This ideal case is the point at which an end is reached in the fight between homogeneous and empty time, which is materialized in the uniformity and regularity imposed on and through the laboring process, and the diverse times materialized in the concrete labor of the laborer. "Being of capital," that is, "refers to the structural logic of capital ... the state when capital has fully come into its own."[29]

The nation that Anderson talks about, as Partha Chatterjee emphasizes, "inhabits" this "utopian time of capital."[30] This is the nation that has fully come into its own. The question of difference is not on its agenda, as if this were left behind. Drawing on Chakrabarty's "being of capital," therefore, I call the nation as discussed by Anderson in *Imagined Communities* the "being of nation" insofar as it "refers to the structural logic" (of nation).

1.2.2.2 Becoming of Nation, or Nation in Heterogeneous Times

Once the homogeneity of the nation is posited, heterogeneity becomes a problem. The tension is irreducible, as Chatterjee argues:

> People can only imagine themselves in empty homogenous time; they do not live in it. Empty homogenous time is the utopian time of capital ... But empty homogenous time is not located anywhere in real space—it is utopian. The real space of modern life consists of heterotopia ... Time here is heterogeneous, unevenly dense ... To ignore this is, I believe, to discard the real for [the] utopian.[31]

Anderson shows in *Imagined Communities* that nation is imagined in homogeneous and empty time, yet he does not appear so concerned with how this imagination manages to survive and further reproduces its internal coherency despite the actual, visible diversities at its core. He does not show the same sort of interest in the serious challenge that the heterogeneity of national space and of times poses to the idea and functioning of the homogeneous or the empty time of deep horizontal comradeship or the way that this challenge is settled within the analytical horizon of "being of nation."

That means imagining the nation cannot be limited only to imagining being of nation. Nationalism, especially in its state-nationalist form, cannot avoid facing up to the diversities at the core of the nation. It has to recognize and define differences and approach them with different policies without undermining the unity of nation posited by being of nation. Therefore, nation also needs to be imagined as some sort of unity in diversity and a taxonomy "mapping differences."[32] In other words, in its search for producing nation, "states both operationalise the grammar of difference (addressing people in their categoric identities) and articulate conceptions of how all these differences fit together—the unity of the nation."[33]

To make sense of how "being of nation" handles the problem of heterogeneity at its core, my suggestion is to look at how historicism and its linear time conception are rendered into tools of power by totalities built on homogeneous and empty time:

> Homogenous time has the present as its axis. It is not that the past and the future are completely denied, but the past and especially the future are subservient to the present: the past is understood as the pre-history of the present, and the future is conceived as the pre-visible extension of the present. Time is seen as a linear movement between past and future.[34]

That is to say, homogeneous and empty time renders diversities that resist being incorporated/assimilated into national totality into unevenly developed and "incomplete" or "lacking" entities that are supposed to come into full being by leaving or "by the addition of certain elements in the chronological time."[35] The name Chakrabarty gives to this transition process in his discussion of capital is "becoming." The becoming of capital "refers to the historical process in and through which the logical presuppositions of capital's "being" are realized. "Becoming" is not simply the calendrical or chronological past that precedes capital but the past that the category retrospectively posits."[36]

My argument, therefore, is that imagining nation cannot be reduced merely to imagining being of nation. It also has to be imagined as a becoming, as an unevenness and hierarchy. Drawing on Chakrabarty's "becoming of capital," I refer to the transition process imposed on diversities by being of a nation as "becoming of nation," which "refers to the historical process in and through which the logical presuppositions of 'being of nation' are realized."

1.2.2.3 Further Deductions on Becoming of Nation: Resistance

The reduction of space to time, subsuming spatial difference into the logic of a modernist, uneven development narrative, is not completely attainable. Thus, a certain resistance to the reduction is an intrinsic part of becoming of nation.

To make sense of the form of the resistance taking place at the very center of becoming of nation, the categorical distinction Homi Bhabha makes between pedagogical and performative representations of nation can be useful. Regarding the pedagogical representation of nation—here, the becoming of nation—Bhabha refers to the representation of nation as an object moving in the past-present-future linearity. It is pedagogical in the sense that it speaks with this authority, based on the "a priori historical presence," which is the "pre-given or constituted historical origin" of nation.[37] Regarding the performative aspects of nation, which takes place at the level of "being of nation," on the other hand, Bhabha refers to the fact that "the people are also the 'subjects' of a process of signification" and "constructed in the performance of narrative, its enunciatory 'present' marked in the repetition and pulsation of the national sign."[38] This performative character of nation, the role of the people as subjects in the performance of nation, opens a place for "the discourses of minorities, the heterogeneous histories of contending peoples, antagonistic authorities and tense locations of culture,"[39] which cannot be objectified in the linearity of the pedagogical representation of the nation:

> Because of the necessity for the performance of the nation's signs by the people as "subject", the pedagogical ideal of the homogenous people can never be realized. This is because the performative necessity of nationalist representations enables all those placed on the margins of its norms and limits ... to intervene in the signifying process and challenge the dominant representation with narratives of their own.[40]

The methodological implication of these arguments for my research is that nationalist motives and stances may take shape, like a pedagogical tune in political discourse, project, or policy, which may not easily reveal itself to an analytical gaze looking for the overt forms, symbols, and languages of nationalism. That is to say, resistance to nationalism may occur in forms that are not political in the usual sense of the word. Everyday dissatisfactions and sabotages may not be apparent in the public realm of formal engagements. Discourses and practices that undermine and disrupt linear transition and "becoming" narratives may be manifestations of a quotidian resistance to nationalism carried out in everyday forms.

1.2.2.4 Further Deductions on Becoming of Nation: Assimilation/ Nation-Building

At a less abstract and more political level, becoming of nation corresponds to the politics of assimilation/nation-building. To expand on this argument, the following two quotations from Anderson and Giorgio Agamben, respectively, are pertinent:

> -[Nation] is imagined as sovereign because the concept was born in an age in which Enlightenment and Revolution were destroying the legitimacy of the divinely-ordained, hierarchical dynastical realm.[41]
> -The sovereign is the one with respect to whom all men are potentially *homines sacri*.[42]

If nation "is imagined as sovereign" and "the sovereign is the one with respect to whom all men are potentially *homines sacri*," it means that nation is imagined above bare life. Yet the "inclusive exclusion" of bare life is not peculiar to the national form of political community:

> The expulsion of someone who used to have rights as a citizen, or simply to categorize some individuals in a society as a form of life that is beyond the reach of dignity and full humanity and thus not even a subject of a benevolent power, is the most elementary operation of sovereign power—be it as a government in a nation-state, a local authority, a community, a warlord, or a local militia.[43]

We should take a step further then to gain a better grasp of the historical specificity of nation: The peculiarity of nation lies in its very attempt at overcoming of bare life rather than mere exclusion of bare life; nation is assimilative in character.[44] The following two arguments are instructive in this regard, first from Anderson and then from Claude Lefort:

> -The nation is imagined as limited because even the largest of them, encompassing perhaps a billion living human beings has finite, if elastic, boundaries beyond which lie other nations.[45]
> -The modern democratic revolution is best recognized in this mutation: there is no power linked to a body. Power appears as an empty place and those who exercise it as mere mortals who occupy it only temporarily or who could install themselves in it only by force or cunning. There is no law that can be fixed, whose articles cannot be contested, whose foundations are not susceptible of being called into question . . . With totalitarianism an apparatus is set up which tends to stave off this threat, which tends to weld power and society back

together again, to efface all signs of social division, to banish the indetermination that haunts the democratic experience. But this attempt . . . itself draws on a democratic source, developing and wholly affirming the idea of the People-as-One, the idea of society as such, bearing the knowledge of itself, transparent to itself and homogenous, the idea of mass opinion, sovereign and normative, the idea of the tutelary state.[46]

The People-as-One—that is, the nation of the nation-state—is not just another sovereign that can be compared to a warlord or a local militia. It is rather a totalitarian answer given within the borders of a particular territory to the radical indetermination of modern society. It is an attempt to return to the realm of the social its lost unity. Nationalist ideology, as John Breuilly argues, "is neither an expression of national identity . . . nor the arbitrary invention of nationalists for political purposes"; rather, it "arises out of the need to make sense of complex social and political arrangements."[47] This means that nationalist ideology does not make any room for the duality of nation and *homo sacer*. To use Zygmunt Baumann's terminology in *Modernity and Ambivalence*, nationalism does not have any tolerance for the "strangeness" posed by *homo sacer* to the single duality recognized and required by the Oneness of People. With "friends" denoting the People-as-One, "enemies" are Other(s), the exporter and communicator of all conflicts and divisive practices in the midst of the otherwise unitary people. In other words, the nation-state is structurally inclined to classify *homo sacer* as either "enemies" to kill or deport or otherwise eliminate from the nation-state territory or else as potential "friends" and try to assimilate them into the nation.[48]

Leaving the issue of extermination of "enemies" aside for the moment,[49] the assimilation of *homo sacer* into the nation, which is the distinctive feature of nationalism of incorporation, works in two ways. Because the nation is imagined as People-as-One, the disciplinary training of *homo sacer* to the norms of this Oneness becomes internal to all assimilation processes. In other words, one aspect of assimilation, to use Michel Foucault's term, is "normation,"[50] through which the "deviant behaviors and identities" of *homines sacri* are corrected. Although Foucault did not specify the nation-state as a site of disciplinary normalization, it is evident from the following definition that it is a site of disciplinary normalization:

> Disciplinary normalization consists first of all in positing a model, an optimal model that is constructed in terms of a certain result, and the operation of disciplinary normalization consists in trying to get people, movements, and actions to conform to this model, the normal being precisely that which can

conform to this norm, and the abnormal that which is incapable of conforming to the norm.[51]

Assimilation and nation-building processes, however, have an additional procedure to the disciplinary one. The transformation of *homo sacer* into *homo nationalis* (sovereign) not only occurs through the disciplinary normalization of *homo sacer*, since the basic human needs of *homo sacer* also need to be properly met to save him from a way of life in which his biological existence faces constant threat and take him beyond a minimum, a bare way of life. Agamben explains the contemporary obsession with development thus:

> In Rome, the internal division of the people was juridically sanctioned by the clear division between *populus* and *plebs*, each of which had its own institutions and magistrates ... But starting with the French Revolution, when it becomes the sole depositary of sovereignty, the people is transformed into an *embarrassing* presence, and misery and exclusion appear for the first time as an altogether *intolerable* scandal. In the modern era, misery and exclusion are not only economic or social concepts but eminently *political* categories ... In this sense, our age is nothing but the implacable and methodical attempt to overcome the division dividing the people, to *eliminate radically* the people that is excluded ... The *obsession* with development is as effective as it is in our time because it coincides with the *biopolitical project* to produce an undivided people.[52] [emphasis added]

To sum up, we can identify three simultaneous moments of assimilation:

1. *The sovereign moment of assimilation*: The nation as a People-as-One is imagined and practiced as sovereign over *homo sacer* imagined and treated as bare life;
2. *The disciplinary moment of assimilation*: The disciplinary normalization of *homo sacer* is applied in which surveillance, control, and other techniques of the security system, education, and law turn *homo sacer* into *homo nationalis*;
3. *The biopolitical moment of assimilation*: The living conditions of *homo sacer* are improved for a way of life liberated from its mere determination by biological survival.

As discussed above with reference to Billig, nationalism is usually identified only or primarily with the first two of these, the sovereign or disciplinary moments of nationalism, and thus reduced either to a body of extremist practices and ideas or else to a visible pedagogical violence imposing the national norms. Adding the biopolitical moment of assimilation to the other two moments of assimilation is simply the recognition of "soft power," that ordinary public services, social policy, and the public investment of the state, which in themselves and at first sight appear to have nothing to do with nationalism or assimilation, may indeed function as an instrument of incorporation of the non-national. This is the first methodological implication of addressing three moments of assimilation and the primary focus of this work. In order to understand how the state's provision of ordinary public services, social policy, and public investment function as a means of nationalist interpellation, and this is the second methodological implication of addressing three moments of assimilation, one also needs to analyze the three moments of assimilation in relation to one another to see the whole.

1.3 Fieldwork: Field and Methodology

This section provides a description of the basic characteristics of the field and the methodology applied in the fieldwork. Comprising the province of Hakkâri—specifically, its three main urban settlements—the field is introduced here through overviews of the physical and political geographies, a history of village evacuation, urbanization, and infrastructure issues, and an outline of the local economy. The methodology is introduced through a review of the author's personal entry to the field, together with details on data collection, sources used, informants met, and specific research sites attended, with a focus also on some limitations of the methodology.

1.3.1 Hakkâri: Basic Characteristics

The fieldwork for this study was carried out in the main urban settlements of Hakkâri, namely the provincial capital, Hakkâri itself, Yüksekova, the largest and most populated district, and Şemdinli. As per the standard system of Turkish place-naming, these places have the same names as the areas of which they are the administrative center; Yüksekova town is in Yüksekova district, for example. Similarly, the province has the same name as its center; thus, "Hakkâri," in this case, refers to the province, the center district, and the district town, or "city." While the fieldwork on doctors and other health personnel was designed to reach health professionals employed in health institutions in all three settlements, the fieldwork on patients was limited to those in Hakkâri city.

1.3.1.1 Hakkâri, Province of Mountains

Hakkâri is a small, mountainous province located at the southeastern corner of Turkey at the juncture with Iraq and Iran.[53] During my research period, the province (*il*) was divided into four districts. In addition to Hakkâri itself, (Kurdish: Colemêrg, the provincial capital), Yüksekova (Kurdish: Gever, the largest district), and Şemdinli (Kurdish: Şemzînan), which comprise the main band of the provincial territory, there is Çukurca (Çelê), to the southwest (Figure 1). Derecik was only divided from Şemdinli and made into a separate district in 2018; henceforth, therefore, all references to Şemdinli as a district include present-day Derecik.

Lying at an elevation of about 5,500 ft (1,700 m), the province of Hakkâri is mostly (some 90 percent) high mountain.[54] Inevitably, this mountainous landscape has played a decisive role in the formation of the territory's settlement patterns, seasonal conditions, and economic activities—including transport and communication. Until the 1940s, for example, Hakkâri had no road connections (for use by motor vehicles) linking it to places outside the province. The road between Hakkâri and the nearest big city, Van, was only opened in 1945—and since this passed through high mountains, it would be closed during the cold, snowy winters.[55] Even today, more than 70 years after the construction and opening of the route for modern traffic and following numerous improvements, the road remains far from the national standard. The 210-km journey from Van to Hakkâri was taking four torturous hours by bus in 2014.

Another natural feature of the mountainous landscape is the scarcity of agricultural land and the abundance of meadows and range. Due to this topography, farming has never had more than a marginal place in the peasant economy. Husbandry—sheep and goat rearing—used to provide the main source of livelihood for Hakkârians. That was until the early 1990s, when most villages were evacuated by the army as a counter-insurgency strategy.[56]

"Kurds have no friends but the mountains" says one famous Kurdish proverb. Until the 1970s, the mountains of Hakkâri hosted many bandits. They might escape to the mountains fleeing from the rural (military) police, the gendarmes, after shooting someone dead over this or that dispute, which most often had to do with family and tribal feuds bursting out or simmering over generations.[57] The bandits used to survive by smuggling and robbery, with the gendarmerie (*Jandarma*) their perennial enemy. Looking through the local newspapers of

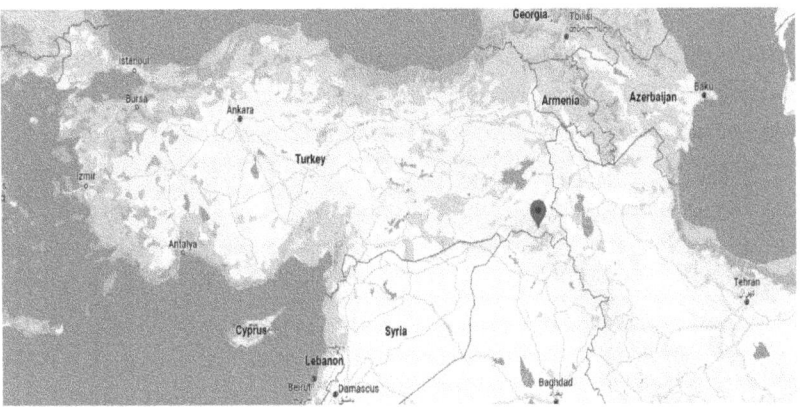

Figure 1a. Regional Location of Hakkâri.
Source: Google Maps

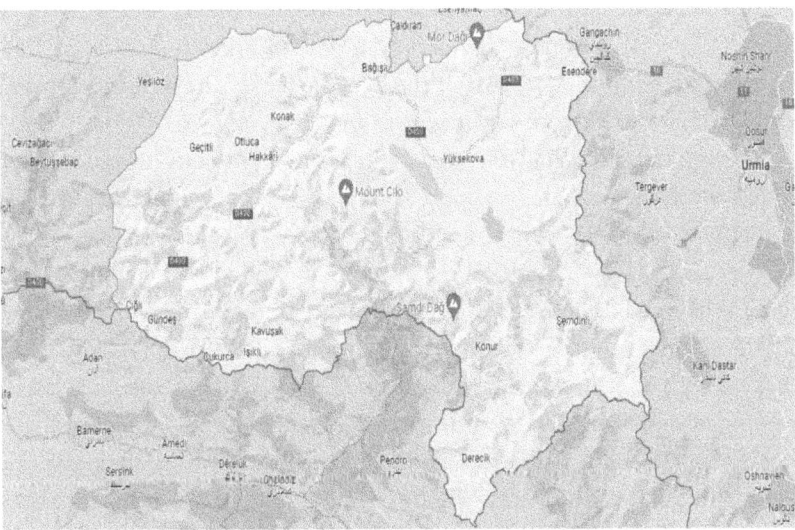

Figure 1b. The Province and Main Settlements of Hakkâri.
Source: Google Maps

Hakkâri from the 1960s and 1970s, one sees that they were full of news stories reporting clashes between the bandits and the gendarmerie.

The same mountains have been hosting PKK guerillas since 1982–83. Using the mountainous landscape as the terrain for their insurgence, the PKK forces waged a major asymmetric war against one of the biggest armies of NATO through the 1990s, which has continued to the present in the form of sporadic actions—even against overwhelming state power and ongoing military operations and notwithstanding PKK ceasefires, the abduction and capture in 1999 of their leader (Abdullah Öcalan), and an alternative strategy now of local autonomy rather than nation-state building.[58] Violent and deadly PKK attacks on military targets have thus continued throughout the AKP era, so within the timeframe of this study, such as ambushes of police border checkpoints and isolated Turkish army outposts situated, like proverbial sitting ducks, alone in the mountains— including those of Hakkâri.

1.3.1.2 Political Geography of Hakkâri: A History of Displacement

One cannot understand the material realities of Hakkâri in the twenty-first century without first reviewing the history of Turkish nation-building. This has included the deportation of heretic Assyrians from Hakkâri during the foundation of the Republic, the construction of national borders hindering the free movement of people, animals, and commodities, and the evacuation of villages during the mid-1990s as a key part of the state's general counter-insurgency strategy employed in the Kurdish region.

According to official statistics, the population of Hakkâri toward the end of the time period covered here was approaching three hundred thousand people— just under two and three-quarter hundred thousand, to be more precise (it is just a little over that now, c. 280k). Of the 273,041 individuals officially recorded as resident in the province in 2013, distributed between urban and rural settlements at a 55-to-45 ratio, 116,327 were living in Yüksekova, 80,497 in Hakkâri district, and 60.616 in Şemdinli, with 15.601 in Çukurca.[59] This population was strikingly homogeneous with regard to ethnicity and religion. Other than a portion of those (civil servants and military personnel) posted there by the state, the (local) population of modern Hakkâri is wholly Kurdish and Sunni Muslim.[60] This was not the case until the early 1920s, as Table 2 shows.

As a result of imperialist rivalry, Islamist policy of the Ottoman state, and regional conflicts between tribes, there was already a growing polarization between the Assyrians and Kurds of Hakkâri in the late nineteenth century. The tensions dramatically escalated in 1915 when Assyrians, regarded as collaborators of the Russians, were subjected to deportation and massacres carried out as part of a population engineering led by the Committee of Union and Progress (CUP, İttihad ve Terakki Cemiyeti). Thousands of Assyrians were killed and thousands more fled to Iran. When a group of Assyrians returned to Hakkâri in 1924, they

Table 2. Population of Hakkâri Districts and Province in 1891 by Religious Belonging

	Muslims	Gregorian Armenians	Assyrians	Chaldeans	Jews	Total
Hakkâri	16,900	2,000	15,000	—	—	33,900
Şemdinli	15,270	—	3,000	—	200	18,470
Yüksekova	14,700	1,900	9,000	300	300	26,200
Çukurca	11,930	—	31,960	—	—	43,890
Total	58,800	3,900	58,960	300	500	122,460

Source: Yurt Ansiklopedisi (1982).

were not welcomed by the army of the newly founded Turkish Republic and promptly re-deported.[61]

The construction of national borders separating Hakkâri from its immediate environment that ensued as part of the postimperial process of nation-state building divided peoples. Some families of a tribe found themselves on the Turkish side of the divide, while other families of the same tribe were on the Iraqi or Iranian side. Although the people and groupings continued to maintain their connections via marriage, sanctioned and illicit visits, and cooperation in cross-border exchanges (goods, produce, etc.), the partition nevertheless inflicted a heavy blow on the societal organization of Hakkârians around tribes. The national boundary also led to the emergence of illegal border trade. Sheep has always been the most common item of illegal border trade, yet the list of items subject to smuggling ranges from guns, tobacco, and diesel fuel to tea, cigarette, and sugar, and nowadays cell phones.

The recent intervention of the Turkish state in the local settlement patterns constituted a further nation-building policy in Hakkâri. Until the mid-1990s, the majority of Hakkârians were dispersed among hundreds of small and tiny rural settlements; the PKK guerillas effectively took advantage of the absence of the state and its consequent lack of control over these rural settlements in the war waged against the Turkish army. The massive village evacuation operations that followed, carried out by the army in Hakkâri in 1995 as part of the counterinsurgency strategy, was aimed at organizing the political geography to make it compatible with the spatial requirements of the nation-state. As a result, thousands of Hakkârians had to leave their homes, often with little or no warning and never with state support or facilities offered for rehousing or even directions where they should go. The spontaneous urban migration routes that developed thus led mostly to Hakkâri city and Yüksekova, in the first instance, and then Van and Mersin (and further afield, especially to Ankara, Istanbul and the West, i.e., western Turkey, in the years that followed). The population of Hakkâri city, for instance, rose from 30,000 to 80,000 with the displacement of the villagers.[62]

1.3.1.3 Village Evacuations, Urbanization, and Infrastructural Problems

The village evacuations of the 1990s have had a decisive impact on the current urban reality of Hakkâri. As shown in Figure 2, Hakkâri underwent a very speedy process of urbanization.

The rapid urbanization entailed significant infrastructural problems in the urban settlements of Hakkâri, and the everyday lives of Hakkârians were beset by many novel problems. Because the water supply network of Hakkâri city had been designed for a population that was less than half of its new number, for years, tap water was only available for 3–4 h every 2 days by the 2010s. In the bathrooms and toilets of each home in Hakkâri city, you would see dozens of big, plastic jerry cans full of water to use during the water cuts. The sewage system now covered just 40 percent of the provincial capital. The rest of the city used either septic tanks or drained its sewage directly to the small Katramas brook, which passes through the city. People around 30 years of age would say that they used to play in the Katramas in 1980s when they were children and it was clean;

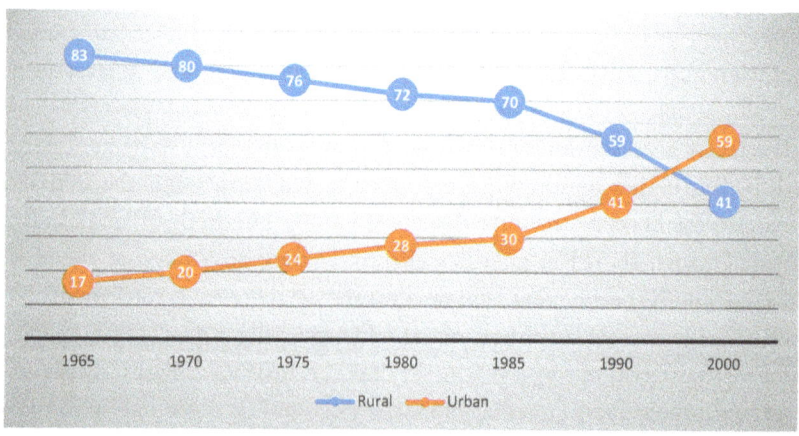

Figure 2. Rural and Urban Population in Hakkâri (1965–2000).
Source: Based on State Statistical Institution (Devlet İstatistik Enstitüsü, 2000) population census.

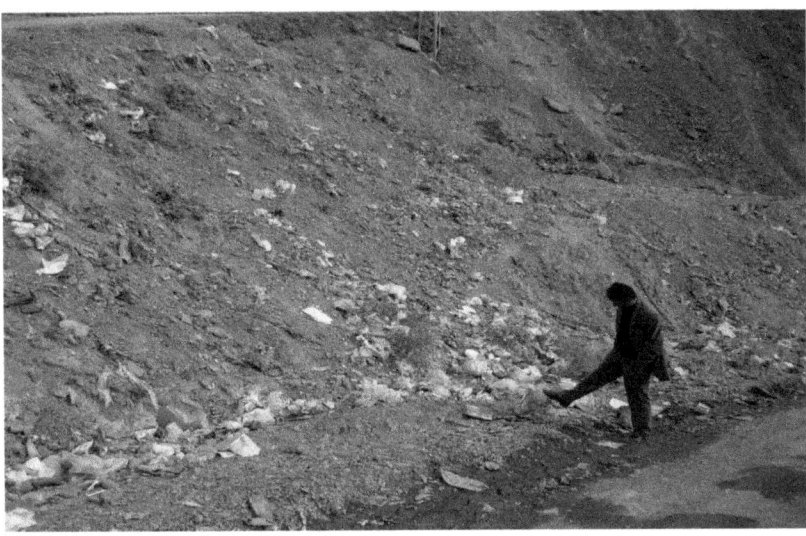

Figure 3. Kicking Garbage or Cursing His Fate? A Man Wanders the Hakkâri City Neighborhood of Keklikpınar, Formed by Village Evacuees.

now, it was more like a natural sewage system than a stream and posed a serious threat to health, especially for the children playing around it. Yüksekova, meanwhile, did not even have a sewage system in 2014, despite the fact that more than 60,000 people lived there.

Air pollution in Hakkâri city also became a terrible side-effect of the village evacuation, displacement, and rapid urbanization. Surrounded by high mountains, the city smoke produced by a dense population, most of whom used poor quality coal distributed by the state to the poor, did not easily disperse, and breathing became very difficult during the winter. Insufficient municipal services, garbage heaps at every corner, streets covered by dust and dirt in the summer and mud on rainy days can also be added to the long list of infrastructural shortcomings that helped to make Hakkâri an unhealthy city.

1.3.1.4 Economy

The economic structure of Hakkâri has been shaped by several factors. In addition to the lack of good roads connecting Hakkâri to other provinces, these have included the harsh physical geography of the province generally and remoteness of the province to main ports and the industrial centers located in western Turkey, as well as the extension of state activities through local employment and financial and other supports (old-age pensions, social aid, etc.)—and then the forced displacement of villagers in 1990s. The local economy has thus become based on animal husbandry, petty commodity production, the illegal border trade, and state salaries and social assistance payments. The unemployment rate in Hakkâri has been among the highest in the country.

Putting animal husbandry and the illegal border trade aside and focusing on the economic structure of urban settlements of Hakkâri, the site of the fieldwork carried out for this study, we can speak of a relatively unchanging reality. This local economy is principally made up of small enterprises and shops, which employ few workers and are largely alien to the logic of the extended reproduction of capital. In 1980, for instance, the number of workplaces in Hakkâri classified as under the manufacturing sector was 67, and 64 of these employed no more than four workers.[63] Nothing had substantially changed by the 1990s, other than the influx of labor. In 1994, there were no private enterprises operating in the manufacturing industry that employed more than ten workers.[64] Even in 2002, of the 2,236 economic units in Hakkâri, all but 43 were small-scale concerns (i.e., employing no more than nine workers).[65] The economy of Hakkâri remains based on small-scale economic enterprises, except for a few local agencies of the larger, nationwide businesses, like banks, mobile operators, and providers of consumer durables.

One can assert that the public enterprise policy followed in Hakkâri by the Turkish state has never been a factor greatly upsetting the prevalent relations of production and employment. In fact, less than 90 people were employed by the grand total of just three public enterprises opened in Hakkâri throughout the entirety of Republican history prior to this study, the first in 1977 and the last in 1986.[66] And these were either closed or privatized during the 1990s and the neoliberal consensus on the retreat of the state from the economy as an enterprise owner-operator.

Given the scarcity of employment opportunities offered by the economy of Hakkâri, it is not surprising that the village evacuations and rapid urbanization during the mid-1990s resulted in fractured communal support systems, poverty, and serious unemployment. Much of the unemployment went unrecorded. Even so, the official rate of unemployment more than trebled in a decade, rising from 3.8 percent in 1990 to 12.2 percent by 2000,[67] thus persisting as one of the highest rates in the country and leading to emigration from the region.

1.3.2 Fieldwork and Methodology

The history of the ethnographic research carried out in Hakkâri for this project dates back to 2007. In a short visit to Yüksekova that year facilitated by the contacts provided by a friend, I entered the field, made my first observations, listened to people, and witnessed their responses. From there, I was able to establish further contacts and develop connections in the area.

The main body of the ethnographical material used in the book was collected during the two-year period between September 2009 and September 2011. However, since I continued my work in Hakkâri that I had started in October 2009 until April 2014—as a research assistant in the Department of Management at the university there—I continued to conduct interviews, make new observations, and extend the field notes.

The material collected came from five main sources: semi-structured interviews conducted with GPs, medical specialists, and other healthcare staff; the illness and treatment narratives of Hakkârians; my field notes and participatory observations; a questionnaire-based study implemented in family health centers in Hakkâri city; and archival studies in the Prime Ministry State Archives and the National Library in Ankara.

There were two main groups of informants, the healthcare staff, especially doctors, and the ordinary users of the public hospital, health posts, and family health centers in the city. During the fieldwork with healthcare staff, information, views, and stories were provided by provincial healthcare directors along with administrators, doctors, nurses, midwives, ambulance drivers, pharmacists, and medical secretaries working in health institutions in urban Hakkâri (city), Yüksekova and Şemdinli.

Most of the doctors in Hakkâri were there to do compulsory public service. This compulsory service was a posting required as part of the qualification and initial employment system of the Turkish state in the fields of medicine and education; broadly, it was (and is) used to fill positions in the less desired areas of the country, since professionals have a tendency to originate from and aim for a more comfortable life in the west of the country. Enacted in 2005, the law requiring newly qualified GPs and medical specialists to fulfill their public service duty in "underdeveloped regions" was introduced as an instrument of the benevolent assimilation strategy. During the period studied, therefore, thousands of doctors fulfilled their compulsory service in the Kurdish region. The experiences and discourses of these doctors have much to tell us about the shortcomings of and subjectivities generated by the new strategy.

For a breadth of input and since the numbers of doctors in each district were not so high, I reached out to doctors across the province. Since Çukurca did not have a hospital but only a healthcare post (where no more than one or two GPs were employed), I met with doctors working in hospitals and healthcare posts in Hakkâri city, Yüksekova, and Şemdinli. In sum, I conducted interviews with 46 GPs, 53 specialists, and dozens of other healthcare workers. All of these interviews were in Turkish.

Most of the interviews with doctors were conducted in their examination rooms and mostly immediately after the end of the working day when done in hospitals. In the healthcare posts, which did not have many visitors, interviews were generally conducted during the day. I would show the one-page permission document taken from the provincial directorate of health before being asked for it. Some doctors would say "No, no, it's unnecessary; we can talk freely," others would read the document carefully to the end and even might ask me for my ID card given by the University of Hakkâri.

I asked the following list of questions in all interviews with the doctors:

- Was Hakkâri on your preference list, or were you appointed to Hakkâri by chance?
- How did you feel when you learned of your appointment to Hakkâri, and how did your family respond to the appointment?
- Where are you staying, and how did you arrange accommodation?
- What is an ordinary day in Hakkâri like?
- What do you do at weekends and in your leisure time?
- Do you spend time just with your colleagues or do you also have some friends from Hakkâri?
- How many patients do you see in a day on average?
- Have you ever been the subject of a complaint from any of the patients you have examined through the patient rights unit; if yes, what was it?
- Does the social tension prevailing in the city have any impact on your relationship with the patients?
- What do you think about the level of patient satisfaction with the medical establishment?
- Is it difficult to meet the expectations of patients?
- How do you communicate with patients who do not know Turkish?
- How would you evaluate your Hakkâri experience with respect to its impact on your plans for professional development, your view of the region and Hakkâri, and suchlike?

In addition to doctors, interviews were also conducted with leading figures of the local health bureaucracy, nursing and midwifery professionals, and other health professionals (ambulance drivers, medical secretaries, health clerks, etc.). Between 2009 and April 2014, there were five provincial directors of healthcare, four of whom were interviewed.

The fieldwork with patients was limited to Hakkâri city rather than extended to the whole province both to avoid risking its quality and diluting it with repetition given the similarity of the urban settlements with respect to economic development, demographic composition, and political outlook. Actually, the choice was between Hakkâri city (the provincial center), and Yüksekova, because the improvement of the medical establishment in the province was most noticeable in these two places. The main factor that pulled me to Hakkâri city and away from Yüksekova was the fact that it was more hospitable for a Turkish researcher. Doing ethnographic research in Yüksekova as a Turkish researcher would have had two limiting factors.

One was that the everyday reality of Yüksekova as a border settlement sustained by border trade, including heroin, was much more clandestine and relied on fewer contacts with civilian Turks as compared to the everyday reality of Hakkâri city, which, as the provincial capital hosting the central buildings of the local state institutions, was more familiar with and accessible to civilian Turks, who worked in the state institutions. Added to this was the difference between Yüksekova and Hakkâri city with respect to the level of political radicalism; in comparison to Hakkâri city, the political climate in Yüksekova is harsh, and one encounters a more suspicious stance regarding one's unusual presence in the town, which sometimes may take a threatening form.[68]

My fieldwork on Hakkârians proceeded mainly through contacts I could make through my position at the university as a research assistant. These contacts can be classified into three groups. The first group refers to actors in the immediate environment of the university, such as students and staff. As a newly founded university whose staff and students were largely from the area, the University of Hakkâri was a good point of access to different segments of the local society. Hakkârian students and employees agreed to be involved in the research either directly or via the participation of their friends and families. As I did not have an administrative position or work as an instructor grading students, there was no explicit hierarchical relationship between us that obviously harmed the quality of our conversations, ethically or ethnographically.

The second group refers to contacts passed on by key informants at the university. Colleagues who were ideologically close to the Kurdish movement and convinced of the genuineness and importance of the research introduced me to their personal contacts and directed them to cooperate with me. Some of these were important figures of the local Kurdish movement who, in turn, afforded further contacts in the Kurdish movement and NGOs led by the movement.

As well as directly and indirectly enabling these connections and contacts, the university also provided me with a legitimate position in the eyes of both the public authorities and Hakkârians who, after long years of war, tended to be suspicious of a researcher asking questions. As Hakkârians traditionally have great respect for teachers (*mamoste*), I could go into any shop and attempt to talk with the owner and people working there about their experiences with and ideas on healthcare provision in the city. Similarly, I never had to devote too much time and energy to convincing NGO administrators, former mayors, journalists, and businessmen to talk and have their comments recorded.

Methodologically, illness and treatment narratives are central to the ethnographic research devoted to understanding patient subjectivities generated by the ongoing improvement of healthcare provision in Hakkâri. To share their experiences with the medical establishment in Hakkâri city, patients most often told illness and treatment narratives, starting in Hakkâri and mostly ending up in Van, Ankara, or Istanbul. Most of these narratives were in Turkish, although a few were in Kurdish, especially those told by informants over 60. In sum, 90 interviews were conducted and countless exchanges engaged in with the local people on various aspects of health services in Hakkâri and their sociopolitical context. Archival work was also an invaluable input for a sense of the subjectivities of Hakkârians. The Prime Ministry State Archives houses official documents on Hakkâri and neighboring cities, especially Van, while the National Library in Ankara has copies of the local newspapers published between the early 1960s and late 1990s—like the *Hakkâri*, *Hakkâri Ekspress* and *Hakkâri'nin Sesi* (The Voice of *Hakkâri*). The National Library also had back copies of the leading Turkish national newspapers, like *Cumhuriyet*, *Milliyet*, and *Tercüman* (Republic, Nation, and Interpreter), giving insights into the issues featured on Hakkâri over the past 40 years and how they had been represented in the mainstream national media.

Apart from archival documents, I also used the official documents of the medical establishment in Hakkâri. These included working reports, statistical tables, and Provincial Directorate of Health presentations, along with certain other official documents obtained through the 2003 Freedom of Information Act (Bilgi Edinme Hakkı Kanunu, Law 4982). Together, these documents facilitated a better grasp of the actual situation of the medical establishment in Hakkâri.

Usage of the Freedom of Information Act was frequently required to gain information from the relevant official authorities. The AKP enacted this legislation in the first year of its rule, when it was committed to the EU membership process and thus to ensuring the transparency of the state and making it a more fully accountable entity. The Act endows Turkish citizens with the right to petition the units of state administration for information on non-private aspects of its operations. To support the ethnographic findings with quantitative data on the performances of the health institutions in Hakkâri, I submitted many petitions to the local health bureaucracy, from the provincial directorate to the public hospitals. However, the way the petitioning process actually proceeded was substantially different than as delineated on paper.

Through a process of trial and error, it became very clear that the nature of my personal contact and prior negotiations with the staff of the unit from which I was requesting information would determine first, whether a response to a petition would be elicited and second, the quality (relevance, usefulness, etc.) of that response. In almost every application made, and again at nearly every step of the process, the gatekeeping officials needed to be convinced both that sharing the data requested was not illegal and also that I would use it in a responsible way. The major consideration was not to cause problems. Effective employment of the Freedom of Information Act, that is, required the expenditure of a kind of affective labor.

This situation was not only related to the political and everyday atmosphere of Hakkâri and nor was it simply a matter of addressing the personal worries of the staff concerned about possible legal-administrative risks they might face in case I turned out to be the wrong person to share data with. Rather, less dramatically but more deeply, the personal worries of the staff concerning possible legal-administrative risks they might face had to do with the wider and more nebulous potential risk of sharing information: blurring the boundary between the domain of the state and society by democratizing official administrative data otherwise monopolized by the empowered bureaucracy and allowing it to be used in unpredictable, unintended, and even challenging ways.

In other words, there was a profound nervousness about giving away state control (i.e., to an outsider, someone not employed by and thus unaccountable in the hierarchy of authority). What I had to prove through the affective labor at every single stage of applications citing the Freedom of Information Act, therefore, was that I would not abuse the democratic potential of the freedom awarded by employing it against the state.

1.3.2.1 Methodological Limits of the Research: Not-So-Militant Anthropology

> My particular sympathies are transparent; I do not try to disguise them behind the role of an invisible and omniscient third-person narrator. Rather, I enter freely into dialogues and sometimes into conflicts and disagreements with the people of the Alto, challenging them just as they challenge me on my definitions of the reality in which I live. To use a metaphor from Mikhail Bakhtin (1981), the ethnographic interview here becomes more dialogic than monologic, and anthropological knowledge may be seen as something produced in human interaction, not merely "extracted" from naive informants who are unaware of the hidden agendas coming from the outsider. (Nancy Scheper-Hughes, 1992) [69]

There were elements to the researcher role I was playing that demanded attention. Indeed, my field experience in *Hakkâri* did lead me to critically reflect on what I was doing, how it was being received, and the wider context in which it was situated. I considered the methodological suggestion from Nancy Schepher-Hughes quoted above, which she describes as "militant anthropology."[70]

In the course of gaining permission for the fieldwork and later in conducting interviews with doctors, I found it impossible to act as a politically and morally engaged ethnographer who might "enter freely into dialogues and sometimes into conflicts and disagreements ... challenging them [the doctors] just as they challenge me."[71] In other words, I could not have completed the part of my fieldwork on doctors had I not maintained the image in the eyes of the local health bureaucracy and doctors of a naive Turkish social-scientist engaged in "neutral" scientific research. Crucially, what this meant in practice was that I was to act more or less in accordance with the expectations of Turkish state-nationalism.

This was made manifest early in the research, during the application to the Ministry of Health (MoH) in Ankara for permission to conduct the interviews in Hakkâri. "But, you are politicizing the issue" was the response of the MoH Head of the Department of Public Hospitals. In fact, it was the proposed title of the project that was the problem: "State, Citizenship and Health Services: Compulsory Public Services of Doctors in the AKP Period." Having predicted such concerns, I had already revised the original title by removing the word "Kurd" and adding "citizenship" and "state," but this was evidently insufficient. A problem remained: the reference to the "AKP Period."

I decided to use personal contacts that might facilitate access to the field site. The governor of Hakkâri at the time was from the same area as my father, making them, thus me, *hemşeri*, people from the same *memleket*. The origins of place with its communal implications of shared roots are a crucial feature of Turkish culture—and others, of course, including Kurdish—and this traditional claim-making for assistance on the basis of geographical, family bonds remains effective in all walks of life. Thus, I asked my father's help in making contact with the governor. It worked, and I succeeded in gaining permission from the local health bureaucracy authorizing me to conduct interviews with doctors and other healthcare staff. Meanwhile, the title of the project needed another adjustment allowing for political sensitivities, to just "Compulsory Public Service, Doctors, and Health Services."

Thus, a form of self-censorship developed, which had to be continued during the interviews with the doctors. Working in a city like Hakkâri led the majority of doctors to adopt a particularly cautious and distant stance toward all beyond their immediate milieu, which was almost exclusively composed of their colleagues. Because I was a PhD student abroad (meaning in the West—Europe or America—Budapest, in fact), a graduate of Istanbul's Bosphorus (Boğaziçi) University, the most prestigious university in Turkey, and a middle-class Turk—and had official permission—it was relatively easy for me to engage with the doctors. We could comfortably "speak the same language," as it were. Yet, I was nevertheless tested at the beginning of almost every interview.

"Where are you from?" the doctors would ask. "Are you from Hakkâri?" This can be read simply as "Are you Kurdish?" Then, "Why did you choose Hakkâri" and "Why this topic?" This questioning of motive and real interest can be rendered, "Do you have a hidden agenda?" Other questions would follow, like "Where did you graduate from?" and "Where are you studying now?" Education is a key indicator of background and perspective; the real question was "Are you reliable?" Or, in an atmosphere of suspicion and concern for their well-being—fear for their lives and their livelihoods, even, the doctors' questions all amounted to one query "Can I trust you?"

The dialogue between us was fragile. It began tentatively and continued that way. Most often, it was just not possible to "enter freely into dialogues and sometimes into conflicts and disagreements," let alone "challenging" one another on our lived realities. Specifically, I did not insist on questioning the terminology they used to refer to the Kurdish issue, words like "terrorism," "underdevelopment," and "ignorance" (the latter two implying the thesis that Kurdish resistance to the Turkish state was a product of the traditional socioeconomic structures still in place, that the lack of modern development and education were the root causes of the problem manifesting as Kurdish violence).

For my part, I tended toward more neutral, "value-free" language. Inspired by medical terminology, for example, I often used the term "the level of social pressure [*toplumsal tansiyon*] in the city" to refer to the extra-ordinariness of everyday life in Hakkâri. While transcribing the interview records, I would notice my avoidance of the terms "Kurd" and "Kurdish," like the doctors.

Thus, it was difficult to ask doctors whether the fact that they did not know Kurdish (i.e., the language) affected the quality of healthcare they provided to old men and women. Obviously it might, since the elderly typically had little Turkish as they had not been to school, where Turkish was the medium of education, or their schooling had only lasted until the beginning of adolescence, and they had long since forgotten any Turkish they had learned. As a result, instead of a straightforward question about the doctors' lack of Kurdish, a version of this became standard: "How does the language issue affect your job?"

The ethnographic cost of adopting such a reticent stance is clear: The information that could have been gained from doctors would certainly have been different and maybe more illustrative than that extracted from the position of a middle-class, "Turkish" researcher had I attempted to appear as a critic of Turkish state-nationalism rather than as an "invisible" and "omniscient" third-person narrator.

Was this ethnographic cost unavoidable or just a preference? I still cannot give a clear-cut answer. I might state that there were gains as well as costs, which is true (see below). On the other, though, the question might rather be reformulated, thus: Is the gesture of carrying out an ethnographic study without having to "disguise" any particular "sympathies" behind the role of the supposedly invisible and omniscient third-person narrator an option equally available for all anthropologists in all situations?

1.3.2.2 Methodological Limits of the Research: Abstractions and Stigmatizations

In order to uncover another constraint of this ethnographic study, it is instructive to consider the resistance of Hüseyin (pseudonym, an informant) to being my ethnographic object. Hüseyin was a village evacuee from Çukurca. Although he had defended his village against the PKK for years as a member of the state-instituted paramilitary the Village Guards (*Türkiye Güvenlik Köy Korucuları*), he was humiliatingly disarmed by the army forces, labeling him as unreliable, when his village was evacuated in 1995. When I met him in 2009, he was a leading figure of the neighborhood of Bilen (not the real name) and made a living selling smuggled items.

I met him in front of the small shanty structure he used as a shop, and we headed off to Bilen to talk with the people living there. Bilen was situated at the foot of Hakkâri Castle, which had been occupied by one of the special police force teams on the pretext of ensuring security since the beginning of the 1990s. Although it is an old neighborhood, evacuees arriving from the villages of Çukurca in the mid-1990s had radically altered its composition. During the period of my fieldwork, like other neighborhoods settled by the victims of village evacuations, it would transform into a battlefield on special days in the Kurdish (political) calendar, with children, teenagers, and young men on one side and special police forces on the other. Indeed, home raids, arrests, gas bombs, armored police vehicles patrolling the streets, and demonstrators throwing stones and chanting illegal slogans were ordinary, mundane aspects of everyday life in the Bilen neighborhood.

I was asking Hüseyin about the neighborhood as we walked, and when we arrived at Bilen, he took me to a man sitting outside his shanty-like house. The man welcomed us and offered tea with the usual hospitality of Hakkârians, and we started discussing health issues, including doctors, the hospital, and his specific health problems. Just a few minutes had passed when a sudden explosion boomed, interrupting our conversation. I spun around to see a smoking object flying through the air. Others followed it. The police were throwing tear-gas bombs from the special police force station. The target was 200 m away, though buildings prevented me from seeing what was going on there.

"Come on, we're going" said Hüseyin and stood up, in a tone that left me no choice but to follow. We began to proceed toward the target of the missiles. We turned a corner, our eyes started tearing up, but we kept on. Meanwhile, Hüseyin was restlessly repeating: "Do you see anybody there? Do you see anybody there? There is nobody at all, you see!" Indeed, there was not.

The rain of gas bombs did not stop for a moment during our walk. Fumes spread over the whole neighborhood, and it became impossible to carry on any further. "Let's stop Hüseyin" I said. "I can't go anymore. I can't breathe. Let's turn back."

The impression that most etched itself into my mind during those difficult moments though was the absence of any sign of panic in the faces and movements of the people around, still going about their daily business as though nothing was happening. Women were washing clothes while wiping the tears from their eyes, and children were running around like normal, as if the whole neighborhood was not being terrorized. I asked the children if I could take their photograph but was declined. An eight- or nine-year-old girl told me that she did not trust me with the words "You aren't trustworthy!" (*Size güven olmaz*).

Who was this "you"? As a Turk walking the neighborhood streets, I was suspicious. Then, I spoke to the girl in Kurdish. I told her that I was not a police officer, I was a teacher in the University of Hakkâri—but she did not agree to have her photo taken, and I did not insist any further. While leaving the street to go to Hüseyin's house to continue talking, Hüseyin said "You saw it, right? There is no one around. Did you see anybody there? No, you saw it!" And then he added in a tone implying some distrust, "You didn't take any photos of the gas bombs. Why not?"

"How could I take photos?" I responded. "The fumes choked me."

"Then take my photo," he said and posed for the camera, rubbing his eyes as if still affected by the tear gas (Figure 4).

Hüseyin's daughters and an old man were in the house when we arrived. Later three men, all from the villages of Çukurca, joined us. Hüseyin got straight to the point: "The Turks don't believe me if I tell them what happened a few minutes ago, but now you've seen it all. You, as a Turk, wouldn't have believed in my words if you hadn't witnessed what just happened."

Certainly, the knowledge that led Hüseyin to have me witness the truth for myself rather than wasting time trying to convince by telling stories was

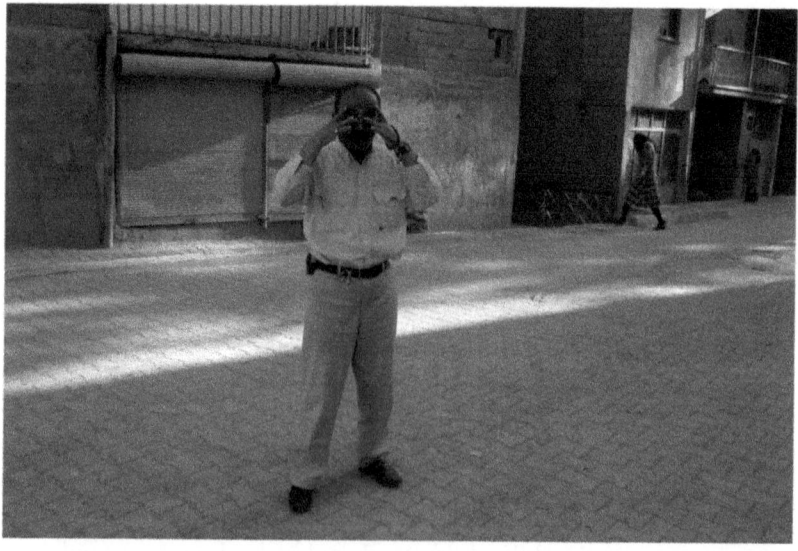

Figure 4. Showing the Effects of Tear Gas (Hakkâri City).

conditioned by the history of the established patterns of relationship between Hakkârians, Kurds, and the Turkish state. My own individuality was lost under the burden of this history. In Hüseyin's eyes, I was abstracted as a Turk identified with the Turkish state, which has always imprisoned the voices of Kurds into a narrative of terrorism. Our encounter was placed within a reality full of abstractions, stereotypes, and stigmatizations.

Similarly, during my first days in Hakkâri, a taxi driver unconsciously approved my initial impressions of the city by saying with a military reference (in Turkish), "Yes, commander" (*Evet, komutanım*). The equation in his mind here was similar to that of the small girl declining my request to take her photo: if you speak fluent Turkish, seem like a middle-class Turk (have such a habitus), and you have short hair, no beard or mustache, then you are presumably a military officer (thus, outsider). The equation was not accurate in my case, but it hints at how my Turkish informants, the GPs, medical specialists, and other health professionals, would perceive me as "one of their own" and feel at liberty to express their sometimes racist and stigmatizing ideas without hesitation while the recorder was on, even after the series of questions listed (above).

Again, inevitably, this reality carried its ethnographic cost. Instead of speaking from within their own particular experiences and with their own words, some of my local informants preferred speaking through an abstract political space of Kurdishness. In other cases, for a sincere conversation to develop, especially with those informants who had greatly suffered from state violence in the past, some issues had to remain unspoken and unaddressed. This occurred, for example, in my interview with the head of an association close to the Kurdish movement.

Q: I understand you've lived through many tragic events?
A: I don't want to talk about it. Otherwise, we won't be able to talk properly. All that was done to me was done in the name of Turkishness, and the people doing all those things did them as Turks, not as civil servants (*memur*).

With the word *memur* here, he referred to the security forces (police, gendarmes, soldiers, etc.). They may have been employed by the state, but they had abused that power as Turks, just as he had been abused as a Kurd, not as a citizen.

1.4 Overview

The organization of this work as an anthropology of policy is guided by the methodological argument conceptualizing "policy as a relation between, first, political programs and justifications for particular ways of exercising power ('political rationalities'); second, everyday practices and methods introduced to govern particular people in particular ways ('governmental technologies'); and, third, the perceptions, experiences, and conduct ('subjectivities') of the people towards whom these rationalities and technologies are directed."[72] In other words, the book examines healthcare provision in Hakkâri in 2003–14 as a privileged instrument of state-nationalism by focusing on the political rationalities imposed, governmental technologies used, and subjectivities constructed and de/reconstructed through healthcare provision in the province.

The book is composed of five main chapters (i.e., other than the introductory and concluding chapters—Chapters 1 and 7). Chapters 2 and 3 provide a historical background of the state-citizen relations in the Kurdish region with a focus on Hakkâri. In Chapter 2, the state-citizen relations in Hakkâri and the Kurdish region generally in the pre-AKP period, that is, Kemalist Turkey, are reviewed, largely as characterized by sovereign violence. Based mainly on archival work, this chapter argues that the Turkish state of the young Kemalist Republic lacked the capacity to carry out an effective program of state-nationalism in the Kurdish region, including Hakkâri. Instead, therefore, the Turkish state had to content itself with instituting its sovereignty in the region and defending it against threats, like the illegal border trade and the PKK, by relying on collective punishment as a deterrent.

Chapter 3 considers a different aspect of the state-citizen relations in Hakkâri in Kemalist Turkey. Introducing the term "indirect state racism" and relying mainly on archival work, this chapter shows that the Turkish state did not or could not expend sufficient effort and reserve sufficient resources to overcome the "underdevelopment" of Hakkâri. A description and analysis of the poverty of healthcare provision in Hakkâri in Kemalist Turkey stands at the center of the chapter.

The fourth chapter focuses on the political rationality of the state-nationalism of the AKP and the technologies, strategies, and instruments employed to practice this rationality in Hakkâri. This chapter identifies the specific nature of nationalism enacted by the AKP and uncovers its historical continuity with the Turkish nationalism of Kemalist Turkey through an analysis of the AKP's discourses on the Kurdish issue. It shows that the state-nationalism of the AKP between 2003 and 2014 was a version of Turkish nationalism aiming to contain Kurdish unrest through the simultaneous use of coercive and benevolent instruments of power. This nationalism embraced Kurds as individual citizens of the one nation, which was Turkish, and as bodies, as service-beneficiaries worthy of care, while criminalizing Kurdishness as the basis of a right to separate polity. It is argued that the simultaneous use of benevolent and coercive instruments to refashion the nation in this way was performed in a more Islamic, less ethnically marked way, but still on a Turkish basis. It is also shown that the effectiveness of the approach of developing a community of service-beneficiaries satisfied with the ever-increasing quality of life built on economic growth and development has been limited. Importantly, this proved insufficient to overcome Hakkârians' firmly established conviction that their lives count for little in the eyes of the state.

In Chapter 5, the focus is placed on the experiences of Hakkârians with the medical establishment in the context of its major improvements during the period. At the center of the examination stands the persistent, massive dissatisfaction of Hakkârians with the quality of healthcare provision despite its upgrading. Based on ethnographic findings, the chapter shows that the persistence of patient dissatisfaction in Hakkâri in the period had to do with two outcomes of the history of state-citizen relations there: the well-established conviction on the part of the local people that their lives counted for little in the Turkish Republic, and the strong political sensitivity and intolerance of Hakkârians to discrimination, to not being treated as fully-fledged citizens.

Chapter 6, which is also based on ethnographic work, looks at the other side of the encounter of Hakkârians and the medical establishment, making its focal point the GPs and medical specialists serving in the health institutions in Hakkâri. Using Henry Lefebvre's approach to the production of space, this chapter reveals that most of Turkish GPs and medical specialists fulfilling their compulsory service experienced life in Hakkâri as an endurance. Their lack of attachment to the province and tendency to keep to the instrumental rationality of day-counting deprived them of the capacity and real contacts through which to empathize with Hakkârians still dissatisfied with their new, improved healthcare provision.

Finally, the Conclusion elaborates on the limits of Turkish state-nationalism carried out in the Kurdish region during the first decade of AKP rule, reflecting upon the gap between Hakkârians still dissatisfied with healthcare provision and Turkish GPs and medical specialists incapable of making sense of this in the face of the material progress made. Through this discussion and with reference to other national experiences, I derive further conclusions which may be useful for analyses of the use of social policy for the containment of ethnopolitical challenges in different multiethnic settings.

Notes

1. Cris Shore and Susan Wright, "Policy: A New Field of Anthropology," in *Anthropology of Policy: Critical Perspectives on Governance and Power*, ed. Cris Shore and Susan Wright (London and New York: Routledge, 1997), 18.
2. See Erdem Yörük, "The Politics of the Turkish Welfare System Transformation in the Neoliberal Era: Welfare as Mobilization and Containment" (PhD diss., The Johns Hopkins University, 2012).
3. See Cemil Koçak, *Umumi Müfettişlikler, 1927–1952* (İstanbul: İletişim, 2003).
4. Tozun Bahcheli and Sid Noed, "The Justice and Development Party and the Kurdish Question," in *Nationalisms and Politics in Turkey: Political Islam, Kemalism and the Kurdish Issue*, ed. Marlies Casier and Joost Jongerden (London and New York: Routledge, 2011), 106–7.
5. Daniel Béland and André Lecours, *Nationalism and Social Policy: The Politics of Territorial Solidarity* (Oxford and New York: Oxford University Press, 2008), 21.
6. Ibid., 138.
7. Ibid.
8. See among others, Nicola McEwen, *Nationalism and the State: Welfare and Identity in Scotland and Quebec* (Brussels: Peter Lang, 2005); Regis Dandoy and Pierre Baudewyns, "The Preservation of Social Security as a National Function in the Belgian Federal State," in *The Territorial Politics of Welfare*, ed. Nicola McEwen and Luis Moreno (London and New York: Routledge, 2005); Michael Keating, "Social Citizenship, Solidarity and Welfare in Regionalized and Plurinational States," *Citizenship Studies* 13, no. 5 (2009).
9. "Seçimler," Yüksek Seçim Kurulu (Supreme Electoral Council), accessed January 15, 2022, http://www.ysk.gov.tr/ysk/GenelSecimler.html.
10. After the building of the AKP provincial organization was bombed by the PKK in 2008, the party could not find a place for rent for several months due to the unwillingness of the supporters of the Kurdish movement and the fear of material and personal damage on the part of property owners. In the end, they rented a place in a building belonging to Hakkâri Provincial Special Administration, where they continued to work after the building was transferred to the University of Hakkâri. Thus, the provincial organization of the government party could only find a place to rent in a public institution. The building had two entrances for two sections of the building, and in front of the entry of the section in which the AKP provincial organization worked, there was a Special Police Force station with sandbags and automatic weapons. When I studied at my University office at night, I had to use

this entrance, which meant a short interrogation each time the duty roster changed. When the building had to be vacated in 2012 due to refurbishment, the AKP was not able to find a place until the following year, which was only enabled with the moderation of the political atmosphere with the Kurdish Opening (see Section 4.2).

11 Cengiz Güneş, *The Kurdish National Movement in Turkey: From Protest to Resistance* (New York: Routledge, 2012), 22.
12 Etienne Balibar and Immanuel Maurice Wallerstein, *Race, Nation, Class: Ambiguous Identities* (London and New York: Verso, 1991), 93.
13 Michael Billig, *Banal Nationalism* (London and Thousand Oaks, CA: Sage, 1995), 5.
14 Benedict R. O'G Anderson, *Imagined Communities: Reflections on the Origin and Spread of Nationalism* (London and New York: Verso, 2006), 5.
15 Billig, *Banal Nationalism*, 8.
16 Anthony D. Smith, *Nationalism: Theory, Ideology, History* (Cambridge: Polity Press, 2010), 83.
17 Jon E. Fox and Cynthia Miller-Idriss, "Everyday Nationhood," *Ethnicities* 8, no. 4 (2008): 537.
18 Smith, *Nationalism*, 84.
19 Fox and Miller-Idriss, "Everyday Nationhood," 537–8.
20 Béland and Lecours, *Nationalism and Social Policy*, 19.
21 Nicola McEwen and Luis Moreno, "Exploring the Territorial Politics of Welfare," in *The Territorial Politics of Welfare*, ed. Nicola McEwen and Luis Moreno (London and New York: Routledge, 2005), 3.
22 Béland and Lecours, *Nationalism and Social Policy*, 219.
23 George Steinmetz, "Introduction: Culture and the State," in *State/Culture: State-Formation after the Cultural Turn*, ed. George Steinmetz (Ithaca, NY: Cornell University Press, 1999), 9.
24 Shore and Wright, "Policy," 3–4.
25 Michael Hechter, *Containing Nationalism* (Oxford and New York: Oxford University Press, 2000), 62.
26 Dipesh Chakrabarty, *Provincializing Europe: Postcolonial Thought and Historical Difference* (Princeton, NJ and Oxford: Princeton University Press, 2008), 62.
27 Ibid., 51.
28 Ibid., 54.
29 Ibid., 62.
30 Partha Chatterjee, *The Politics of the Governed: Reflections on Popular Politics in Most of the World* (New York: Columbia University Press, 2004), 6.
31 Ibid.
32 John Clarke, "Welfare States as Nation States: Some Conceptual Reflections," *Social Policy and Society* 4, no. 4 (2005): 412.
33 Ibid., 413.

34 John Holloway, *Change the World without Taking Power* (London and Sterling, VA: Pluto Press, 2002), 58.
35 Chakrabarty, *Provincializing Europe*, 249.
36 Ibid., 62.
37 Homi K. Bhabha, *The Location of Culture* (London and New York: Routledge, 2004), 208, 211.
38 Ibid., 211.
39 Ibid., 212.
40 John McLeod, *Beginning Postcolonialism* (Manchester and New York: Manchester University Press, 2000), 119.
41 Anderson, *Imagined Communities*, 7.
42 Giorgio Agamben, *Homo Sacer. Sovereign Power and Bare Life*, Meridian (Stanford, CA: Stanford University Press, 1998), 84.
43 Thomas Blom Hansen and Finn Stepputat, "Introduction," in *Sovereign Bodies: Citizens, Migrants, and States in the Postcolonial World*, ed. Thomas Blom Hansen and Finn Stepputat (Princeton, NJ: Princeton University Press, 2005), 17.
44 Nicos Poulantzas also asserts that the assimilative aspect of nation is its distinct feature. See Nicos Poulantzas, "The Nation," in *State/Space: A Reader*, ed. Neil Brenner et al. (Malden, MA: Blackwell, 2003), 65–83.
45 Anderson, *Imagined Communities*, 7.
46 Claude Lefort, *The Political Forms of Modern Society: Bureaucracy, Democracy, Totalitarianism* (Cambridge: Polity Press, 1986), 305.
47 John Breuilly, *Nationalism and the State* (Manchester: Manchester University Press, 1993), 63.
48 Zygmunt Bauman, *Modernity and Ambivalence* (Ithaca, NY: Cornell University Press, 1991).
49 For a comprehensive study on the causality between the emergence of popular sovereignty and ethnic cleansing, see Michael Mann, *The Dark Side of Democracy: Explaining Ethnic Cleansing* (New York: Cambridge University Press, 2005).
50 Michel Foucault, *Security, Territory, Population: Lectures at the CollèGe De France, 1977–78*, ed. Michel Senellart (Basingstoke and New York: Palgrave Macmillan, 2007), 85.
51 Ibid.
52 Agamben, *Homo Sacer*, 100–101.
53 See "Hakkari," in *Yurt Ansiklopedisi: Türkiye, il il* (Istanbul: Anadolu Yayıncılık, 1982), 3291.
54 Ibid.
55 Hüseyin Atmaca, *Bir Köy Çocuğunun Serüveni: Köy Enstitüsünden Parlamentoya* (Ankara: Abis, 2009), 180–82.
56 Enver Özkahraman and Nasrullah Müezzinoğlu, *Hakkari 94* (Ankara: Erk Yayıncılık, 1996), 51–65.

57 Ahmet Özcan, *"Ama Eşkiyalık Çağı Kapandı!": Modern Türkiye'de Son Kürt Eşkiyalık Çağı (1950–1970)* (İletişim: Istanbul, 2018).

58 Joost Jongerden and Cengiz Gunes, "A Democratic Nation: The Kurdistan Workers' Party (PKK) and the idea of nation beyond the state," in *Beyond Nationalism and the Nation-State: Radical Approaches to Nation*, ed. İlker Cörüt and Joost Jongerden (London: Routledge, 2021), 3–22.

59 Türkiye İstatistik Kurumu [Turkish Statistical Institute], *Seçilmiş Göstergelerle Hakkari 2013* (Ankara: TÜİK, 2014), 97.

60 Parallel with the general rise in the education level of people in the Kurdish region since 1990s, there has been a growing trend of Kurdification of local state personnel in recent years; indeed, this was one of the biggest fears of Kemalists, as can be seen in the classified reports listing measures necessary to be taken for Turkification of Kurds.

61 David Gaunt, "The Complexity of the Assyrian Genocide," *Genocide Studies International* 9, no. 1 (2015): 92–94.

62 Dilek Kurban et al., *Coming to Terms with Forced Migration: Post-Displacement Restitution of Citizenship Rights in Turkey* (Istanbul: TESEV, 2007), 277–311.

63 Devlet İstatistik Enstitüsü [State Statistical Institute], *1980 Genel Sanayi Ve İşyerleri Sayımı* (Ankara: DİE, 1983), 1–21.

64 Devlet İstatistik Enstitüsü [State Statistical Institute], *Ekonomik Ve Sosyal Göstergeler* (Ankara: DİE, 1998), 242.

65 Türkiye İstatistik Kurumu [Turkish Statistical Institute], *Genel Sanayi Ve İşyerleri Sayımı, 2002* (Ankara: TÜİK, 2006), 69.

66 Cemil Kutbay, *Kalkınmada Öncelikli İllerde Sanayii Tesisleri* (Ankara: Başbakanlık Devlet Planlama Teşkilatı, Kalkınmada Öncelikli YÖreler Dairesi, 1993), 15.

67 Devlet İstatistik Enstitüsü (State Statistical Institute), *2000 Genel Nüfus Sayımı: Nüfusun Sosyal ve Ekonomik Nitelikleri, Hakkari*, 52.

68 Once, I went to the Iran Bazaar in Yüksekova, where oriental items were sold. I entered a shop selling mostly blankets. There was no shopkeeper, but a youngster of around 14 years old was dealing with the customers. I had a look at some blankets and asked their prices. When I was about to leave the shop, the youngster said "When our time comes, we'll settle the score with you," which, in the face of my surprised bemusement, he repeated. The shopkeeper next door, who had witnessed the dialogue, intervened and asked me to forgive the boy's disrespect, saying he was just messing about. Most probably, the lad thought I was from the police or similar. This incident cannot be easily dismissed as the insolent and foolish talk of a youngster, however. A year later, on September 27, 2011, Engin Yıldırım, a chemical engineer in Kocaeli accompanying his wife who had been appointed to Yüksekova as a primary school teacher, was shot dead after being mistaken for a policeman.

69 Nancy Scheper-Hughes, *Death without Weeping: The Violence of Everyday Life in Brazil* (Berkeley: University of California Press, 1992), 25.

70 "The Primacy of the Ethical: Propositions for a Militant Anthropology," *Current Anthropology* 36, no. 3 (1995).
71 Ibid.
72 Gritt B. Nielsen, "Peopling Policy: On Conflicting Subjectivities of Fee-Paying Students," in *Policy Worlds: Anthropology and the Analysis of Contemporary Power*, ed. Cris Shore, Susan Wright, and Davide Però (New York: Berghahn Books, 2011), 69.

2

The Kurdish Question, Sovereign Violence, and Hakkâri

In order to inquire into the nature of state-citizen relations in Hakkâri in the first decade of the AKP period, it is necessary to provide a context by reviewing them prior to that, in the pre-AKP period of Kemalist Turkey, and by situating these relations within the larger context of the Kurdish question. Through detailed archival work, this chapter shows that these relations were determined by the Turkish state's lack of capacity to control and colonize daily life in Kurdish provinces generally. Thus, it was not able to effectively assimilate Kurds into Turkishness, as was planned, particularly in the eastern and rural parts of the region, including Hakkâri. Thus, while the primary principle structuring the way in which the Turkish state ruled in most parts of Kurdish region was that of the constitution and defense of state sovereignty, the main mechanism deployed for this purpose was the continuous collective punishment of the population.

2.1 Historical Background of the Kurdish Question

The last hundred years of the Ottoman Empire was a history of the disintegration of a multiethnic and multireligious empire. The Empire had to leave most of its former lands, first in the Balkans through the nineteenth century and then in the

Middle East after the defeat of the Triple Alliance with which the Ottomans had allied in the First World War (WWI). The Treaty of Sèvres (August 10, 1920), the post-WWI pact between the victorious Allied powers and the Ottoman state, "left the Ottoman Empire only a rump state in northern Asia Minor with Istanbul as its capital."[1]

The gradual disintegration had resulted in two parallel processes: an Islamization of the population[2] and concomitant political adoption of Islamism in the Hamidian Era and the development of Turkish nationalism, which became a ruling strategy after the Balkan Wars (1912–13).[3] The establishment by Christian subjects of their own nation-states in the Balkans in the nineteenth century, the migrations of Muslim subjects to Anatolia (from the Balkans in the northwest after the Balkan Wars and from the expanding Russian Empire in the northeast, including Crimea and the Caucasus, after the Russo-Ottoman War of 1877–78), the migration of non-Muslim subjects in Anatolia to Europe and America, and the massacre of the Armenian population in 1915 by the ruling CUP were the main features of the Islamization process. The Anatolian population became almost wholly Muslim, with the exception of Greeks.[4] On the eve of the national struggle (1919), therefore, the population of what was to become Turkey was mainly composed of Turks and Kurds.

As for the ideological transformation, even though Ottomanism as the embracing and umbrella ideology of the 1908 Constitutional Revolution replaced the modernist Islamism of Sultan Abdul Hamid II, the disintegration of the Empire could not be prevented. Gradually, the CUP gave up on the imperial ethos—under duress following WWI—in favor of Turkish nationalism and secularism. Nevertheless, it was the Muslim composition of the population and cementing power of Islam that determined the ideo-political orientation of the national struggle.

The national struggle led by the former Ottoman commander Mustafa Kemal took place between 1919 and 1922, largely against Greek forces, which occupied the Aegean region of western Anatolia. The goal of the struggle as formulated by the leadership was "to preserve national independence and to protect the sultanate and caliphate."[5] The nation whose independence was sought was not (yet) declared to be the Turkish nation. As expressed by *Mustafa Kemal* in a speech in the assembly on May 1, 1920, "[W]hat is intended here is not only Turks, not only Circassians, not only Kurds, not only Lazes, but the Islamic ethnic elements comprising all these peoples . . . [that together constitute] a sincere community."[6]

During the national struggle, warm messages concerning the ethnic rights of Kurds were many times given by the Kemalist leadership. As the logical result of this Islamic understanding of nation, the majority and minorities were defined with respect to their religious belonging in the Peace Treaty of Lausanne of 1923, which established the Republic of Turkey as an internationally recognized sovereign state.[7] Jews, Greeks, and Armenians were given minority status and hence the right to open their own community schools, as during the Empire, but under the strict control of the Ministry of Education.

The turning point for Turkish-Kurdish relations was the Sheikh Said rebellion in 1925. The abolition of the caliphate and the visible Turkish (modern nationalist) orientation of the Kemalist leadership in 1924 following the consolidation of Kemalist leadership in the elections held after the victory in the Independence War triggered widespread discontent, especially among the Kurdish intelligentsia. Organized by the Kurdish nationalist Azadi (Freedom) society and led by Sheikh Said, a leading figure of the (Sunni Sufi) Naqshbandi order—making it ethnoreligious, or partly (Kurdish) nationalist in character—a major uprising developed in the Kurdish region. It was harshly suppressed. The leaders were executed and thousands of Kurds were deported to the west of the new country.[8] Other revolts were to follow, including the Mount Ağrı and Dersim rebellions of 1927–30 and 1937–38, respectively, which were also dealt with.

The lesson drawn from the post-independence Sheikh Said rebellion by the Turkish nationalist elites of the ruling Republican People's Party (Cumhuriyet Halk Partisi, CHP) led by Mustafa Kemal was not the necessity of the destruction of the Kurdish population, although this was considered.[9] Rather, it was taken to demonstrate the urgency of a systematic assimilation (*temsil*) program. The CHP leadership mostly believed that Kurds, along with other non-Turkish Muslim ethnicities, could be assimilated since the constitutive assumption of Turkishness in the establishment of the Republic was its Islamic character. It was necessary to be Muslim to be eligible for Turkishness, as *Soner Çağaptay* shows through an analysis of cases of naturalization and denaturalization; while non-Turkish Muslims, such as Bosnians or Albanians, were granted Turkish citizenship, Orthodox Christian Gagauzian Turks were not.[10]

"How happy is the one who calls himself a Turk" was the motto of this conflated, ethnoreligious understanding of the nation, grounded in a kind of imperial inclusiveness (in the sense of being open to Muslim subjects of the Ottoman Empire irrespective of ethnicity) but expressed through a restrictively interpreted modernist definition (under the ethnocultural hegemony of Turkishness)—and increasingly so by the hard-line "Kemalists," as they became known. This understanding set the policy to be followed by the Turkish state until the early 1990s.

Essentially, the separate existence of Kurds as an ethnicity was denied while the Turkishness of the Kurds was asserted.

2.2 Sovereign Violence and State Incapacity

Numerous reports were submitted to the top ruling cadres to assist with the assimilation of Kurds. The Eastern Reform Plan (Şark Islahat Planı), prepared immediately after the Sheikh Said rebellion, was particularly important. The measures it recommended formed the framework of Turkish assimilation strategy and also the basis of later texts devoted to this task.[11] One of the measures suggested in the Plan was control of the Kurdish region by emergency rule. Demographic engineering was another. The deportation of unreliable Kurdish families to the west of the country and Turks to the Kurdish region was suggested. Cultural assimilation via boarding schools and the banning of Kurdish was also a central plank of the strategy, as was the integration of the region into the rest of the country, both through effective border policing, which would de-link it from Iraqi and Iranian Kurdistan, and by the construction of roads and railroads. The need to establish an effective surveillance system was also mentioned. Last and by no means least, an empowerment of the state capacity and ensuring of its autonomy from local dynamics and actors via staffing of the state bureaucracy in the region with competent and well-paid *Turks* was also suggested in the Plan.[12]

As is evident from the articles of the Plan, it focused on the manufacture of national identity, institution of national sovereignty, and construction of an autonomous state apparatus as necessary for the accomplishment of these tasks. Other than the construction of roads and railroads—which also had central control and security implications (since they enabled the movement of troops and weapons, etc.)—developmental issues, like the establishment of public enterprises, incentives, and initiatives to promote agriculture and animal husbandry and the economy as a whole, were not central to the Plan—a lack that included or extended to the non-existence of health investments or consideration of wellness issues generally.

The Plan and its succeeding, derivative plans could not be accomplished adequately, however. The manufacture of national identity was not achieved or the sovereignty of the state institutionalized. Neither did it prove possible to construct an autonomous and effective state apparatus, a recurring item of the assimilation programs of the Republic.

The state did, it must be admitted, face a huge challenge. For one thing, the overwhelming majority of the population in the Kurdish region, as in the whole country, lived in rural settlements which lacked any road connection to the nearest town or city and were thus inherently inaccessible. Furthermore, the manufacture of national identity through literacy was critical for promoting Turkish nationalism. Turkish nationalism was inculcated through the education system, but most people in the Southeast were still illiterate villagers after the Second World War (WWII). Half of the population in the eight provinces of the geographically, state-defined Southeastern Anatolian Region (Güneydoğu Anadolu Bölgesi), which intersects with Turkey's Kurdish Southeast, was still illiterate going into the 1980s, and half of the population in Hakkâri remained unable to read and write in 1990 (Table 3).

The transformation of the demographic landscape for the Turkification of the region proved quite unobtainable (Table 4). Despite some attempts, like the enactment of the Law Regarding the Transportation of Certain People from the Eastern Region to the Western Provinces (No. 1097) in 1927 and The Settlement Act (No. 2510) in 1934, the proportions of Kurds in the Kurdish provinces remained unchanged.

As for the level of development, the biopolitical aspect of nationalism, the proportion of villages in the Kurdish region without electricity, telephone, or road connections by 1984 is a striking indicator of the poor developmental performance of the Republic there. At the beginning of 1984, when the PKK launched its guerilla war against the state, six in every ten Kurds in the Kurdish provinces were living in rural settlements, and these were still poorly connected to the urban centers. The proportion of rural settlements with electricity, telephone,

Table 3. Illiteracy Rate in Southeastern Anatolia Region and Hakkâri, 1950–1990 (%)

	1950	1955	1960	1965	1970	1975	1980	1985	1990
Hakkâri	91.59	88.39	88.57	82.39	77.14	73.94	68.38	54.15	47.71
Southeastern Anatolia Region*	85.92	81.55	81.28	74.40	67.96	58.91	56.67	43.84	39.55

Sources: State Statistical Institute (Devlet İstatistik Enstitüsü, DİE), SEAP (Southeastern Anatolian Project) Provincial Statistics, 1950–95[98] and DİE, 2000 Census of Population.
*Adıyaman, Siirt, Diyarbakır, Batman, Şırnak, Mardin, Gaziantep, Şanlıurfa.

Table 4. Proportion of Kurdish Population in Kurdish Provinces, 1935–1990 (%)

	1935	1990
Ağrı	72.1	70.45
Diyarbakır	72.8	72.78
Mardin	63.8	74.84
Muş	69.1	67.75
Siirt	79.5	78.78
Van	72.4	70.7
Bingöl	n/a	76.63
Bitlis	n/a	64.03
Hakkâri	n/a	89.47
Tunceli	n/a	55.9

Sources: General Directorate of Statistics, 1935 Population Census[99] and Servet Mutlu, *Ethnic Kurds in Turkey*.[100]

and asphalt, stabilized or graded road links were 24.6, 16.8, and 64.8 percent, respectively. In Hakkâri, the situation was worse.

Some 70 percent of Hakkârians were living in rural settlements in 1984. Of these settlements, only one in ten had electricity, less than a quarter had a telephone line, and under two-thirds had a passable road in and out which were closed for weeks and months during long-lasting winters.

In addition to the failure to manufacture a Turkish national identity and the poor developmental performance in the region, the institution of state sovereignty also was not properly accomplished. The mountainous landscape of the border zone made effective border policing impossible, and the illegal passage of people, commodities, and animals could not be prevented. Nor could the state monopoly of violence be ensured. Until the late 1980s, most people in the Southeast lived in its thousands of scattered hamlets, villages, and uplands, which were typically quite beyond the state's effective reach. Therefore, it was not state courts and the legal process that were decisive in the settling of disputes but rather deterrent power, which meant having guns and the backing of a large family or tribe. Large-scale military operations were occasionally organized in the region to confiscate people's weapons, as done in the "commando operations" of the early 1970s.[13] These had very limited success in disarming the people. Indeed, the guerilla war launched in 1984 by the PKK and the paramilitary forces armed by

Table 5. Provincial Proportions of Villages with Electricity, Telephone, and Road and of Rural Population in Kurdish Provinces at the End of 1983 (%)

	Villages with electricity	Villages with telephone	Villages with road link (Asphalt, stabilized or graded)	Proportion of population of rural settlements (1985)
Ağrı	20.4	33.0	82.1	66
Bingöl	38.0	16.1	53.1	75
Bitlis	27.5	29.2	63.8	60
Diyarbakır	20.1	5.9	69.1	49
Hakkâri	10.5	22.9	64.3	70
Mardin	24.7	10.4	78.8	63
Muş	26.1	12.2	93.6	77
Siirt	22.8	7.4	39.7	55
Tunceli	25.2	10.4	42.5	72
Van	31.1	31.1	79.5	65
AVERAGE	24.6	16.8	64.8	61.7

Source: Constructed based on data at State Planning Organization (Devlet Planlama Teşkilatı, DPT), Priority Development Regions Report No. 5.[101]

the state in 1985 against the PKK almost wholly canceled out the state's (formal) monopoly of violence.

It is similarly impossible to speak of much success in the construction of an autonomous and efficient state apparatus since neither the social nor working conditions were sufficiently improved to make postings in the region attractive, especially in Hakkâri. The inevitable outcome of this negligence, discussed in the next chapter with reference to "indirect state racism," was expressed in the day-counting of civil servants lacking motivation, work discipline, engagement with the city, and respect for its citizens.[14] The local newspapers of Hakkâri, for instance, were always full of calls made to civil servants in the province, requesting them to work more efficiently and approach citizens in a more understanding manner.

The impact of tribes on the state apparatus in the Kurdish region, especially after the transition to a multi-party period in 1946, also considerably diminished the autonomy of the state apparatus. Among the most dramatic and striking evidence of the power of tribes and the limits of the autonomy of the state was the armed conflict between the Jirki tribe and the gendarmerie in a village of Beytüşşebap district of Hakkâri in 1975. It resulted in the immediate deaths of Ahmet Agha, the head of the Jirki tribe, and eight soldiers, and later, a state prosecutor.

According to the nephew of Ahmet Agha, he was a deserter, like many Hakkârians in those years, and the gendarmerie commander in Beytüşşebap ignored the case, taking the fragile situation in the province into consideration. The newly appointed prosecutor did not tolerate this, however, and ordered the commander to arrest Ahmet Agha. According to the nephew again, the commander informed the prosecutor about the special conditions of the region and was even able to manage the case for a while. In the end, though, on the order of the prosecutor, he had to mobilize a group of soldiers and go to Ahmet Agha's village, Tuzluca, to take him into custody. They came across Ahmet Agha near the village.

The nephew recounts that Ahmet Agha extended his hand to shake the prosecutor's hand, but the prosecutor declined and instead slapped Ahmet Agha in the face. When Ahmet Agha tried to attack the prosecutor, the prosecutor ordered the soldiers to shoot. Villagers witnessing the killing of their Agha responded to the attack with automatic rifles and killed eight soldiers. The commander and the prosecutor managed to escape (the latter to be killed 2 months after), and the state transferred commando brigade to the town.

Guessing the likely results of the action, the men and young lads of the tribe escaped to the mountains, leaving the women and children behind. They remained there for the next 10 years, until 1985, when the state and Tahir Adıyaman, brother of Ahmet Agha and the new leader of Jirki tribe, came to an agreement. According to this agreement, the state would not arrest Tahir Adıyaman and other Jirki members involved in the murder of soldiers, and Tahir Adıyaman would cooperate with the state against the PKK.

One may view the incident and its victims as the cost of a blindness to the gap between the compromise on the ground and the autonomous logic of the normative-legal requirements of the state. There were alternative accounts of the incident, however. It was said that there had already been conflicts among Ahmet Agha, the public prosecutor, and the administrative head of Beytüşşebap, the trio who together ruled the area. The public prosecutor, the claim goes, used a complaint made by a Syriac villager against Ahmet Agha, who was already deserter, to arrest him.[15]

In this case, the alternative account of the incident, it is reasonable to suppose that the normative-legal requirements of the state were employed by the public prosecutor for his own purpose, turned into a personal instrument for use in power struggle. Certainly, his slapping Ahmet Agha suggested the issue had a personal aspect beyond enforcing the law. We do not know exactly what led the prosecutor to act as he did, yet, one thing is evident: the state as enacted in the region, especially Hakkâri, was not an overarching, translocal, "spatially encompassing reality"[16] capable of acting independently of local dynamics and power balances. On the contrary, it was clearly enabled via specific compromises and enacted by personal relationships on the ground.

In short, we should not be constrained by the vocabulary of the nationalist elites and their numerous plans and reports and should rather conclude that relations between the state and "its" Kurds, Hakkârians, specifically, in the period of the Republic until the PKK insurgency were too static to be considered as instantiating any type of fully-fledged assimilation or story of "becoming." Beyond its motivations and aims, the state lacked the necessary capacity.[17]

Beyond facts and statistics, the inability of the Turkish state to insert the people into a narrative of becoming through the ideals of a modern nation-state can be best followed through examples from everyday responses and knowledge of the people. We can find such examples in the interviews Marxist intellectual and publisher Muzaffer Erdost conducted with villagers of the Şemdinli district in the early 1960s.

The following exchange between Erdost and a 25-year-old young woman living in a border village of Şemdinli took place in 1963 or 1964 with the help of a translator. It shows that even 40 years after its foundation, the Republic had changed practically nothing in the everyday life of a Kurdish woman living in the border zone (which, as a politically sensitive area, might be expected to have been of particular interest to the state). The woman did not have even any sense of calendrical time, let alone a sense of becoming or transition:

Q: Have you ever seen a car or truck or jeep?
A: No, I've never seen one.
Q: Have you ever heard of refrigerators?
A: No, I haven't.
Q: Have you ever seen money?
A: No, I haven't.
Q: Never?
A: I have never seen it.

Q: Do you know which day of the month it is today?
A: I don't know.
Q: Which year are we in?
A: Really, I don't know.[18]

The other interviews reported by Erdost confirm that the woman was not exceptional. The answers he received from primary school pupils were similar to those of the woman. Some of them had never heard the name of Mustafa Kemal Atatürk, the founder of the Republic. When asked what the biggest province of Turkey was, some gave the name of Zive, a district in Iran. Some did not even know the name of the country. Almost none had seen money or cars before.[19]

It would be, therefore, more realistic to portray state-Kurds relations until the mid-1990s as a repetitive encounter and only nominal control. This was especially the case in the mountainous and border areas of the Kurdish region. Most Kurds lived in rural areas, they enjoyed *de facto* autonomy and collectively violated essentials of state sovereignty via illegal border trade and by bearing arms, with the military rule having little capacity in an alien and mountainous landscape.

The Turkish state-Kurdish people relations was not only a failure of assimilation, however. Rather than focusing on lacks and absences, this work is concerned with the positivity of the encounter: the rationality, tactics, strategies, and practices enabled by this sort of encounter. The tactics, strategies, and practices facilitated by the encounter of Kurds with the military rule encumbered by weak infrastructural power were not, in fact, categorically different from the instruments and rationality employed by "traditional," "despotic," "premodern" states in their encounters with their subjects. This is to underline a modality of power that is common to infrastructurally weak states, those lacking "the capacity ... to actually penetrate civil society, and to implement logistically political decisions throughout the realm."[20] The features of this genre of power and their particular reflections in Hakkâri may be identified in three ways.

First, and fundamentally, the goal of sovereign power is nothing but the defense and maintenance of its sovereignty against threats posed by other sovereigns. A "self-referring circularity"[21] is at work in sovereignty. It is neither in search of the transformation or assimilation of its outside nor infrastructurally able to achieve this. To use Anthony Giddens' words, in the eyes of the "traditional state," as he calls it, "it is not really relevant what the rest of the population do in their day-to-day lives, so long as they do not rebel and are compliant in respect of the payment of taxes."[22]

To transpose that argument to this investigation, by claiming that the Turkish state acted in Hakkâri and the Kurdish region within the ideo-political matrix of sovereignty I intend to say that the military rule acquired a distinct, self-referring logic and was not a means of anything outside itself. Unlike the intended role of the Eastern Reform Plan and succeeding plans, the military rule in Hakkâri and the Kurdish region ought not to be considered as a moment of assimilation. A brief and very striking expression I would hear in Hakkâri summarized the self-referring circularity in this regard. People would point out a patrolling military vehicle or building and say, "Here the state protects itself, nobody else."

Second, the sovereign enjoys a great deal of discretionary power: *L'État c'est moi*. The answer given by a public defender to anthropologist Victoria Sanford's complaint about the humiliating behavior of professional soldiers of the Colombian army at a security checkpoint sheds light on the logic behind this discretionary power very well: "The problem is, they believe they can do whatever they want, because they can."[23]

That is to say, it is the fact of not being delimited by anything that defines the sovereign. This is why Foucault defines the sovereign as the one who enjoys "the right to *take* life or *let* live" (emphasis original).[24] Even the law of the sovereign does not form a limit to the sovereign, let alone the lives of its subjects, for the sovereign is above the law and free to "decide on the state of exception."[25]

The practices of the gendarmerie throughout the history of the Turkish Republic and later the army and special police teams, especially after 1984 and until the annulment of the state of emergency in early 2000s in Hakkâri and the Kurdish region in general exemplify how large was the range of arbitrariness that the "security forces" enjoyed as sovereigns. In these practices, the lines between criminals and the security forces frequently became blurred. Killing, torturing, beating, degradation of citizens, confiscation of their property and animals by the armed forces of the state were the rule, not the exceptions, in Hakkâri.

Third, collective punishment emerges as an expression of the infrastructurally weak despotic power. Defined as "a form of reprisal that seeks to inflict pain on a particular group or population for crimes supposedly carried out by one or more of its members,"[26] collective punishment is oriented to the "conduct of conduct"[27] of the subjects, enacted when the infrastructural power of the state fails at an individual level.[28] As a totalizing form that the state as sovereign adopts in eliminating a threat when its infrastructural power is insufficient to individualize the threat and break it into its elements, it ensures self-discipline at a community level. Thus rendered an undifferentiated mass, those who are collectively punished become a worthless mass in the eyes of punishers—as Kurds have been in the eyes of the Turkish state in most periods of the history of the Republic (see below).

As a form of "rough justice," the enactment of punishment at the level of the collective requires that the punishment of individual "innocents" along with individual "criminals" does not pose a major ethical problem for the sovereign—which becomes a source of deep discontent, further distancing the people from the state and thus exacerbating the problem that prompted the collective approach in the first place insofar as it promotes resistance of various kinds—which again has been evident in Turkey's "Kurdish problem." The circularity of failure—wherein collective punishment performed as "necessity" through a lack of state control further diminishes its control in the long run by undermining its moral claim to power.

One can see some of the most striking examples of collective punishment of modern times in European colonies. There, it was not only a part of counter-insurgency operations, as in the British measures taken against the *Mau Mau* uprisings in Kenya in 1952,[29] but also an ordinary instrument of the legal system used to ensure public order. This is evident in the Collective Punishment Ordinances enforced in Nigeria, Kenya, Northern Rhodesia, Nyasaland, Somaliland, and elsewhere.[30] The circularity of failure was eventually recognized in these cases by decolonization—by independence claimed, sometimes fought for, sometimes granted, but either way won.

Village evacuations during the first half of the 1990s were the most obvious example of collective punishment in Hakkâri. Thousands of rural settlements were brutally depopulated throughout the Kurdish region to make it more difficult for rebels to propagate the guerilla war. Establishing border areas as forbidden zones as a measure against smuggling beginning in 1956 was another example of collective punishment. For the people living in settlements within and around border areas, these forbidden zones meant the material restriction of goods they could take into the settlement, the need to gain permission every time they returned to their village, and a ban on grazing, in addition to the psychological pressures of facing constant gendarmerie suspicion and the threat of ad hoc detainment.

Another example of collective punishment in the region was the purchasing restriction placed on the inhabitants of rural settlements at the height of the clashes between the army and the PKK in the 1990s. Attempting to thwart the logistics of guerilla warfare, the state set quotas for each consumption item in the shops in towns, which would prevent the villagers from buying more than they could consume. A ban on uplands was another instance of collective punishment.

Beginning from the late 1980s, the Turkish state started to forbid villagers in Hakkâri from using the high mountain land. The goal was to deprive the PKK guerillas of the opportunity of easy access to food and shelter, but the local people needed the uplands for summer grazing, their primary source of livelihood.

Security checkpoints should also be named as instances of collective punishment. During the 1990s, there were more than ten security checkpoints along the Hakkâri-Van road, and even in 2009, when the emergency rule was already lifted, cars and buses would all be stopped at three or four security checkpoints where, especially during the 1990s, passengers were interrogated, sometimes arrested, and routinely insulted.

To sum up, even if it was not totally independent of the character ascribed to Kurds, neither was collective punishment just the totalizing outcome of a hatred and exclusionary stance toward them. Rather, it was a method of eliminating a threat and forcing people to practice self-discipline given that the individualizing capacity of the state was extremely poor and the status of Kurds in the eyes of the Turkish nation-state was too low to require a careful distinction between "innocent" and "terrorist."

2.3 Dehumanization: Sovereign Violence and the Official Discourse on Kurds

> *"Kurd" is not a noun; it is an adjective.*
> Abidin Özmen, Inspector of the First General Inspectorate[31]

Addressing the question of how the Turkish state reconciled its claim to be a modern state obeying the rule of law with a "premodern" sovereign violence of collective punishment, the punishment of innocents along with "criminals," and the systematic violation of basic human rights can afford a better understanding of that sovereign violence and hence the nature of state-Kurd relations between 1923 and the 1990s. In this regard, Dipesh Chakrabarty provides a good point of departure:

> The person who is not an immediate sufferer but who has the capacity to become a secondary sufferer through sympathy for a generalized picture of suffering ... occupies the position of the modern subject. In other words, the moment of the modern observation of suffering is a certain moment of self-recognition on the part of an abstract, general human being. It is as though a person who is able to see in himself or herself the general human also recognizes the same figure

in the particular sufferer, so that the moment of recognition is a moment when the general human splits into the two mutually recognizing and mutually constitutive figures of the sufferer and the observer of suffering.[32]

According to this argument, dehumanization is inherent in modern cruelty.[33] For the modern subject to cause intentional suffering without feeling any twinge of guilt, he must already have canceled the commonality between himself and his victim, the fact of being human. For Herbert Kelman, this refers to having an identity and independent will and being a member of a community.[34]

If one aspect of the collective punishment of Kurds by the Turkish state was the state's insufficient disciplinary capacity to individualize, its other side was the official nationalist discourse between 1925 and the 1990s that dehumanized. Although this was implicit rather than overt, as Kurds were legally Turkish, it devalued them as people and left them short of the full status, respect, and rights due to them as human beings. The usual official discourse on Kurds did not attribute to Kurdishness any community status and viewed ordinary Kurds as the serfs of feudal landlords and slavish followers of sheiks, not as individuals with personal authority, making choices, and exercising agency.

According to the official discourse, Kurds were Turks in origin, yet due to their geographical isolation from the rest of the country by mountains, interaction with Persians and Arabs, and control by sheiks and feudal landlords, they had fallen away from the Turkish nation.[35] What was implied but not explicitly declared in this discourse was that Kurds as Kurds embodied degeneration. Kurdishness was a worthless amalgam of Turkishness with those designated by Turkish nationalism as its other: Arabic, Islamic, feudal cultures, and the like. The Kurdishness of Kurds was not recognized as a positive entity and a separate ethnicity and thus deprived of any national status. That is why, for example, local Hakkârian newspapers of the 1960s and 1970s, which were under strict control of the authorities, characterized Hakkârians as dumb (*dilsiz*) and called for the Turkish civil servants in Hakkâri to have a more understanding stance toward them. They were simply not capable of articulating their problems in a proper (civilized, Turkish) way. The anecdote shared by an older middle-aged Hakkârian teacher when we were chatting in the office of the left-wing and pro-Kurdish Education and Science Workers' Union (Eğitim ve Bilim Emekçileri Sendikası, Eğitim-Sen) serves as a striking indicator of how the official stance toward Kurdishness until early 1990s was one of humiliating indifference:

When the coup happened in 1980, I was working as a teacher at the Public Education Center in *Hakkâri*. The military regime appointed Yunus Güçel, a retired general, to Hakkâri as the governor. One day, we were informed by the governorship that the governor would visit the Public Education Center to witness the works of the center and congratulate the teachers on their good performance. Anyway, he came to the center that day as scheduled. We welcomed him, started to show him our classrooms, and briefed him about the activities of the center. While he was touring the center, he turned to an old man who was one of the students to ask him whether he was satisfied with the activities of the center. The man did not know Turkish well and could only say to him that he did not know Turkish well. I will never forget the answer given by the governor to him: "Do not say that 'I don't know Turkish'; rather say that 'I don't know how to speak'". For him, for the state on behalf of which he spoke, Kurdish did not have the status of language.

The reduction of Kurdishness to some sort of degeneration meant that Kurdish individuals were deprived of full human status. This is evident in the lines written by a Kemalist, Naşit Hakkı, after the Dersim massacre in 1938. In this passage, the Kurd is likened to grass and hence reduced to a mere biological existence, or, to use Agamben's phrase, to bare life:

> A man who is rooted to the land as grass is called as "Kurd". A Kurd is bought and sold with the land, and he is the commodity of he who owns the land ... A Turk is honorable. He never accepts to be a slave. It is necessary to "Kurdify" a Turkish village in order to dominate it.[36]

If we adopt Herbert Kelman's perspective on dehumanization as defined by discourses and practices depriving the individual of identity and community, it is clear that the usual Turkish approach toward Kurds was a dehumanizing one. Yet, one also needs to add, and unlike some explicitly racist cases of dehumanization, such as in the portrayal of the Japanese as rats in the United States media during WWII[37] or the description of Tutsis as cockroaches during the genocide in Rwanda,[38] the difference of Kurds, the Kurdishness of Kurds, was almost never underlined and belittled in Turkish public. The Kurdishness of Kurds was rather something Turkish nationalism had a clear, negative idea about but preferred to remain silent on, as if such a thing did not exist.

In fact, the Turkish nationalist conviction that Kurds formed a degenerated community below human society was not the only conviction of Turkish nationalism about Kurds. The degeneration did not go so far as to terminate the potential and original *Turkishness* of Kurds and render them into *incorrigible* degenerates. In other words, Turkish nationalism put its emphasis not on degeneration (the Kurdishness of Kurds), and thus the necessity of deportation or annihilation of Kurds, but rather on the lack (still recoverable Turkishness of Kurds) and thus the necessity of the assimilation of Kurds (into Turkishness). The duty of Turkish nationalism, therefore, was to emancipate Kurds from the traces of Middle Eastern culture and remind them of their somehow forgotten Turkishness.

This optimistic aspect of the official approach to Kurds as "future Turks"[39] is well observed in the title of the memoirs of Sıdıka Avar, a teacher who worked as a Turkish missionary after the Dersim massacre to gather Kurdish girls for boarding schools. The name of the memoirs is "My Mountain Flowers."[40] The Kurdish children of Dersim gathered by Avar to be assimilated in boarding schools were conceived of as mountain flowers, as an uncultivated beauty waiting to be refined in the hands of teachers committed to the cause of Turkish nationalism.

Nevertheless, in all cases, the place reserved for Kurds by official Turkish nationalism did not go beyond bare life, being grass to be cut and mountain flowers to be cultivated and refined. The Kurd as such was a degeneration to be eliminated, and the Kurd as future Turk was a potential to be educated and disciplined. In no cases were Kurds in their actuality considered worthy of recognition. It was this unworthiness of Kurds that normalized the collective punishment, made it ideologically tolerable and even desirable in the eyes of the state agents.

2.4 Sovereign Violence in Hakkâri

As mentioned (above), despite all the assimilationist rhetoric, the years passing under military rule were too repetitive to be described by a linear becoming and narrative of assimilation. Rather than acting as the signifier of a somewhat transcendent story, the military rule embodied the self-referring circularity of a constant search for the establishment, maintenance, and defense of itself. The collective punishment of Hakkârians for the enforcement of the border to prevent illegal trade and in the fight against the PKK was the main manifestation of the sovereign violence characterized by this self-referring circularity.

2.4.1 Collective Punishment in Hakkâri or Rendering All Citizens into Suspects

It must be acknowledged that the region under my administration does not resemble to any part of the country in any respects and that its government by laws employed in other parts of the country would not establish the desired peace, silence and assimilation in the region ... If a man planning to go at banditry knows that his children and wife he would leave behind in the village and those who would protect and help him would be immediately annihilated, it is certain that the number of those who would go at such awful things would decrease.
Abidin Özmen, Inspector of the First General Inspectorate[41]

My observations in Erzincan have convinced me to the necessity of disciplining ... the villages of Aşkirik, Gürk, Dağbey, Haryi, which considerably damage the economy and threaten the public order of the province. To have a [deterring] effect on all Kurdish villages in the province ... and also to institute the sovereignty of the state, it would be appropriate to damage these villages by an air fleet that would be sent to Erzincan.
Marshall Fevzi Çakmak, Chief of General Staff[42]

"Illegal and unreasonable gendarmerie oppression must be abolished."[43] This was one of the demands in the list of demands of Hakkâri sent to the Prime Minister's Office in 1966. In the answer to the petition from the Office, the petitioners were informed that "all authorities were warned to correct the false impression that [gendarmerie] stations are places of torture and beating."[44]

Indeed, gendarmerie oppression in Hakkâri went far beyond a false impression that could be easily corrected. On the contrary, the systematic use of violence has been the norm in Hakkâri throughout the whole history of the Turkish Republic. Extraordinary forms of rule in Hakkâri began in 1925 when the government promulgated the Law for the Restoration of Order (1925-1927) against the Sheikh Said Revolt in the Kurdish region. The establishment of the First General Inspectorate in 1927 followed the Law. Its task was to integrate the Kurdish region into the nation-state (in terms of economy, culture, security, transportation, and language, etc.).

The First General Inspectorate was de facto abolished by the CHP in 1947 when Turkish politics had already acquired a competitive character with the foundation of the Democratic Party (Demokrat Parti, DP) in 1946. No special legislation was issued for the period between 1947 and 1979, but this by no means indicated a return to a normal form of rule in Hakkâri. Being accused of violating forbidden zones declared after 1956 as a measure against smuggling, peasants living along the Iraqi and Iranian border were routinely exposed to gendarmerie oppression as part and parcel of everyday life. Commando operations carried out in 1970 in the name of seizing people's guns and fighting against banditry were another instance of the extraordinary methods of rule in which the basic rights of the people were systematically suspended. In 1979 Hakkâri was added to the list of the 13 provinces ruled under martial law. Authoritarian doses of martial law increased when the military came to power in 1980 and extended martial law to the whole country. Martial law lasted until 1987, when it was replaced by emergency rule.

No period in the history of Hakkâri and the Kurdish region during the Republican period, except perhaps the period of the General Inspectorate, can be compared to the emergency rule in terms of the degradation of lives, that is, the reduction of people to a disposable bare life. This was effected through village evacuations, thirty-day detention periods in which suspects were systematically tortured, murders of political opponents by the Gendarmerie Intelligence and Counterterrorism Organization (Jandarma İstihbarat ve Terörle Mücadele Teşkilatı, JİTEM) and special police forces, degrading behaviors and arbitrary detentions in military checkpoints, and the complete suspension of the right of assembly and free speech—a list that can be continued.

Above all, sovereign violence in Hakkâri took the form of collective punishment. The following sections analyze two forms of collective punishment of Hakkârians. First, the use of collective punishment as a measure against the illegal border trade is considered. Then I analyze the technologies of collective punishment employed against the Kurdish insurgency led by the PKK.

2.4.1.1 Illegal Border Trade and Collective Punishment of Border People
Thirty-three Bullets
They applied the decree of death
They stained
The half-awakened wind of dawn
And the blue mist of the Nimrod
In blood
They stacked their guns there
Searched us
Feeling our corpses
They took away
My red sash of Kermanshah weave
My prayer beads and tobacco pouch
And left
Those were all gifts to me from friends
All from the Persian lands
We are guardians, relatives, tied by blood

We exchange with families
Across the river
Our daughters, these many centuries
We are neighbors
Shoulder to shoulder
Our chickens mingle together
Not out of ignorance
But poverty
We never got used to passports
This is the guilt that kills us
We end up
Being called
Bandits
Killers
Traitors . . .
Kinsman, write my story as it is
Or they might think it a fable
These are not rosy nipples
But a dumdum bullet
Shattered in my mouth

Ahmet Arif[45]

Illegal border trade in the Kurdish region is coeval with the division of historically Kurdish lands between Turkey, Iran, Iraq, and Syria following the disintegration of the Ottoman Empire. Since the Turkish state could not integrate the region into the national market and lacked the capacity to police the border and given that the people had no difficulty in establishing cross-border connections due to their kinship networks, the illegal trade has commonly been both the sole economic way of accessing basic convenience goods and also a somewhat profitable enterprise.

According to the nationalist elites of the early Republican period, illegal cross-border trade was not an ordinary crime but rather a huge problem concerning the assimilation of Kurds to Turkishness. Thus, in 1931, Minister of the Interior Şükrü Kaya told İbrahim Tali Bey, first head of the First General Inspectorate, that smugglers should be regarded as traitors and the fight against smuggling as a national struggle.[46] It was no accident that this war on trade was also addressed in the Eastern Reform Plan, the guiding text of the Turkish assimilation strategy.

The danger posed to the assimilation policy by the illegal border trade had two key elements. First, the plan to integrate the region into the Turkish economy by cutting the region's cross-border links was threatened by illegal border trade. In fact, the fight against this trade was regarded in terms of the loyalty of the people. In a classified report submitted to the Prime Minister İsmet İnönü in 1931, the Minister of the Interior Şükrü Kaya said that:

> It is our right to demand the deportation from the border zone of the people who are occupied with both political banditry and smuggling, like Dashnak leaders and smugglers in Qamishli ... They both threaten the security of our borders and also use smuggling for their political attacks. Habituating aghas, tribal leaders, and transporters who could not be deceived so far by political propaganda to smuggling, they gain their loyalty.[47]

One can see similar remarks in the local *Hakkâri* newspaper in 1983, just a year after the first PKK guerilla groups began entering the province and visiting hamlets and villages for reconnaissance and propaganda. In a circular on illegal border trade written by the gendarmerie, it was mentioned that "destructive and divisive ideologies" were imported by smugglers who inevitably had contact with "armed anarchists."[48]

The second danger to the Turkish state by the illegal border trade was the considerable income it provided the PKK "taxing" illicit items to finance its war. Sarı Baran, a PKK guerilla who was active in mountains of Hakkâri during 1990, told Aliza Marcus that they used to seize 3 percent of each herd as tax to let smugglers pass through.[49] According to a report submitted to the Van Gendarmerie Command of Public Security in 1999, the PKK used to raise some 1.5 trillion TL (equivalent at that time to around 3.5 million USD) annually from animal smuggling.[50]

As a province with districts situated along the border, Hakkâri has had illicit trade as one of its major economic activities since the institution of the barriers to traffic. With the modern state enforcement of the Ottoman-Iran border in the second half of the nineteenth century,[51] non-taxed cross-border trade in Hakkâri became criminalized, and smugglers there and their illegal trade began to be documented by the officials.[52] After the Treaty of Ankara (1926), which drew the present-day border between Turkey and newly established Iraq, smuggling activities in the province further extended to the Iraqi border.

Due to the large share of animal husbandry in its local economy, livestock was the preferred item of business. In 1940, for instance, it was decided by the Ministry of Finance to reward the governor of Hakkâri with a letter of appreciation recognizing his successful struggle in cooperation with colleagues in Mosul and Erbil against the illegal border trade of livestock.[53] In the local newspapers of Hakkâri of the 1960 and 1970s, one can see countless cases of armed conflict between gendarmes and livestock smugglers. The following case reported by the *Hakkâri* in November 1962 was typical:

> The gendarmerie learned that Ömer and his friend from Hetris village of Beytüşşebap and Mustafa from Uruzi village of Iraq, who have collected 2,500 purple sheep from the Beytüşşebap area for three-to-four months, take sheep to the Iraqi border. Upon the denunciation, gendarmes ambushed these two people, and while bandit Ömer was killed, his friend Mustafa surrendered to the gendarmes at the end of the conflict.[54]

During the conflict-ridden 1980s and 1990s, the illicit trade in livestock continued unabated; if anything, in fact, it increased—to the extent that the illegally imported livestock was carried across the border in trucks.[55]

The illegal border trade in Hakkâri has never been limited to the livestock trade. In Şemdinli, for instance, the illegal border trade of tobacco always had an important place in household economies,[56] just as did the heroin trade in Yüksekova. The unlawful cross-border trade of fuel in Hakkâri, especially in its former district of Başkale, was at such a high level in 2010–11 that thousands of people subsisted on it, directly and indirectly. The volume of trade of daily consumption items like sugar, tea, and cigarettes in Hakkâri was also massive.

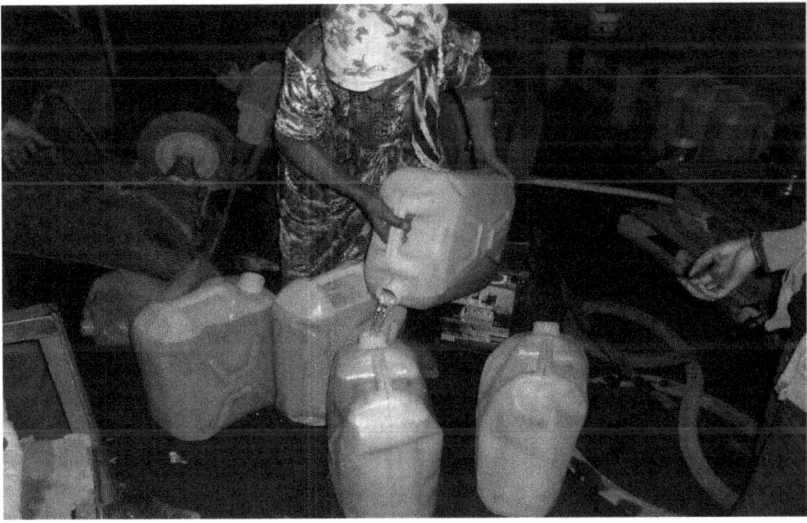

Figure 5. A Shanty Hut Filled with Smuggled Fuel (Şemdinli).

Illegally imported packets of cigarettes were sold in streets of Hakkâri without any police intervention.

The role of illegal border trade in the economy of Hakkâri can be clearly followed in the statistics provided by annual reports prepared by the Department of Anti-Smuggling and Organized Crime. According to the 2011 report, which ranked provinces in terms of the amount of illegally imported items seized by police, Hakkâri ranked third with 4,163,652 packets of cigarettes, first with 1,110,336 kilos of tea, second with 13,900 kilos of meat, and third with 430 kilos of heroin.[57]

As an infrastructurally weak sovereign entity incapable of meting out individualized treatment, the way the Turkish state responded to illegal border trade was to render all local population suspects. The violent character of the totalizing view of border people was apparent during the rule by the General Inspectorate between 1927 and 1946. The massacre of 33 peasants accused of being livestock smugglers in the Özalp district of Van by the order of General Muğlalı in 1943—the subject of Ahmet Arif's poem (above)—was the most brutal instance of the stance taken during the single-party period.[58] This massacre was perpetrated as an exemplary punishment intended to send a message to the larger Kurdish community, making clear the consequences they would face if they continued smuggling.

With the transition to a multi-party period and the DP taking power from the CHP in 1950, border people could relax to some extent, yet they continued to be targets of the totalizing gaze rendering them suspects. The measure taken by the DP against illegal border trade was to declare security zones in border areas and restrict the flows of people, animals, and commodities through them. In August 1956, the DP issued the Law on the Modification of Some Articles of the Law on the Prevention and Prosecution of Smuggling (No. 1918) and the Supplementation of New Articles to the Law. Through this legislation, the government was authorized to declare security zones on border areas, nationalize lands in security zones, and also deport and settle those settled in security zones to other regions.[59]

In its meeting in November 1956, the Council of Ministers prescribed the border areas of Hatay, Gaziantep, Urfa, Mardin, and Hakkâri as security zones. In another meeting of the Council of Ministries held 3 weeks later, the items subject to permission were specified. Taking the following items into the security zone required the permission of the units authorized by the Ministry of the Interior and the Ministry of Customs and Monopolies: sheep, goats, and cows; all sorts of animal and vegetable oils; cotton seed, and sesame; leather, wool, goat hair, intestines, and eggs; wheat, barley, rye, rice, pistachio nuts, and cotton; and oak gall, and wood coal.[60] The citizens living in security zones were not allowed to stockpile these items beyond an amount exceeding their half-yearly needs.[61]

Taking the practice of this decision into account, a new and more realistic notice was issued in November 1957. With the new notice, the security zone and list of items subject to permission were divided into two. In the area up to 10 km from the border, the strict policy of the previous notice was maintained and tightened further. While in the previous notice, the citizens in the security zone were allowed to stockpile the listed items according to their half-yearly needs, the new notice did not allow them to have more than their personal, familial, or professional needs, which would be set by the governor responsible for the security zone. For the area ranging from 10 to 25 km inside, a more moderate policy was adopted. The items subject to the permission of the governor and the declaration were restricted for this area to just sheep, goats, and cows.[62]

In December 1962, the Council of Ministers took a new decision concerning security zones. In the new decision, the security zone was redefined and narrowed. Now, the area ranging from the border to 5 km inside was designated as the security zone and the next 5 km a precaution zone. In the security zone, the restrictions prescribed in the previous regulations were maintained. The citizens in the security zone were not allowed to stockpile the items subject to permission. In the precaution zone, a smuggling commission was to be formed, which would be authorized to impose the same sanctions imposed as in the security zone if deemed necessary.[63]

In March 1981, another regulation concerning the security zone was enacted. Following this decision of the Council of Ministries, the security zone was broadened to 10 km and the term "precaution zone" annulled. Those living in the security zone were still not allowed to have those items addressed in the previous regulations or any to be fixed by the Provincial Commission of Smuggling above amounts set by the Commission.[64]

The policy of declaring security zones was an instance of *preemptive* collective punishment. All border people were thus criminalized and rendered suspect. This meant constant tension between border people and gendarmes. One of the major manifestations of this tension centered on the livestock grazing in the security zone. It was stated, for instance, in the *Hakkâri Sesi* of June 1977 that there were "at least fifteen or twenty villages which are fifty meters from the border and subsist wholly on animal husbandry"; since the gendarmerie troops "do not let the citizens' livestock graze in the forbidden zone," it was rhetorically asked, "What should then the peasants who live on the border do?"[65] According to the *Hakkâri*

Sesi, most of the citizens' uplands and pastures were in the security zone, and the peasants had no alternative but to graze their livestock there because of the difficulty of finding available pasture land.[66]

Apart from the issue of grazing, the border people of Hakkâri, especially those of Çukurca, suffered from the bureaucratic procedures concerning the declaration of items they bought from the provincial capital. One can read numerous complaints in the *Hakkâri Sesi* about the need to attain permission for the items restricted by the law and the Hakkâri Provincial Commission of Smuggling. For instance, it was stated in the February 1975 *Hakkâri Sesi* that "it is shameful that Turkish citizens have to take permission from the authorized units to take a pouch of flour and sugar into Çukurca."[67] There were also some complaints in November 1974 that "the local people [of Çukurca] cannot take even the three-monthly, half-yearly or yearly needs of their children into [Çukurca] without permission from the governorship or district governorship."[68]

Another manifestation of the conflicts between the border people of Hakkâri and gendarmes was that the border people of Hakkâri would be exposed to gendarmerie violence in the security zone. Mikail İlçin, the deputy of Hakkâri, described the gendarmerie violence in the security zone in the Assembly in Ankara thus:

> It is a fact that by the decision no. 10 issued in 1956, smuggling could not be prevented. From the very beginning of the implementation of the aforementioned decision, our poor citizens who live in security zone and zone of precaution have been exposed to all sorts of illegal and arbitrary treatments, have been beaten, insulted, and killed. Peasants living in the villages where the decision has been implemented have been thus deprived of their freedoms.[69]

Referring to the cases of gendarmerie violence in the security zone, İlçin asked the Minister of the Interior, "What are the measures taken to prevent gendarmes on duty along the border from implementing the law of the jungle?"[70]

2.4.1.2 Collective Punishment as Emergency Rule

Aside from the forbidden and security zone and usual patterns of gendarmerie violence, officially, there was no extraordinary form of rule in *Hakkâri* between 1950 and 1979. However, following the Alevi pogrom in Kahramanmaraş by ultra-nationalist militants in December 1978, one of the high points of polarization during the 1970s, martial law was proclaimed in 13 provinces where the political tensions were high, and later in the Kurdish provinces. This included Hakkâri, even though there was no significant political polarization there.⁷¹ Martial law was extended to the whole country after the coup d'état in September 1980. Yet, while it was gradually annulled in the western provinces of the country in parallel with the pacification of the socialist movement, in Kurdish provinces, as of July 1987, it was replaced by the rule of Emergency Governorship. This was due to the biggest Kurdish rebellion yet, under the leadership of the PKK in 1984. Hakkâri was ruled by Emergency Governorship until July 2002.

Between 1979 and 2002, especially after 1984, Hakkârians were the target of collective punishment methods employed by the state against the threat posed by the PKK guerillas, whom the local people en masse were presumed to support. As an infrastructurally weak entity neither able to individualize, to distinguish "terrorists" from "normal citizens," nor to police and control the hundreds of scattered rural settlements in the province, the Turkish state refashioned sovereign technologies of power that had been already in use.

The village evacuations, the most comprehensive form of collective punishment employed in Hakkâri and the Kurdish region generally, were intensified in the first half of the 1990s as part of the army's counter-insurgence strategy. Until 1993, the Turkish army lacked any well-defined counter-insurgence strategy against guerilla forces relying on the facilities and logistics enabled by thousands of dispersed and weakly controlled rural settlements on a largely mountainous landscape. Joost Jongerden describes the situation thus:

> The Turkish military took up defensive and static positions, especially at night, when soldiers were thought to be safe in their enclosures. Garrisons were built and fortified, and army units confined themselves to these garrisons. Operations were carried out, but units returned to their barracks before dawn. The Turkish armed forces had decided to concentrate on the defense of larger settlements and to refrain from nocturnal operations, which gave the PKK considerable freedom to establish control in the smaller settlements and to move by night.⁷²

The success of the PKK between 1987 and 1991 attained such a level that it completed the stage of strategic defense, the first phase of its Maoist insurgency war strategy, and moved to the second stage, toward strategic balance, which meant establishing liberated zones.⁷³ Above a picture of marching PKK guerillas, for instance, the headline of *Serxwebun*, PKK's underground paper, on September 1991 read "Botan-Behdinan: We are Walking Toward the War Government."⁷⁴

The announcement of the "field domination doctrine" by the Turkish General Staff in 1991 and its implementation by 1993, however, changed the dynamic of the war. According to Jongerden, "The objective of the new doctrine was the destruction of the PKK environment, both by contraction (resettlement of the population) and penetration (deployment of special forces, applying the principles of a war of movement, and penetrating the spaces of the PKK, as well as drafting the civilian populations in PKK areas into the village guard system)."[75]

Village evacuations were one of the most decisive policies of this field domination doctrine. In a speech delivered to military officers, Osman Pamukoğlu, the commander of the Hakkâri Mountain and Commando Brigade between 1993 and 1995, was referring to Hakkâri when he stated that "In this province, there are 674 villages and hamlets," which he characterized as forming "the spider's web in which the PKK feeds itself"; then, he suggested, "[W]hy don't we concentrate all [villagers] in two or three main settlements?"[76] As is apparent in these words, what was aimed by village evacuations was to render guerilla tactics logistically difficult.

By the start of the village evacuation policy, peasants were forced to make an ultimate choice between fighting against the PKK as paramilitary village guardians or leaving their villages.[77] At the end of 1995, the peak year of evacuations in Hakkâri, most of the villages in Hakkâri city and Çukurca districts and some villages in Yüksekova and Şemdinli were evacuated (see Appendix 1).

The dramatic demographic effects of village evacuations in Çukurca, the district most affected by village evacuations along with Hakkâri city, can be traced in the statistics provided by the DİE. The rural population of Çukurca declined from 14,271 in 1990 to 3,609 in 2000.[78]

Another instance of collective punishment in Hakkâri and the Kurdish region was the treatment of civilians as supporters and collaborators of the PKK. This led to a standard critique that the armed forces failed to "distinguish terrorists from normal citizens" during the rule by Emergency Governorship. There were four main reasons for this.

First, as stated, the state simply lacked the infrastructural capacity to individualize and to distinguish "terrorists" from "normal citizens." Second, the unworthy status of Kurdishness as a degenerated community in the eyes of the Turkish nation-state normalized collective punishment, making it acceptable and even desirable in the eyes of the state agents. Third, the PKK attained such organizational power that there were objective limits to the distinction of those who were from those who were not PKK affiliates. Fourth, the members of special police teams working in the region and in Hakkâri were mostly militants of ultranationalist parties like the Nationalist Action Party (Milliyetçi Hareket Partisi, MHP) and Great Union Party (Büyük Birlik Partisi, BBP). The right-wing MHP and BBP were ideologically biased against Kurds, and governments understood that their militants could be used against the PKK.

These four factors combined to render all Hakkârians into potential PKK affiliates in the eyes of the state and its formal and informal allies. Thus, they could be legitimately killed, tortured, beaten, and insulted. In short, terrorization of the masses was adopted as a counter-terror strategy by the state. A parliamentary question asked by Cumhur Keskin to the Minister of the Interior concerning the murder of a child by the armed forces in a village in the district of Çukurca in June 1988 reveals the event as an ordinary symptom of the terrorizing, totalizing gaze of the armed forces toward the people:

> On the night of 30.06.1988 Ramazan Dağ, who was a thirteen-year-old child, was shot dead by the gendarmerie in Uzundere village of Çukurca district of Hakkâri while he was returning from a neighbor's home to the house where he lived with his father . . . Is it true that a curfew is imposed in the provinces under emergency rule and that it has become almost a rule that the citizens who do not obey the curfew are arbitrarily fired upon . . . ? It is obvious that Ramazan Dağ was a thirteen-year-old child, used to live in Uzundere village, and was shot dead without any warning to stop being made. What questions have been raised so far about those who prepared the official reports which showed him as a "PKK militant captured dead at the end of the clash"? [. . .] When will arbitrary searches, detentions, and the practices that humiliate human dignity come to an end in the region?[79]

The massacre of three peasants from Yoncalı village in July 1989 by a commando troop was another tragic result of the totalizing gaze. According to Keskin, on the day of the massacre, a group of peasants were mowing grass. Due to an ongoing feud issue, they had arms with them. When they noticed a group of soldiers in search of a PKK group approaching the place they were mowing, they tried to hide the arms, in panic. Without any summons, the officer, a major, ordered his men to fire at the peasants with rockets, automatic guns, and a howitzer. Three peasants were killed and their corpses were burned. Later, it was announced that three PKK militants had been captured dead.[80]

There were countless such examples of the mistreatment, abuse, and worse of Hakkârians. Hakkârians were not allowed to walk together in groups in the streets. When they did so as more than three or four individuals, they would be humiliated and beaten by members of special police teams. The special police teams would arbitrarily fire for hours without any target in the streets; this might continue throughout the night until morning. The special teams would also raid weddings so as to prevent local singers from singing Kurdish songs. It was routine for Hakkârians to be made to wait for hours at the numerous roadside security checkpoints, where they would be required to show their IDs, open their luggage and bags, and answer the roughly asked questions in a demurring way. To put it succinctly, all Hakkârians, except for the village guards, were treated as potential terrorists and PKK affiliates during the emergency rule.

Forced disappearances and extrajudicial killings of Kurdish activists must also be addressed when considering the collective punishment methods employed in Hakkâri and the Kurdish region. The following case is typical of the political murders committed by the special units of the Turkish security forces during the 1990s and early 2000s:

> A: I was playing backgammon with Yaşar in the coffee house next to the municipality. Then I noticed that some people were wandering around us. I said to Yaşar, "Yaşar, they're here either for you or for me." "No," he said, "They're trying to find a seat to play backgammon as well." I repeated: "Yaşar, they're here either for you or for me. I'll go to one side, and you go to the other. Let's see who they've come for." We left our backgammon game, climbed up the stairs, and then I walked toward the Kıran neighborhood while Yaşar walked toward the Rectorate. Later I heard that he had been taken into custody, put into a panzer [armored vehicle], and taken to Şine. Then they had shot him dead by twenty-five bullets to his head.
> Q: Was he politically engaged?
> A: Yes, but not so much ...

The victim of this brutal murder was Yusuf Yaşar. The killing was done in 2005, 3 years after the annulment of emergency rule.[81] His was one of the numerous political murders known in Turkey as "murder by unidentified assailants" (*faili meçhul cinayetler*). The victims were often enough unidentified also, as the corpses would be disposed of casually in the countryside, thrown like rubbish in a desolate spot and left to rot or else buried in shallow graves that are still being found with only bones to speak of what happened. Much of this dirty war remains undisclosed; however, the murder of Kurdish activists by the state in Hakkâri and the broader Kurdish region was admitted by the former governor of Hakkâri.[82]

Although forced disappearances and extrajudicial killings seem at first glance as an individualizing form of state terror, it is indeed another form of collective punishment. This has been discussed, for example, in the extensive literature on cultures of fear and the dirty war methods of military regimes in Latin America.[83] It is not the immediate victim of the murder or disappearance who is really targeted by those who employ such violence but rather the wider community. The real intention is to spread fear and intimidate through the shock of the disappearance.

The aim of this collectivization of fear was the inculcation of a sense that anybody could fall victim at any moment, without any procedural judgment, evidence, or record. What takes place in forced disappearances is the "instrumentalization of fear" as a "mechanism of social discipline."[84] The policy of "this murder by unidentified assailants" did not merely eliminate a particular threat, it served the cause of ensuring self-discipline.

Thirteen forced disappearance cases involving the deaths of 38 people occurred in Hakkâri so far.[85] The most severe of these was in Şemdinli, in July 1994. On the day of the disappearances, gendarmes forcibly collected all the men of Ormancık village, who were village guards then, at the helicopter landing pad laid out in the village. They shot dead one villager who resisted, and they caused two pregnant women to have miscarriages by beating them. The men were stripped naked and beaten harshly. Then, the gendarmes took 12 village guards into custody, accusing them of being PKK affiliates, and interrogated them at the Derecik military base. They were never seen again.

Military officials claimed that the gendarmes released the detainees after the interrogation.[86] However, according to a soldier who completed his military duty in the Derecik military base in the years in question, they were interrogated and tortured for 5 days by JİTEM members who tried to extract information on local PKK guerillas, and then they were shot dead. According to the soldier, the corpses were buried on the grounds of the military base.[87] It would not be wrong to conclude that both these forced disappearances and extrajudicial killings—and the message delivered through the victims of these cases to Hakkârians—functioned as exemplary punishment at the height of the armed conflict between the PKK and the army.

Another form of collective punishment, widespread both in the Kurdish region in general and in Hakkâri at the height of the armed conflict between the PKK and the army, was the imposition of food restrictions on villages. The official name given to this was "controlled food transfer" (*kontrollü gıda sevkiyatı*). The rationale guiding the policy of the food embargo was simple. The state was unable to control and police the villages, which were central to the logistics of the guerilla war. Given that the state was unable to identify which villagers gave support to the PKK, in addition to its inherently anti-Kurdish mindset, it was not surprising that it considered all villagers as suspects, as potential PKK affiliates. To show how this controlled food transfer was implemented in Hakkâri, the words of a present-day grocer in the Hakkâri city serve well. This man was a child in the early 1990s, when the food embargo was strictly implemented by the armed forces. This is what he said:

> During the 1990s—1993, 1994, 1995—flour sacks coming to the shop used to be counted [by special police teams]. Special police teams would count flour sacks when they were carried from the truck to the shop like they were the owners of the shop. After I sold the flour sacks, I'd take the invoices to the police. They'd count the invoices as well and say "You had 250 flour sacks, but there's only 240 invoices here. Where are the invoices of the ten flour sacks?"

A taxi driver listening to the grocer confirmed how strictly the food embargo policy was implemented in Hakkâri in these years:

> There was a security check point in Katramas. It was removed in 1998. I was a taxi driver then. The special police teams waiting there would take note who was taking how much foodstuff home: " ... one flour, one sack of pasta ... " The person they noted who had taken one flour sack to his house wouldn't be allowed to take another home before a month had passed.

Exclusion from uplands has been mentioned (above) as another instance of pre-emptive collective punishment. Just as the villages in the Kurdish region were largely outside the control of the armed forces, so too were the higher mountain lands and pastures. In the uplands, PKK guerillas used to spread their message freely and could easily take sheep, goats, and animal products from the villagers. To deal a blow to the logistics of the guerilla war, therefore, people were banned from the uplands throughout the Kurdish region from the late 1980s. This exclusion persisted even after the abolition of emergency rule. The villagers of Hakkâri were not allowed to use most of their uplands until 2012, in fact. Data obtained from the Hakkâri Provincial Directorate of Food, Agriculture, and Livestock through the Freedom of Information Act gives the numbers of banned uplands and meadows in Hakkâri between 2008 and 2011 as generally in excess of 100, giving an indication of the real and dramatic consequences of this form of collective punishment on Hakkârians and the local economy of Hakkâri (Table 6). Not only had animal husbandry always been the primary economic activity, but transhumance activity and mountain life constituted an integral part of the village existence, determining lifestyles, relationships, and societal dynamics.

Table 6. Number of Banned Uplands and Meadows in Hakkâri

	Hakkâri City	Yüksekova	Çukurca	Şemdinli	TOTAL
2008	19	15	20	64	118
2009	25	16	31	67	139
2010	11	20	28	44	103
2011	5	8	11	25	49

Source: Hakkâri Provincial Directorate of Food, Agriculture and Livestock.

2.5 Privatization of Sovereignty in Hakkâri

> *Our province is not a colony of the Republic.*
> Celal Çeliker, Head of the Van Provincial Organization of the CHP [88]

Sovereign violence meted out to Hakkârians did not only take the form of collective punishment methods employed to institute and defend Turkish sovereignty in the region. Almost as a rule, members of the armed forces there applied their sovereignty over the local people as a means of instituting their personal authority. Borrowing the concept elaborated by Achille Mbembé,[89] I define this usage of institutional sovereignty as the "privatization of sovereignty."

The privatization of sovereignty was a constant phenomenon in Hakkâri and the Kurdish region throughout the history of the Republic. It was originally performed by the gendarmerie and later continued with the participation of paramilitaries after 1985. We do not have records, documents, and memoirs to shed light on how it developed in Hakkâri during the era of the General Inspectorate in the single-party period (1925–46). However, the reports sent by the heads of the Van provincial organization of the CHP during the early 1940s may be used to gain an understanding of the situation in Hakkâri in those years. There was, then, little that distinguished Hakkâri from its neighboring province of Van with respect to geography, demographic structure, and social structure: both were border provinces populated overwhelmingly by Kurds organized around tribes and largely settled in rural areas.

From one of the reports sent by the head of the Van CHP to the General Secretary of the Party in January 1946, it is evident that the members of state armed forces in Van used to use their state power as mere criminals:

> We witness that armed forces burn vineyards and gardens of the people and burgle one or two houses a night, and that these things are not prevented by the commanders of the armed forces ... In September, a peasant in Binçeva village in Muradiye who had just been demobilized from the army was bayoneted by soldiers just because he asked the soldiers who tried to confiscate his cows to allow him to release his load beforehand. In the Balçıklı village of Özalp, [gendarmes] took forty of Hüseyin's sheep ... from his flock because he had refused the demand of the local troop commander to give him butter free of charge. When Hüseyin followed his sheep, he was caught by the gendarmes, his hands were tied, and he was beaten seriously and then taken to court with a claim based on a fabricated official report accusing him of smuggling sheep to Iran ... If we add to this atrocity, which includes issues that are not limited to just a few reports and pertain even to chastity, the awful events of the past—especially mass murders, exiles, robberies, and imposition of forced labor beyond the peasants' capacities ... carried out by the former governor Hamit Onat and his friends—one can understand the excessive suffering of our province and its people.[90]

The abolition of the General Inspectorates with the 1946 transition to a multi-party system, coupled with an emerging sensitivity to the demands of the people due to the competitive terrain of electoral democracy, reduced gendarmerie pressure on the people in the period between 1950 and 1979. Hakkârians continued to live in extraordinary conditions, however. The reduction was only a comparative one, and the difference was too slight to conclude that having been disposed of at will during the extraordinary days of General Inspectorate, Hakkârians became citizens of a democratic republic with its abolition and endowed with inalienable rights in the following decades. Mikail İlçin, the mayor of Hakkâri between 1963 and 1968, complained in a press conference he held in Ankara in 1966 that "in the East the law of the jungle prevails." According to İlçin, the region was used as a place of exile and punishment for the corrupt civil servants:

> The administrators and gendarmes appointed to the region under these conditions take out their anger on the citizens and inflict unimaginable cruelty on them, thinking that "they cannot be exiled any further."[91]

In Hakkâri, the continuity with respect to gendarmes' suspension of basic human rights can also be followed in a case reported by a correspondent of the prestigious Kemalist *Cumhuriyet* newspaper (first issued in May 1924). Reporting from the Yüksekova district of Hakkâri in September 1968, the correspondent mentions a case of complaint he witnessed while talking in the district governor's office with the district governor and the former mayor Mikail İlçin about the problems of the province and the region. The complaint was made by the *mukhtar* of Ginyanis village about the gendarmes' misconduct. The *Cumhuriyet* correspondent reports his address to the district governor (Caimacam [Kaymakam]) before going on to record İlçin's view:

> "Dear Caimacam Pasha. We peasants have all died. Gendarmes come to the village and seize our money and belongings. If we don't give them anything, they beat us, they kill us. We ask for your help, Caimacam Pasha."
>
> The former mayor of Hakkâri municipality Mikail İlçin said "The peasants have been left wholly at the mercy of the gendarmerie here. They face illogical accusations due to even a minor resistance or complaint: they are labeled as Kurdist, rebel, or smuggler. In the eyes of the peasants, the biggest authority, after God, is the gendarmerie . . . That is to say, here the people don't have any right to petition."[92]

Rather little changed since the 1940s, one might say. In Hakkâri in 1968, peasants were still devoid of the right to legal remedy against the gendarmerie in practice. The state they knew was a military apparatus, such that the only authority left to resort to, the head of the administration of a district, could be imagined only in the form of military commander and addressed as "Pasha," a title of respect for high-ranking military officers. And not did the gendarmerie-citizen relationship alter greatly during the following decades.

In August 1981, for example, gendarmes seized 1,140 sheep from peasants in Uludere, claiming that they were grazing in a security zone. Instead of delivering the sheep to the customs officers, the gendarmes took the animals to the gendarmerie troop to kill and eat, for the meat.[93] In a similar case in Başkale, a district in Van on the Hakkâri border, in September 1976, 30 gendarmes tried to lead a herd of sheep belonging to the villagers of Güvenlik, which was just outside the security zone, into the security zone so as to seize the animals. When the villagers resisted, the gendarmes fired at the peasants. The altercation continued for hours; the gendarmes broke the doors and windows of nearby houses and arrested two villagers whom they beat at length.[94]

These cases of the privatization of sovereignty by gendarmes in the 1960s and 1970s show how the gendarmes continued to enjoy great discretionary power over the Kurdish peasants of Hakkâri even after the abolition of the General Inspectorates and the transition to electoral democracy. Neither the bodies nor the belongings of these peasants were safe; everything and anyone was liable to be violated. İlçin described the discretionary power employed by the gendarmerie over Hakkârians in the mid-1970s thus:

> Unfortunately, gendarmerie troops of the Republic in our region, who are in charge of ensuring the interior peace and security and of protecting the life, property, and honor of the citizens—especially those settled at the border zone—somehow could not abandon ... the methods they have been using for fifty years, like insulting and beating and bastinado [caning the soles of the feet], ignoring all laws, internal regulations, and orders given to them.[95]

The period beginning with the 1979 transition to emergency rule, and especially the foundation of the Emergency Governorship in 1987 to deal with the rising guerilla warfare, witnessed the intensification of acts of privatization of sovereignty. These were extended from the state armed forces to the paramilitary village guards after 1985. This was unsurprising in that the extent of sovereign power enjoyed by armed, paramilitary, and other, irregular forces during the rule of Emergency Governorship can only be compared to that enjoyed during the rule of General Inspectorate when Kurds were, in the fullest sense of the word, no more than bare lives to be disposed of at will.

The criminal records of the Village Guards can be taken as a striking indicator of privatization of sovereignty during the rule of Emergency Governorship. Village guards certainly turned the sovereign power awarded to them into a criminal asset. According to the records of the Ministry of the Interior, between 1985 and 1996, village guards in the Kurdish region were involved in a total of 3,498 criminal cases, including 217 of murder and 168 of injury, 13 of rape and 64 of abduction of women, 61 of robbery and burglary and 40 of violation of dwelling immunity, and 65 of the illegal trafficking of narcotics.[96]

The most concrete example of the privatization of sovereignty in Hakkâri with the involvement of village guards during the period of emergency rule was the criminal network known as the "Yüksekova gang."[97] Including actors from all sectors of the armed forces, the Yüksekova gang committed innumerable crimes, ranging from the illegal trafficking of narcotics, arms smuggling through kidnapping leading, affluent figures of society to murder. The 1996 murder of Abdullah Canan, elder brother of the former Hakkâri deputy Esat Canan, was the gang's most notorious criminal act. Because Canan did not withdraw the lawsuit he filed against Mehmet Emin Yurdakul, head of the gang, for damages caused to his village and home during the operation organized by Yurdakul's order, he was simply taken into custody and tortured to death.

2.6 Conclusion

This chapter has provided an examination of sovereign violence in Hakkâri in the pre-AKP period. The Turkish state apparatus in the Kurdish region and especially in Hakkâri was so weak in Kemalist Turkey that it could not effectively apply the state assimilation programs, all of which were classified. Instead, it was mainly limited to instituting Turkish sovereignty.

The state's incapacity to penetrate deeply into the everyday lives of Hakkârians, reinforce the border and prevent illegal border trade, or distinguish "innocents" from the PKK affiliates led to the treatment of all Kurds as suspects and potential criminals. This followed quite "naturally" given the national ordering in which Kurdishness was regarded as degenerate and Kurds less than full human beings.

In practice, this meant the collective punishment of Hakkârians through the enforcement of security zones, forced displacement of villagers, imposing food embargo on villagers, exclusion from uplands, and the systematic terrorization of civilians by the constant threat of abduction, torture, and "disappearance." This, very broadly, comprised the violent history of othering and situation on the ground in Hakkâri and Turkey's Southeast when the AKP came to power in Ankara.

Notes

1 Erik Jan Zürcher, *Turkey: A Modern History* (London and New York: I.B. Tauris, 1993), 147.
2 See Kemal H. Karpat, *Ottoman Population, 1830–1914: Demographic and Social Characteristics* (Madison: University of Wisconsin Press, 1985).
3 See Zürcher, *Turkey: A Modern History*, 76–133.
4 Istanbul retained some multi-ethnicity, with significant numbers of Armenians and also Jews as well as Greeks. Greeks settled outside Istanbul and Turks settled outside Western Thrace were "exchanged" in 1923 by the agreement of the Turkish and Greek governments. See Renee Hirschon, ed. *Crossing the Aegean: An Appraisal of the 1923 Compulsory Population Exchange between Greece and Turkey* (New York: Berghahn Books, 2003).
5 Quoted in Zürcher, *Turkey*, 150.
6 Quoted in Feroz Ahmad, *Turkey: The Quest for Identity* (Oxford: Oneworld, 2003), 81.

7 See Baskın Oran, "The Minority Concept and Rights in Turkey: The Lausanne Peace Treaty and Current Issues," in *Human Rights in Turkey*, ed. Zehra F. Kabasakal Arat (Philadelphia: University of Pennsylvania Press, 2007), 35–56.
8 Zürcher, *Turkey*, 169–72.
9 The minutes of the meeting of General Inspectorates held in 1936 show that the annihilation of Kurds was one of the options voiced and discussed but left aside for the moment. See Bülent Tanık, ed. *Umumi Müfettişler Toplantı Tutanakları-1936* (Ankara: Dipnot Yayınları, 2010).
10 Soner Çağaptay, *Islam, Secularism, and Nationalism in Modern Turkey: Who Is a Turk?* (London and New York: Routledge, 2006), 83.
11 Mesut Yeğen, Introduction to *Kürtler'e Vurulan Kelepçe: Şark Islahat Planı*, by Mehmet Bayrak (Beysukent, Ankara: Öz-Ge, 2009), 11–18.
12 Mehmet Bayrak, *Kürtlere Vurulan Kelepçe: Şark Islahat Planı* (Ankara: Öz-Ge Yayınları, 2009), 125–32.
13 For a serial on commando operations penned by İsmail Cem, who later became foreign minister, see *Milliyet* (1970: 9, 11, 12, 14 June).
14 Selahattin Şimşek, *Hakkâri Dedikleri* (Istanbul: Martı Yayınları, 1990), 74–77.
15 "Tuzluca Olayları Üzerine," Bağımsızlık, Demokrasi, Sosyalizm için Yürüyüş, accessed March 13, 2022, https://issuu.com/solyayin/docs/y_75_029/16.
16 James Ferguson and Akhil Gupta, "Spatializing States: Toward an Ethnography of Neoliberal Governmentality," *American Ethnologist* 29, no. 4 (2002): 981–1002.
17 Metin Heper regards this incapacity as evidence of that the Turkish state did not really attempt to assimilate Kurds. Metin Heper, *The State and Kurds in Turkey: The Question of Assimilation* (Basingstoke and New York: Palgrave Macmillan, 2007).
18 Muzaffer İlhan Erdost, *Şemdinli Röportajı* (Ankara: Onur Yayınları, 1993), 164–65.
19 Ibid., 242–45.
20 Ibid. Michael Mann, "The Autonomous Power of the State: Its Origins, Mechanisms and Results," *European Journal of Sociology / Archives Européennes de Sociologie* 25, no. 2 (1984): 189.
21 Michel Foucault, "Governmentality," in *The Foucault Effect: Studies in Governmentality*, ed. Graham Burchell, Colin Gordon, and Peter Miller (Chicago: Chicago University Press, 1991), 95.
22 Anthony Giddens, *A Contemporary Critique of Historical Materialism*, vol. 2, *The Nation-State and Violence* (Cambridge: Polity Press, 1985), 59.
23 Victoria Sanford, "Contesting Displacement in Colombia: Citizenship and State Sovereignty at the Margins," in *Anthropology in the Margins of the State*, ed. Veena Das and Deborah Poole (Santa Fe, NM: School of American Research Press 2004), 253.
24 Michel Foucault, *The History of Sexuality* (New York: Vintage Books, 1988), 136.
25 Carl Schmitt, *Political Theology: Four Chapters on the Concept of Sovereignty* (Chicago: University of Chicago Press, 2005), 5. See also Giorgio Agamben, *State of Exception* (Chicago: University of Chicago Press, 2005).

26 Leslie Alan Horvitz and Christopher Catherwood, *Encyclopedia of War Crimes and Genocide*, Facts on File Library of World History (New York: Facts on File, 2006), 89.
27 Mitchell Dean, *Governmentality: Power and Rule in Modern Society* (London and Thousand Oaks, CA: Sage, 1999), 20.
28 Douglas D Heckathorn, "Collective Sanctions and the Creation of Prisoner's Dilemma Norms," *American Journal of Sociology* 94, no. 3 (1988).
29 See Huw Bennett, "The Mau Mau Emergency as Part of the British Army's Post-War Counter-Insurgency Experience," *Defense & Security Analysis* 23, no. 2 (2007); David French, *The British Way in Counter-Insurgency, 1945–1967* (Oxford and New York: Oxford University Press, 2011), 105–37.
30 Shane Darcy, *Collective Responsibility and Accountability under International Law* (Ardsley, NY: Transnational Publishers, 2007), 57.
31 Serap Yeşiltuna, ed. *Atatürk Ve Kürtler: Resmi Kanun, Kararname, Rapor Ve Tutanaklarla* (Istanbul: İleri Yayınları, 2007), 248.
32 Dipesh Chakrabarty, *Provincializing Europe: Postcolonial Thought and Historical Difference* (Princeton, NJ and Oxford: Princeton University Press, 2008), 119.
33 Zygmunt Bauman, *Modernity and the Holocaust* (Ithaca, NY: Cornell University Press, 1989), 102–4.
34 Herbert C. Kelman, "Violence without Moral Restraint: Reflections on the Dehumanization of Victims and Victimizers," *Journal of Social Issues* 29, no. 4 (1973).
35 M. Şerif Fırat, *Doğu İlleri Ve Varto Tarihi* (Ankara: Türk Kültürünü Araştırma Enstitüsü, 1981).
36 Naşit Hakkı, *Derebeyi Ve Dersim* (Ankara: Hakimiyet-i Milliye Matbaası, 1939), 17.
37 Ben-Ami Shillony, "The Flourishing Demon: Japan in the Role of the Jews," in *Demonizing the Other: Antisemitism, Racism and Xenophobia*, ed. Robert S. Wistrich (Amsterdam: Harwood Academic, 1999), 293–308.
38 Scott Straus, *The Order of Genocide: Race, Power, and War in Rwanda* (Ithaca, NY: Cornell University Press, 2006), 157–60.
39 Mesut Yeğen, *Müstakbel Türk'ten Sözde Vatandaşa: Cumhuriyet Ve Kürtler* (Cağaloğlu, Istanbul: İletişim, 2006).
40 Sıdıka Avar, *Dağ Çiçeklerim, Anılar* (Ankara: Öğretmen Yayınları, 1986).
41 Yeşiltuna, *Atatürk Ve Kürtler*, 211.
42 Reşat Hallı, *Türkiye Cumhuriyeti'nde Ayaklanmalar 1924–1938* (Ankara: Genelkurmay Harp Tarihi Bşk. Yay., 1972), 35.
43 BCA BMGMK [Catalogue Number: 030 01/120 765 1].
44 Ibid.
45 Written by the famous poet Ahmet Arif on the murder of 33 Kurdish smugglers in the Özalp district of Van on the order of General Mustafa Muğlalı in 1943.

"Thirty-Three Bullets," in *Hasretinden Prangalar Eskittim*, trans. Murat: Nemet Nejat, http://www.siir.gen.tr/siir/a/ahmed_arif/thirty_three_bullets.htm.
46 Hüseyin Koca, *Yakın Tarihten Günümüze Hükümetlerin Doğu-Güneydoğu Anadolu Politikaları* (Konya: Mikro Basım-Yayım-Dağıtım, 1998), 323.
47 BCA BMGMK [Catalogue Number: 030 10/ 180 244 6].
48 *Hakkâri*, January 27, 1983.
49 Aliza Marcus, *Kan Ve İnanç: Pkk ve Kürt Hareketi*, trans. Ayten Alkan (Istanbul: İletişim Yayınları, 2009), 246–47.
50 Erdal Sarızeybek, *Şemdinli'de Sınırı Aşmak* (Istanbul: Pozitif, 2011), 95.
51 Sabri Ateş, *Ottoman-Iranian Borderlands: Making a Boundary, 1843–1914* (New York: Cambridge University Press, 2013).
52 For reports documenting salt and arms smuggling in Hakkâri-Iran border in late nineteenth century, see BOA DH MKT [Catalogue Number: 1646/21] and BOA DH.ŞFR. [Catalogue Number: 148/24].
53 BCA BMGMK [Catalogue Number: 030 10/230 548 10].
54 *Hakkâri*, November 26 1962.
55 Sarızeybek, *Şemdinli'de Sınırı Aşmak*, 94–97.
56 Erdost, *Şemdinli Röportajı*, 185–86.
57 KOM Department, *Turkish Report of Anti-Smuggling and Organized Crime 2011* (Ankara: KOM Publication, 2012), 10–35.
58 See I'smail Beşikçi, *Orgeneral Mustafa Muğlalı Olayı* (Istanbul: Belge-Uluslararası Yayıncılık, 1991).
59 Republic of Turkey, *T.C Resmi Gazete*, no. 9401, September 7, 1956.
60 *T.C Resmi Gazete*, no. 9495, December 28, 1956.
61 *T.C Resmi Gazete*, no. 9529, February 7, 1957.
62 *T.C Resmi Gazete*, no. 9763, November 22, 1957.
63 *T.C Resmi Gazete*, no. 11330, February 9, 1963.
64 *T.C Resmi Gazete*, no. 17303, April 7, 1981.
65 *Hakkâri Sesi*, June 27, 1977.
66 *Hakkâri Sesi*, January 10, 1975.
67 *Hakkâri Sesi*, February 1, 1975.
68 *Hakkâri Sesi*, November 23, 1974.
69 Republic of Turkey, *Millet Meclisi Tutanak Dergisi*, term 4, session 132, vol. 20, September 14, 1976.
70 Ibid.
71 Zafer Üskül, *Siyaset Ve Asker: Cumhuriyet Döneminde Sıkıyönetim Uygulamaları* (Ankara: İmge Kitapevi, 1997), 276.
72 Joost Jongerden, *The Settlement Issue in Turkey and the Kurds: An Analysis of Spatial Policies, Modernity and War* (Leiden and Boston: Brill, 2007), 66.
73 Ümit Özdağ, *Türk Ordusu Pkk'yı Nasıl Yendi? Türkiye Pkk'ya Nasıl Teslim Oluyor* (Ankara: Kripto, 2010), 81.

74 *Serxwebun*, September 1991.
75 Joost Jongerden, *The Settlement Issue in Turkey and the Kurds* (Leiden and Boston: Brill, 2007), 91.
76 Osman Pamukoğlu, *Unutulanlar Dışında Yeni Bir Şey Yok: Hakkari ve Kuzey Irak Dağlarındaki Askerler* (Istanbul: Harmoni, 2004), 59–60. Quoted and translated by Jongerden, *The Settlement Issue in Turkey and the Kurds*, 43.
77 In fact, threatening of the peasants of *Hakkâri* pushed them into taking part in the war against the PKK in order to stay in their villages following the establishment of the Village Guard system in 1985. In a gathering held in Çukurca in September 1989 with the attendance of the governor, the commander of the Hakkâri Mountain and Commando Brigade, the provincial police chief, and the regiment commander, according to Cumhur Keskin, Hakkâri deputy of the governing Social Democratic People's Party (*Sosyaldemokrat Halkçı Parti*, SHP), the *mukhtars* of the villages of Çukurca and leaders of the tribes who were also present were all threatened. One of the officials was reported to have said, "This is my last warning. Take up arms. You have one week to come to a decision. If you don't take up arms and become village guards, we'll consider you PKK supporters. Keep this in mind when making your decision." The official warned the people that they "may face the similar things to those taking place in Iraq" if they did not take up arms. See Republic of Turkey, *T.B.M.M Tutanak Dergisi*, term 18, session 19, vol. 33, October 19, 1989.

Regarding the comparison to Iraq, the people of Çukurca were being explicitly threatened by genocide, like that which occurred in Halabja in March 1988. Most probably in the same meeting, Mustafa Zeydan, the leader of the North Pinyanişi tribe and collaborator of the state, said to the villagers "You either will take up arms or go to the mountains. You don't have any alternative." Ormanlı, Çimenli, and Kelatan villages were completely evacuated because the inhabitants refused to sign the document concerning their taking up arms. See *Serxwebun*, January 1990.
78 Devlet İstatistik Enstitüsü (State Statistical Institute), *2000 Genel Nüfus Sayımı: Nüfusun Sosyal ve Ekonomik Nitelikleri, Hakkari.*
79 Republic of Turkey, *T.B.M.M Tutanak Dergisi*, term 18, session 6, vol. 14, September 29, 1988.
80 *T.B.M.M Tutanak Dergisi*, term 18, session 27, vol. 33, November 7, 1989.
81 Although emergency rule in Hakkâri was abolished in 2002, a few months before the AKP came to the power, its methods were only curtailed after 2006, when two members of the Gendarmerie Intelligence were caught in Şemdinli in the act of attacking the shop of a leading Kurdish activist with hand grenades.
82 *Star*, August 30, 2011.
83 See Kees Koonings and Dirk Krujit, *Societies of Fear: The Legacy of Civil War, Violence and Terror in Latin America* (London and New York: Zed Books, 1999) and Linda Buckley Green, *Fear as a Way of Life: Mayan Widows in Rural Guatemala* (New York: Columbia University Press, 1999).

84 Norbert Lechner, "Some People Die of Fear: Fear as a Political Problem," in *Fear at the Edge: State Terror and Resistance in Latin America*, ed. Juan E. Corradi, Patricia Weiss Fagen, and Manuel A. Garretâon Merino (Berkeley: University of California Press, 1992), 32.

85 For the details of these cases of disappearances, see "Zorla Kaybedilenler Veritabanı," Hafıza Merkezi, accessed May 5, 2018, http://www.zorlakaybetmeler.org/events.php?city.

86 "Case of Meryem Çelik and Others," European Court of Human Rights, accessed February 11, 2022, http://hudoc.echr.coe.int/sites/eng/Pages/search.aspx#.

87 Republic of Turkey, *T.B.M.M Tutanak Dergisi*, term 23, session 50, vol. 59, January 20, 2010.

88 *BCA CHP* [Catalogue Number: 490 01/490 1976 1].

89 Achille Mbembé, *On the Postcolony* (Berkeley: University of California Press, 2001).

90 *BCA CHP* [Catalogue Number: 490 01/490 1976 1].

91 *Hakkâri*, December 19, 1966.

92 *Cumhuriyet*, September 4, 1968.

93 Republic of Turkey, *T.C Resmi Gazete*, no. 20231, June 24, 1989.

94 *Millet Meclisi Tutanak Dergisi*, term 4, session 1, vol. 21, November 1, 1976.

95 Ibid.

96 Republic of Turkey, *Millet Meclisi Tutanak Dergisi*, term 20, session 42, vol. 18, January 7, 1997.

97 See Enis Berberoğlu, *Kod Adı Yüksekova* (Istanbul: Milliyet Yayınları, 1998).

98 Devlet İstatistik Enstitüsü (State Statistical Institute), *Gap İl İstatistikleri 1950–1996* (Ankara: DİE, 1997), 10.

99 İstatistik Genel Direktörlüğü (General Directorate of Statistics), *Genel Nüfus Sayımı 1935* (Ankara: Mehmet İhsan Basımevi, 1937), 144–45.

100 Servet Mutlu, "Ethnic Kurds in Turkey: A Demographic Study," *International Journal of Middle East Studies* 28, no. 4 (1996).

101 State Planning Organization (Devlet Planlama Teşkilatı), *Kalkınmada Öncelikli Yöreler Raporu No: 5* (Ankara: Devlet Planlama Teşkilatı, Kalkınmada Öncelikli Yöreler ve Bölgesel Kalkınma Genel Müdürlüğü, 1987).

3

Indirect State Racism, Healthcare Provision, and Hakkâri

My wife was pregnant, and she was about to give birth prematurely. The doctor examined her and said that she had to go to Van as soon as possible.

Q: When did this happen?

A: It was 1996. The doctor decided to transfer her to Van. Yet we waited for the ambulance for hours. It was nine o'clock when [the doctor] decided to transfer her. My wife was pregnant with twins, and it was the seventh month of her pregnancy. It was a premature birth. She was in labor for hours, but no ambulance was available. In the end, she gave birth here. Immediately after the birth, one of the twins died. The other was still alive and needed to be transferred to Van. We needed to transfer her by ambulance in an incubator. We waited for the incubator for hours. In the end, the incubator became available, but the ambulance didn't have the facilities to work it. We had to cover the baby with cotton, put her into the incubator, which did not work, and transfer her to Van at midnight in the winter.

Q: Did the ambulance come at midnight?

A: Yes. We left for Van at midnight in the winter. It was minus 15 or 20 degrees. By the time the ambulance arrived in Van, the door [of the ambulance] had been opened at least six times [by soldiers] checking if there was really a patient in the ambulance or not. We saw that each time the door was opened the baby was exposed to the cold air. At one in the morning, we managed to get to Van Yüzüncü Yıl Research Hospital.

Q: Couldn't you ask the soldiers not to open the door?

A: Was that possible then? We were living in the emergency region. Frankly, it was a time when specialist sergeants were like generals. Each time the door was opened, the baby was exposed to the cold, and also the incubator did not work. In the end, because of these failures, I lost my other baby as well in the [research hospital]. That's what happened to me. Thousands of people experienced similar things. At the time, I was a civil servant in the provincial Directorate of Health.

When we met, he was the head of a department of the provincial Directorate of Health. He was born and bred in Hakkâri and also the provincial head of the Health and Social Services Employees' Union (Sağlık ve Sosyal Hizmet Çalışanları Sendikası, Sağlık-Sen), which was a member of the government-affiliated Confederation of Public Servants' Trade Unions (Memur Sendikaları Konfederasyonu, Memur-Sen).

This chapter focuses on state-citizen relations in Hakkâri in the pre-AKP period of Kemalist Turkey through an analysis of healthcare provisioning. And this conversation reveals in a very striking manner how, by 1996, the state's attitude toward omissions, shortages, shortcomings, and problems with immediate life-threatening implications in Hakkâri was one of indifference. The health-service issues leading to the babies' deaths were too numerous and structural in nature to be accounted for as mere omissions or shortages. The babies most probably would have been alive today if the Hakkâri Public Hospital had been adequately equipped and staffed to perform medical interventions on time, making the transfer unnecessary. Likewise, the babies could have been saved had fully equipped ambulances been available in sufficient numbers to meet the actual local need on time, or if the one that arrived had at least been functioning properly and capable of activating an incubator, if the road connecting Hakkâri to Van had been better, if Hakkârians had not been collectively criminalized as suspects causing the soldiers at security checkpoint to stop the ambulance and open its door to check, looking for potential terrorists, or if the soldiers at the checkpoints had at least cared enough about the local people to think of or bother to radio to other checkpoints to let the ambulance through.

Inspired by Foucault's "state racism," I use the term "indirect state racism" to point to the huge gap in Kemalist Turkey between the resources and personnel reserved for Hakkâri and those required for the satisfaction of Hakkârians' actual needs. By "indirect state racism," I refer to the likelihood of "exposing someone to death, increasing the risk of death for some people"[1] by not expending sufficient effort, care, and resources to eliminate or reduce sources of risk that threaten lives on the assumption that these lives are not really worth the expenses and effort. The term "indirect state racism" needs further elucidation. This is given below, first by further conceptual explanation and then by quantitative indicators for a comparative analysis of public investments made in Hakkâri in Kemalist Turkey. Finally, again with a focus on Kemalist Turkey, indirect state racism in (toward) Hakkâri is considered by focusing on the poverty of healthcare provision in that period.

3.1 Indirect State Racism

Foucault first formulated the concept of "state racism" in the lectures compiled in the book *Society Must Be Defended*. "State racism" is the answer he gave to his following question:

> [H]ow will the power to kill and the function of murder operate in this technology of power, which takes life as both its object and its objective? How can a power such as this kill if it is true that its basic function is to improve life, to prolong its duration, to improve its chances, to avoid accidents, and to compensate for failings? [...] How can the power of death, the function of death, be exercised in a political system centered upon bio-power?[2]

His answer, which introduced the concept, was as follows:

> Racism makes it possible to establish a possible relationship between my life and the death of the other that is not a military or warlike relationship of confrontation, but a biological-type relationship: "The more inferior species die out, the more abnormal individuals are eliminated, the fewer degenerates there will be in the species as a whole, and the more I—as species rather than individual—can live, the stronger I will be, the more vigorous I will be. I will be able to proliferate." The fact that the other dies does not mean simply that I live in the sense that his death guarantees my safety; the death of the other, the death of the bad race, of the inferior race (or the degenerate, or the abnormal) is something that will make life in general healthier: healthier and purer.[3]

According to Foucault, National Socialism and Soviet Socialism were two prototypes of state racism, albeit with entirely opposite discourses. Both the German fascist and Russian socialist regimes defined their enemies in economic and biological terms. The enemies of each were conceived of as burdens on the resources and economies of the state and as threats to the biological well-being of the nation.[4]

It may be argued that state racism does not really describe the Turkish state's approach to the Kurds and Hakkâri. Even when Kurds posed a threat to the Turkish state via the numerous rebellions, these rebellions were not primarily perceived by the state elites as threats to the welfare and the "well-being" of the nation, at least until the mid-1990s when the economic burden of the war in the Kurdish region on the treasury and economy started to be discussed. Rather, these rebellions were seen as threats to *sovereignty*, to the sovereignty of the state. This means that state racism as defined by Foucault—approaching the "other" as a bio-economic threat to be eliminated for the sake and welfare of the nation—does not fit the Turkish stance toward the Kurds and hence Hakkârians.

Yet the term "state racism" can still be helpful. If state racism means the elimination, for the strength of the nation, of some groups supposed to be economically harmful to it, then the state's negligent withdrawal from reserving and providing the resources necessary for the survival and development of a population group can also be seen as a type of state racism. In fact, Foucault himself acknowledged this possibility:

> When I say "killing," I obviously do not mean simply murder as such, but also every form of indirect murder: the fact of exposing someone to death, increasing the risk of death for some people, or, quite simply, political death, expulsion, rejection, and so on.[5]

This *covert* form of state racism involves the insufficient expenditure of the effort required to counter deprivation and poverty, thereby threatening lives regarded as not economically productive or promising. To distinguish this from overt forms of state racism—the active and direct involvement of the state in the elimination of lives, including those considered economically detrimental—I call the former "*in*direct state racism" and the latter "direct."

In indirect state racism, an economic perspective is implicitly present. While the "other" of direct state racism appears as exploiter and parasite and directly harmful to the national body, in indirect state racism, the "other" appears as high opportunity-cost, an unnecessary burden on resources that can be used more efficiently.[6] The restriction of public resources reserved for unproductive pensioners, the disabled, and the unemployed can be taken as examples of indirect state racism.

Finally here, the concept of indirect state violence can be clarified by a comparison with "structural violence," as described by Paul Farmer.[7] In fact, the large-scale social, political, and economic inequalities and hierarchies making Hakkârians more vulnerable to life-threatening dangers on a daily basis could very well be described as "structural violence." This concept as used by Farmer refers precisely to what is termed "indirect state racism" here, namely, the stances and processes that devalue the lives of the disadvantaged in implicit but by no means less harmful ways that violate the disadvantaged people's right to survive, not openly by the suspension of their civil rights with recourse to sovereign violence, but indirectly, by depriving them of the protective shield of social and economic rights.

The difference between the terms "indirect state racism" and "structural violence" resides not so much in the referents of the concepts but rather in the center of gravity of their different emphases. The main emphasis of "structural violence" is on causality and effects, while that of "indirect state racism" is on political subjectivity and agency. "Structural violence" points to a linkage between social, economic, and political policies that are not obviously violent and immediately life-threatening and their actual, life-threatening results for those systematically experiencing the effects of the policies, especially in the middle- and long-term. From the perspective of "indirect state racism," however, the fact that the violence and life-threatening effects of social, economic, and political policies on certain sections of society occur in indirect ways and after some time does not diminish the issue of agency and make this violence a "structural" one.

Centering on the issue of political subjectivity and agency, the concept of indirect state racism urges us to see the social, economic, and political policies involved in the production and reproduction of inequalities and hierarchies—which *in turn* produce life-threatening effects on some sections of society in the middle- and long-term—as symptoms of a coherent biopolitical stance that does not attribute much value to the lives of these sections of society. The distinction may appear somewhat technical, but what it does is to throw moral responsibility onto the agent, as the perpetrator of the deed, rather than allow the escape into institution, as passive and amoral, afforded by the abstraction of "structure."

3.2 Indirect State Racism toward Hakkâri: Not an Ethnic Phenomenon?

The "racism" in "indirect state racism" does not refer to hatred related to the other in terms of a biological stigmatization of certain human societies as inferior races. Rather, it refers to the indifference toward the needs, even vital ones, of groups (not necessarily ethnic groups) regarded as not economically contributory to the well-being and welfare of the nation. Underlining this point, we can argue that Hakkârians fell victim to indirect state racism in the pre-AKP period not immediately because of their Kurdishness but because of the developmentalist investment preferences of the Turkish governments. The investment preferences of the Turkish governments in the pre-AKP period were almost always determined by overall economic concerns, such as fast growth and economic development.

The governments of the Republic did not follow a public investment policy aiming at a geographically *balanced* growth. The prosperity of the nation did not extend to and incorporate a sense of its equity across the territory and a foregrounding of social justice. This was something that Hakkârians very much needed due to the marginalization and isolation they—their province, the Southeast—were subject to during the process of incorporation into the system of capital and the state's central administrative structure.

This is not to completely discard the role of the ethnic dimension in the historical administration of the Republic and its approach to development. On the contrary, there are at least two major reservations about this in relation to the indirect state racism toward Hakkâri and Kurdish region in Kemalist Turkey that indicate how the specifically ethnic dimension can be understood as having had its roots in the character of the Turkish assumption and aim of assimilationism. These are noted below. First, though, we should take a closer look at the historical economic investment aspect of the issue.

At a world-historical level, the peripheralization of Kurdish region can be traced back to the emergence of a new international division of labor with the rise of a European world-economy.[8] Although the leading port cities of the Ottoman Empire, like Istanbul, Salonika, and Izmir could incorporate the new international division of labor through the nineteenth century, becoming locations for the export of raw materials and the import of manufactured goods,[9] eastern and interior Anatolia could not achieve this. Connecting these areas to port cities could have partially reversed the process of peripheralization of eastern Anatolia and the Kurdish provinces, but the transportation system was wholly structured by the necessities of the new international division of labor. That meant the emergence of a railroad system—what İlhan Tekeli called a "colonial tree scheme"—that is, a railroad system linking the hinterlands to port cities in support of import and export processes.[10]

The logic of this capitalist drive was compounded, however, by the fact that the formation of the nation-state and all concomitant nation-state practices—notably the institution of national borders, deportation and dispossession of so-called non-national groups, and counter-insurgency measures taken to terminate threats to the nation-state—reinforced the peripheralization of the region and especially border provinces like Hakkâri. In other words, attempts to incorporate the region as national substantially deepened the process of peripheralization, as they "preclude[d] the possibility of an economic base to support independent indigenous existence" and "blocked internal economic development" of the region.[11]

The deportation and massacre of non-Muslim populations, especially in the process beginning in WWI, led to a big decline in the region's productive capacity. The massacres and forced deportations, mostly of Armenians but also heretic Assyrians in the Kurdish region and in Hakkâri specifically, resulted in considerable losses with respect to the skilled population of artisan workers and its structures of wealth production.[12]

National borders, meanwhile, uncoupled eastern Anatolia from its immediate economic milieu. The economy of the region became largely disconnected from the Aleppo-centered economic network in the south of the region and also the economic network of Caucasia and Russia to the north.[13] Consequently, the transhumance practices of many nomadic tribes subsisting on animal husbandry and thus going back and forth between historically Kurdish lands to be subsequently demarcated as Iraq, Iran, and Turkey were hit hard by the establishment of national borders.[14]

For İhsan Çölemerikli, a local intellectual known for his historical studies of the province, that led to a serious decline in animal husbandry in the Republican period. Indeed, Hakkâri had been one of the main providers of meat to Mosul and Iraqi Kurdistan in the Ottoman period. The impact of the decline of animal husbandry—especially for Hakkâri—of the creation of national borders following the loss of economic production generally through the population exterminations and migrations was accelerated further by the depopulation of rural areas and exclusions from uplands in the Kurdish region during the counter-insurgency operations against the PKK in the 1990s. That was especially so in Hakkâri where the extent of village evacuations and bans from uplands was massive. Thus, for instance, the number of sheep in Hakkâri declined drastically, more than halving between 1990 and 1995 (dropping, according to official numbers, from 698,170 to 307,240).[15]

But none of this was unknown. In the biopolitical metaphor, the broken bones of Hakkâri could have been repaired and new implants could have nourished the weakened body of Hakkâri. Foucault defines biopolitics as "a matter of organizing circulation, eliminating its dangerous elements, making a division between good and bad circulation, and maximizing the good circulation by diminishing the bad."[16] As described (above), the state attempted to diminish "bad" circulation, that is, the circulation of people and goods supposed to be harmful to the national body. However, it failed to maximize the "good" circulation; it failed to compensate or make a reasonable attempt to compensate for what the province and the region had lost during the development of capitalism and the nation-state.

The logic guiding Turkey's public investment policy was almost entirely an economic-developmentalist one according to which it was not only the case that "resources should be invested in the most productive areas" but also that "projects in the backward regions should be preferred over others *only if* they were at least as good as the others with respect to economic investment criteria" (emphasis added).[17] All development plans between 1963 and 2000 "either explicitly or implicitly professed this criterion," according to Servet Mutlu, one of the main development economists in Turkey; "this was reasonable in the light of the backwardness of the country as a whole, which necessitated that the resources be put to the best use"[18]—but it also deepened regional developmental imbalances inherited from the Ottoman Empire between more urbanized and economically developed Western regions and the rural interior, eastern Anatolia, and the Kurdish region, which had been already poorly linked to the rest of the country even before the radical changes of the twentieth century.[19]

The figures below (Figures 6a, 6b, and 6c), constructed from official data, indicate the share of the total public investment (in education, public works, health, and agriculture) Hakkâri received between 1946 and 2002, the year when the AKP came to power. The public investment data are not available for the period between 1946 and 1960, so the public expenditures data as calculated by Sait Aşgın are used for these years.[20]

In addition to Hakkâri and also the whole of Turkey, the relevant data for four large provinces in eastern Anatolia—Van, Diyarbakır, Kars, and Erzurum—are presented to shed light on to the nature of indirect state racism suffered by Kurds generally. Taking Van and Diyarbakır, two predominantly Kurdish provinces,

Indirect State Racism, Healthcare Provision, and Hakkâri | 91

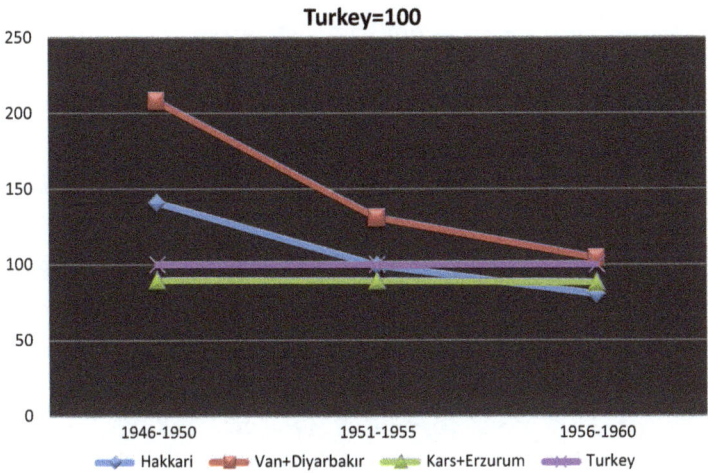

Figure 6a. Public Expenditure Per Capita (Education, Public Works, Health, Agriculture) between 1946 and 1960.
Source: Constructed by the author based on data in *Cumhuriyet Döneminde Doğu Anadolu'ya Yapılan Kamu Harcamaları*.

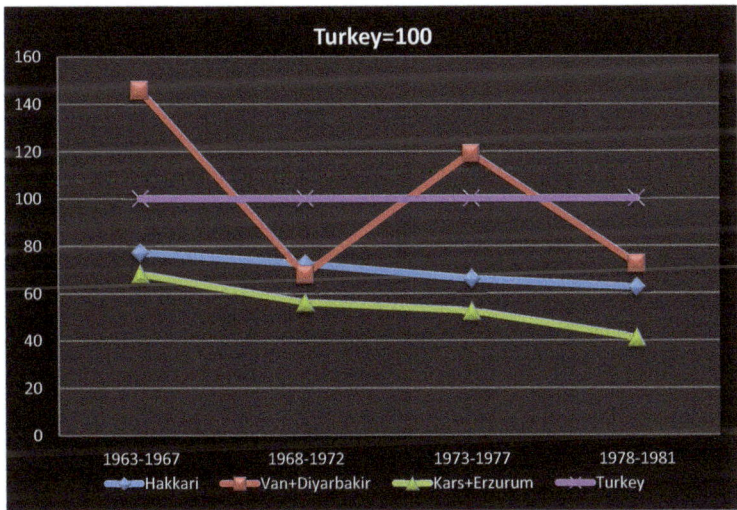

Figure 6b. Public Investment Per Capita between 1963 and 1981.
Source: Constructed by the author based on data in *Kamu Yatırımlarının Kalkınmada Öncelikli İller ve Yöreler ve Diğer İller İtibariyle Dağılımı (1963–1981)*.

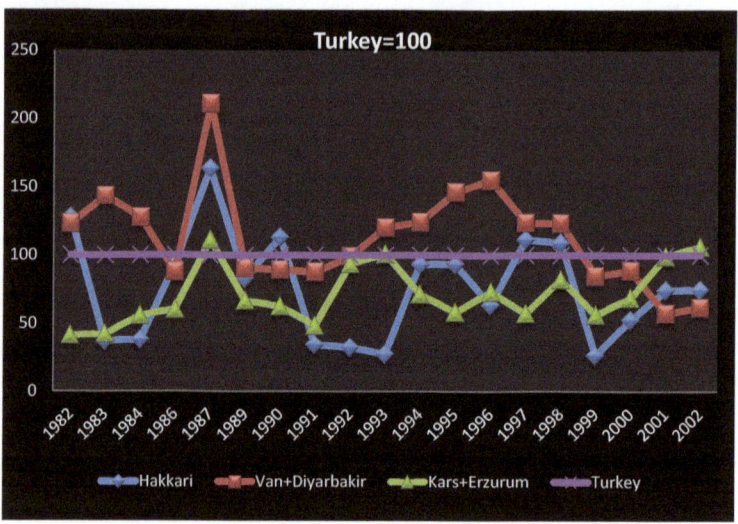

Figure 6c. Public Investment Per Capita between 1982 and 2002.
Note: Calculated based on allocations in the budget program; public investments unclassifiable into provinces not included.
Source: Constructed by the author based on data in public investment reports between 1982 and 2002 (Library of the Strategy and Budgeting Ministry; Strateji ve Bütçe Başkanlığı: Kütüphane website).

as a single unit, and Kars and Erzurum, two demographically heterogeneous provinces, as another, enables this comparative perspective.[21] We are then able to make an assessment of whether or not the structural violence as indirect state racism had an immediately ethnic aspect.

Assuming that public expenditure per capita trends during 1946–60 were largely in parallel with the equivalent public investment trends, we see that public investment per capita in Hakkâri was almost always considerably below the average of pre-AKP Turkey. Yet these figures also prevent us from deriving a hasty conclusion that the systematic neglect of Hakkâri by the state proves a discriminatory stance taken against the Kurds. Public expenditure per capita in 1946–60 and public investment per capita in 1963–81 in the demographically heterogeneous Kars+Erzurum area was even lower than that in Hakkâri (with the single exception of the 4 years between 1956 and 1960); and Kars+Erzurum fared no better than Hakkâri overall between 1982 and 2002 (when the relative fortunes alternated). Moreover, public investment per capita in the Kurdish Van+Diyarbakır area for the period from the end of WWII to the end of the twentieth century was generally a little higher than the average for Turkey as a whole (though by no means so much higher as to allow us to confidently speak of a considerable positive discrimination toward Van-Diyarbakır).

These findings seem to confirm that the discriminatory stance of the state toward Hakkâri with respect to the public investment preferences in the pre-AKP era was economic-developmentalist in character and should be taken as a part of *indirect* state racism posed toward Turkey's East as a whole, regardless of the ethnic composition of the provinces. However, considering the nature of Turkish assimilationism directed toward the Kurds, we should be prudent with these findings and not jump to any conclusion that indirect state racism toward Hakkâri in Kemalist Turkey did not involve any ethnic dimension. There are two reasons for this reservation, both of which have their roots in the Turkish nationalist stance toward Kurds.

First, if public investment strategies of the Turkish governments had been led by the principle of a geographically balanced growth and not by economic-developmentalist criteria, the governments would have had to single out eastern Turkey and develop a special policy set and institutions. The investment in the Kurdish provinces in particular would have needed to be much *higher* than in other provinces in order to bring them up to the levels of prosperity enjoyed elsewhere in the country. That might have served to the assimilation of Kurds into Turkishness as "future Turks," as was repeatedly mentioned in the classified reports of the single-party period, 1925–45. However, that would have involved a violation of the basic gesture of Turkish nationalism toward Kurds: keeping absolute silence on and making completely invisible all signs signifying the exceptional reality of eastern Turkey, most of whose population consisted of Kurds.

Second, the difficulties that Turkish nationalism might have faced had the state established a special regional developmental institution to implement positive discriminative developmental policies in its eastern portion did not only involve an acknowledgment of the exceptional nature of the East, which is predominantly Kurdish. Another question that such a focus on eastern Turkey would have posed to Turkish nationalism was whether the Kurds were worth it. Even if, on the one hand, it was deemed acceptable and even necessary for the Turkish nationalism of Kemalist Turkey that Kurds—as "future Turks"—needed to be positively discriminated for in developmental issues, Kurdishness as such, on the other hand, embodied in the eyes of Turkish nationalism no more than a case of degeneration, a worthless amalgam of Turkishness with those designated by Turkish nationalism as its "other": Arabic, Islamic, tribal and feudal cultures with bandits and lawlessness and all that went with as the very antithesis of the modern, as "development."

Given that the "split due to being in-between East and West is [. . .] constitutive of [. . .] ontology"[22] of modern Turkish identity—that the constitutive gesture of Kemalist Turkish identity with which it approved its Western-European character was the negation of institutions, relationships and traditions associated with the "East"[23]—one may reasonably question whether the persistence of "underdevelopment" of eastern Turkey and its Kurdish region in the pre-AKP period was something *required* by Kemalist Turkish identity and thus intrinsic to Turkish nationalism. This type of othering as a function of nation-state identity is evident in the disciplinary usage of the region for public servants—throughout the history of the Republic, it was used as a place of exile for the most problematic and a boot camp for the least experienced. In short, there is no reason to imagine that Kurds as a degenerate and worthless "under-ethnicity," a representation of Kurds that mostly appeared in the classified documents of the state, guided Kemalist policies toward Kurds any less than did the idea of Kurds as "future Turks," the other and publicly available representation of Kurds.

3.3 Poverty of Healthcare Provision as Indirect State Racism toward Hakkâri

However one defines Hakkârians' experience with the Turkish state in the pre-AKP period, the quality of life of Hakkârians at the turn of the millennium was undisputedly very low. In a report prepared by the United Nations Development Programme (UNDP) in 1998, six provinces in Turkey were given an overall score on the Human Development Index, placing them in the category of "low human development." All were Kurdish; one was Hakkâri, ranked 75th out of the 78 provinces. Life expectancy in the province was just over 60 years, with a fifth of the population not reaching 40 years old, the second-worst provincial performance for this metric. The Kurdish provinces generally filled the bottom positions for all metrics.[24] In another report prepared by the UNDP in 2001, Hakkâri was ranked 77th of the 78 provinces in the Human Poverty Index.[25]

Among other considerations, such as poverty, education, and gender, healthcare provision provided one of the factors in the classification of the term "low human development." Again, the southeastern provinces were the lowest-ranked for this in Turkey at the end of the 1990s. Hakkâri was equal bottom with other Kurdish provinces in the measures for underweight young children (one in five) and for people dissatisfied with the health service (one in three).[26] Here, archival and ethnographic findings are employed to show that the poverty of healthcare provision in Hakkâri in Kemalist Turkey reflected an established lack of will to find ways of ensuring that Hakkârians received sufficient resources, cadres, and care to keep them healthy and alive. First, the situation of the people working in the health sector in Hakkâri is reviewed, with a focus on the Republican history of the employment of doctors, nurses, dentists, midwives, pharmacists, and clerks and the systems used to transfer these professionals to the area of need and provide care in the province.

3.3.1 Health Workforce in Hakkâri

The health workforce in Hakkâri has been characterized by two facts throughout the history of the Republic. The more important of these is the insufficiency of medical personnel, especially GPs and specialists, as can be seen in Table 7, giving the (quantitative) state of the health workforce in Hakkâri between 1955 and 2005. The table shows a very slow improvement beginning in the mid-1960s, before which it is impossible to speak of even a poor presence of medical cadres

Table 7. Health Workforce in Hakkâri (Numbers of State Professionals Employed, Five-Yearly), 1955–2005

	Specialists	GPs	Dentists	Nurses	Midwives	Health clerks	Pharmacists
1955	0	5	0	0	0	4	0
1960	0	5	0	0	1	8	0
1965	1	11	1	9	12	13	0
1970	1	7	2	12	26	30	0
1975	1	13	4	18	40	11	3
1980	7	22	3	45	41	15	4
1985	8	28	5	77	65	38	14
1990	11	53	4	61	91	84	10
1995	19	68	3	105	77	102	13
2000	16	68	5	121	63	108	12
2005	37	68	10	222	80	194	22

Sources: Constructed from health statistical yearbooks prepared by the MoH/ Ministry of Health and Social Assistance (Sağlık ve Sosyal Yardım Bakanlığı, MHSA)[101] and Turkish Statistical Institute (Türkiye İstatistik Kurumu, TÜİK), Regional Indicators 2009: TRB 2 Van, Muş, Bitlis, Hakkâri.[102]

in the province. For the slowness of the improvement, one has to bear in mind also the context of a rising population (around fourfold during the period covered here). Thus, for example, while the number of GPs in Hakkâri increased threefold, approximately, between 1980 and 2000, the general population also increased, by about half (so the proportion of GPs to total patient population only doubled across these two decades, not trebled).

The issues pertaining to the health workforce in Hakkâri have not only involved the insufficiency of numbers: medical personnel in Hakkâri have always been in constant rotation, making for an insufficiency in experience, intimate knowledge of local conditions, patient history, and suchlike. Specialists especially, but also GPs, were employed in Hakkâri only temporarily, either on assigned for a few months or on compulsory service for a longer but still temporary period. The weakness of the engagement of health staff with the province reinforced and reproduced the massive and chronic problems of the health institutions in the province already suffering from the lack of medical personnel.

3.3.1.1 From the Foundation of the Republic to the Early 1960s: The Era of Absolute Deprivation

Healthcare provision in the small provinces and towns of Anatolia and the Kurdish region did not greatly change until the 1960s. In each district, there was a government doctor, on paper at least, who was primarily responsible for preventing the spread of contagious diseases and for constructing the statistical tables of deaths and births in the area. Curative services were of secondary importance and provided only for a few hours in the week on certain days in small clinics (Examination and Treatment Houses [Muayene ve Tedavi Evleri]).

Given that it used to take days and longer to get to the towns from the villages where the majority of the population lived due to the lack of roads and vehicles, in reality, villagers were not covered by the healthcare services provided by government doctors. Only when a contagious disease broke out or the health clerks traveled from village to village on the back of a mule a few times in a year were the villagers able to see a government doctor or health clerk. Hospitals, which were operated by provincial special administrations until 1954 and then transferred to the Ministry of Health and Social Assistance (Sağlık ve Sosyal Yardım Bakanlığı, MHSA), were only in provincial centers and not in all of them (for Hakkârians, as mentioned, the nearest hospital was in Van). Also, curative services were not free of charge; unless patients submitted an official paper to the hospital documenting that they were classified as poor, they would be charged.[27]

Overall with regard to medical personnel, healthcare provision in Hakkâri until the 1960s was not exceptional when compared to the general situation but was nevertheless rather extreme. As Table 7 shows, until the socialization of the health system in Hakkâri in mid-1960s—that is, until the opening of health posts in each district and some big villages of the province—formal healthcare provision was supplied by just a few GPs and health clerks. Until 1965, according to state records, no specialists worked in Hakkâri since there was no hospital treating patients until 1968, and that could hardly be considered a functioning hospital with its lack of personnel and equipment.

Table 7 also shows that in addition to the shortage of medical personnel, there was a lack of pharmacists in Hakkâri until the late 1960s. The only way for patients to access pharmaceutically prepared medicine before then was to buy it from the medicine cabinet of government doctors, provided that there was a government doctor in their district.[28] Selahattin Şimşek, an idealistic primary school supervisor working in Hakkâri in these years, wrote in his memoir that the first question he heard in villages was *Derman hene?*—Do you have medicine? Peasants who went toward him, supposing him to be a doctor, would then slowly leave when they realized that he was not a doctor and did not have any *derman*. In general, village midwives and local herbs provided the folkloric health service in villages—as they had in centuries past.

3.3.1.2 From the mid-1960s to 1981: The Era of Socialization and Rotations of Specialists

The period ranging from the mid-1960s to 1981 needs to be addressed separately in the history of the health workforce in Hakkâri. During this time, the socialization of health services began, resulting in a considerable increase in health staff in Hakkâri. The socialization of health services was a policy reflecting the petty-bourgeois radicalism of lower-rank military officers who took power on May 27, 1960, by a coup d'état.

Aiming to establish access to healthcare provisions as a citizenship right, the new policy approach had as its essence the goal of overcoming the massive unevenness between urban and rural, West and East, rich and poor with respect to access to healthcare provision.[29] In order to achieve this, it was decided that health posts and health stations should be opened throughout the country, beginning in Eastern Anatolia. Health stations staffed with a midwife would be responsible for basic medical affairs, like the maternal and children's health of small rural settlements with a population of no more than 2,500–3,000 people. Health posts staffed with a GP, a midwife, a nurse, a health clerk, a medical secretary, and a driver would be responsible for providing mainly preventive but also curative services to populations of 5,000–10,000. In addition to this, health staff employed in underdeveloped areas would be paid high enough wages to prompt a flow of health workers from developed to underdeveloped areas.[30]

Between the mid-1960s and 1981, in parallel to both the socialization of health system and the opening of the hospital, the number of medical personnel in Hakkâri increased. The numbers given by the MHSA in 1971 confirm the improvement over this period. In Hakkâri, while there were 17 midwives in 1963 but no specialists or dentists and just 5 GPs along with a nurse and nursing assistant and 3 health clerks; in 1970, there were 25 midwives with a specialist and 2 dentists, together with 8 GPs, 4 nurses, 7 nursing assistants, and 18 health clerks.[31]

This appointment of medical personnel to health stations and health posts in Hakkâri, however, did not in any way mean that the health staff needs of Hakkâri were adequately met. Due to the shortcomings of the socialization policy and the fact that nothing had fundamentally changed in Hakkâri to make it attractive to health personnel, the major health staff deficit persisted. According to an article in *Hakkâri Sesi* in February 1973:

> We have constructed many health posts in socialization regions, yet in many of them there are no midwives, let alone doctors. If you do not believe that, please ask about the situation of health posts in Hakkâri to the governor of Hakkâri and learn the truth.[32]

The local newspapers of the period were full of complaints concerning the absence of doctors in the health posts in different parts of Hakkâri. The following quotations from the *Hakkâri Sesi* document the fact that the shortage of doctors in health posts remained a large problem during this period:

> -There have been no doctors in Beytüşşebap and Çukurca for six months. The people cannot even find an aspirin in the health post and have to go to the provincial center, Uludere or Van even for a minor illness ... Aren't the people living or working here human beings as well? The number of doctors in our province does not exceed four. That means that the number of patients per doctor is over 35,000 in Hakkâri, while it is 2,000 in Ankara, Istanbul and Izmir.[33]

> -Çukurca has suffered from the absence of any doctor for a *year* and its roads are about to be closed by the snow. I ask the government to let the people freely go to Mosul and Baghdad in Iraq, as it did in the past, [for them] to get treatment in case of emergency.[34] (Emphasis added)

Indeed, there was a dearth of medical personnel.[35] There were no personnel (GPs, health clerks, nurses, midwives) at all in half (7 from 14) of the health stations in 1973 and no GPs in three of eight health posts (see Appendix 2).

As for specialists, it was only with the opening of the public hospital in the provincial center in 1968 that these began to come and work in Hakkâri. According to the Table 7, until 1981, the year when the law on compulsory service was issued, the number of specialists gradually increased, but only very gradually. While there was only one specialist in Hakkâri in 1970, a decade later, in 1980, there were seven, at least on paper.

The lack of specialists in Hakkâri remained a serious problem. Moreover, these few specialists only used to come to Hakkâri to work for 1 or 2 months; then, they would leave, to be replaced by their newly arriving colleagues. It was almost impossible to see a specialist working for 5 or 6 months in Hakkâri Public Hospital in these years. The shortage of specialists (including surgeons), just as of GPs and other health professionals and administrative staff, was the invariable item in the long complaint and demand lists published in the local newspapers of the period:

> At the present time, specialists and surgeons have been almost entirely concentrated in hospitals of big urban areas. The people in small and border provinces survive entirely by chance. Because specialists and surgeons are absent there, the fittest survive and the weak die.[36]

According to the writer of these lines, the solution to the problem was to impose a compulsory one-year service for specialists and surgeons to work in undeveloped border and small provinces.[37]

A law on compulsory service was not issued until later; instead, between the 1960s and 1980, a rotation system, a short-term version of compulsory service, was adopted. A surgeon and either one or two specialists were appointed to Hakkâri city for a few months at a time during this period.[38] Yet even the rotation system did not work well. Between 1975 and 1980, the MHSA sometimes could not send any specialists or surgeons to Hakkâri city, and the area would go without for several months. The *Hakkâri Sesi* reported a complete lack of specialists and surgeons in the city for the 6 months prior to March 1977, for example.[39] In these periods, when the rotation system failed, patients were taken to other provinces for even simple medical operations—if their families could afford it:

> Our province is, on paper, within the scope of socialization. The governments were to send a surgeon and two or three specialists. Unfortunately, no surgeon

or specialist has arrived in our province for three months. We have to take our patients to Van or Diyarbakır even for births, hernia operations, and appendectomies. There is no specialist in the public hospital, which is equipped with fifty beds. Where is socialization, and where is social justice?[40]

The rotation system was a palliative solution to the shortage of specialists in Hakkâri. Because specialists appointed there for a few months lacked any attachment to the city and its hospital—to the whole region, in fact—they lacked any great commitment to improving things and developing the local capacity for professional service provision. They did not expend much effort on the chronic problems and shortages of the hospital, such as the lack of medical equipment, education of personnel, ensuring hygiene, establishing systems and order:

> Now the biggest problem ahead is to find for our well-constructed hospital a surgeon and internist who are ready to work for one or two years. With the appointment of experienced people to our public hospital, the hospital could operate in an orderly and systematic way, and thus patients would be paid more attention. Today the public hospital lacks even a well-kept register of equipment. The tools and equipment sent for medical operations either have been lost or cannot be found for other reasons. If specialists are appointed to here for two years, such things will not happen. Work concerning the hygiene of the hospital, refurbishment of the building and administration is now carried out in an arbitrary way . . .[41]

Further to this *superficiality*, the rotation system also resulted in negligent treatment practices. We do not know what role the rotationally appointed specialists' sense of cultural superiority might have played in the poor treatment of patients, yet it is certain that their unwillingness to work in Hakkâri was significant. The following complaint about the doctors was rather typical:

> The citizens complain about the public hospital of the province. There are some people coming to our office to complain that neither the chief doctor of the hospital . . . nor the newly appointed, monthly surgeon pay attention to the patients and treat them well.[42]

To summarize, there was a relative increase in the number of health staff in Hakkâri in the mid-1960s to 1980 as compared to the earlier period. The socialization of the health system and the opening of health posts and a public hospital in Hakkâri city played a role in this increase. It was in this period that civil specialists and surgeons came and worked in Hakkâri for the first time. Yet both the persisting insufficiency of health staff and the problems resulting from the palliative character of rotation system—the way of appointing specialists and surgeons to Hakkâri in these years—persisted.

3.3.1.3 Compulsory Service of Doctors and the "Golden Age" of the Health Workforce in Hakkâri: 1981–1995

A committee of the State Planning Organization (Devlet Planlama Teşkilatı, DPT) offered the following snapshot of the health workforce in the Kurdish region and Hakkâri in 1981, a year after the coup d'état of September 12, 1980:

> The major problems of healthcare provision in the provinces visited by us are the insufficiency of medical personnel, especially doctors, and the lack of fully equipped hospitals. Some provinces have [equipped] hospitals but insufficient doctors, and others have neither satisfactory hospitals nor sufficient doctors. It seems that the two-monthly rotation system employed to send doctors to provincial centers is far from bringing a solution to the problem.
>
> It was tried, via health stations and health posts, to provide healthcare to rural areas, but this failed. In many of these [health stations and health posts], even allied health personnel are missing.[43]

The suggestion made by the committee in the face of the shortage of doctors and the uselessness of the rotation system was to introduce a system of compulsory service:

> The number of technical and administrative personnel employed in East and Southeast Anatolia must be increased, and also their problems concerning wage and accommodation must be solved. Staffing these regions ... by appointment of some groups of qualified personnel via compulsory service [law] should be considered.[44]

This suggestion reflected the point of view of the military regime, too. The compulsory service law, which was often discussed in the 1960s and 1970s but could not be enacted due to the political climate of the era, was enacted in 1981 by the military regime with special reference to the shortage of doctors in the East.[45] Thus, both newly qualified GPs and specialists became obliged by the law to do compulsory service in remote areas of the country for 2 years.

In the period ranging from the enactment of the compulsory service law (*Bazı Sağlık Personelinin Devlet Hizmeti Yükümlülüğüne Dair Kanun*) in 1981 to its annulment in 1995, Hakkârians, especially those located in Hakkâri city, could find the specialists they most needed, including gynecologists, pediatricians, internal medicine physicians (internists), and general surgeons. According to the numbers given by the DPT experts, the gap between Hakkâri and the rest of Turkey in terms of patients per doctor declined considerably during these years. The ratio of patients per doctor in Turkey to patients per doctor in Hakkâri fell from approximately 1:6 in 1985 to 1:2 in 1991.[46] One of the administrators of Hakkâri Public Hospital during the late 1980s expressed with a remarkable sense of pride that he remembered quite well when there were 11 specialists in Hakkâri Public Hospital in 1989.

The optimistic atmosphere arising from the relative abundance of doctors in Hakkâri as a result of the compulsory service law can be followed in local newspaper reports of the period. For instance, it was stated in the *Hakkâri Halkın Sesi* in January 1984 that "the specialists appointed to our province in 1983 rendered the public hospital a house of healing"; this, the newspaper article continued, "became a source of hope to the patients and freed them from the need to go to neighboring provinces."[47] It was in this period also that the relative abundance of doctors led people to problematize, for the first time, the lack of an otolaryngologist and an orthopedist.[48] In earlier years, only the appointment of surgeons, internists, or gynecologists had been demanded.

It should be borne in mind that, even in this "golden age" of the health workforce, the numbers of doctors were still too low to meet the actual needs of the province. When *Hakkâri Halkın Sesi* was able to conclude in 1985 that it was the "golden year" of the hospital, it only had five doctors working there.[49] At the time, the population of Hakkâri city district was approximately 44,000: 23,000 in the villages and 21,000 in the city itself. There were no hospitals in Çukurca, Yüksekova, Beytüşşebap, Uludere or Şemdinli in 1985.

The few specialists would tend to take advantage of the opportunities created by being the sole expert in their medical field in the province and develop private practices. This seriously diminished the potential contribution they could give to healthcare provision. They would treat fewer patients in the public facility and instead reserve some of their working time to see patients in their private clinics. As one of the administrators of the hospital in the late 1980s explained, and as can also be seen from the statistical data for the relevant years (Table 10), the numbers of patients examined and in-patients treated in the hospital in these years never exceeded 55,000 and 4,000, respectively.

Another drawback of doctors' involvement in private practice was qualitative rather than quantitative, that they were more concerned with the affairs of their private clinics than those of the hospital or health posts. This resulted in a negligent stance of uncaring toward patients and the hospital that extended to abuse:

> Shouting at patients and keeping them waiting for hours have become normal here. Yet these doctors, who are grim-faced, change in their private clinics and turn into good-humored [people]. Doctors are granted the legal right to open private clinics but are not granted the right to neglect the hospital and outpatient clinics to direct people to their private clinics. They are also not granted the right to start working at 10:00 or 11:00 a.m. when they are obliged to start work early ... We ask the doctors and specialists of the public hospital to take care of the hospital and serve more efficiently. It is necessary to remind the specialists of the need to pay at least as much attention to the hospital as they pay attention to their private clinics.[50]

To summarize, the period 1981–95 was a golden era for the health workforce in the history of Hakkâri when compared with earlier periods. Due to the law on compulsory service issued by the military regime in 1981, specialists in different branches and also GPs had to come to Hakkâri and work more than a year. Yet the improvement was only a relative one, which was still far from meeting the needs of the province.

3.3.1.4 Back to Rotation System: 1995–2001

> *In the so-called intensive care unit, there is no more than a bed covered with a dirty, creased, and rumpled sheet, that's all. There is no intensive care unit equipment in the hospital. There are no pediatricians, nor are there any internists. The number of patients per doctor is 65,000, and 44 more specialists are needed. If you are seriously injured and want to go to another province to get treatment, you cannot do that, either, since Hakkâri is like a semi-open prison after 3:00 p.m. All roads are closed for security reasons.*
>
> Duygu Asena[51]

The insistent demands and struggles of doctors ultimately resulted in the 1995 suspension of the compulsory service duty for specialists and its shortening for GPs.[52] Unsurprisingly, a sharp fall in the number of doctors serving in the province ensued. Between 1995 and 2001, the number of specialists halved (from 19 to 9), while the number of GPs fell by a quarter (from 68 to 50), especially after 2000 when the compulsory service duty of GPs also was suspended.[53]

The solution adopted to deal with the developing crisis was to return to the old palliative rotation system and appoint doctors rotationally for a few months. Hakkâri's health needs were too extensive to be met by any palliative solution.

The head of the non-infectious diseases unit, who worked in Hakkâri for years as a health clerk, offered a dire image of the state of the health workforce during this period:

> Health posts used to work at an occupancy rate of 20–30 percent. Most of the time, we couldn't find any doctors [there]. Sometimes there were two doctors serving in the health post in Hakkâri city, but the health posts and health stations in villages suffered seriously from the lack of health staff ... Most of the time, we couldn't find specialists of even the most important branches. They would come by rotation from other provinces and hospitals for 50 or 60 days, but those doctors appointed by rotation would mostly report as sick immediately after their arrival, spend 45 days on sick leave, and then return back to their home town ... 80–90 percent of patients used to be transferred to the neighboring provinces, mostly to Van.
>
> Q: Which specialists used to come through the rotation system?
> A: Only those from major branches, gynecologists, internists, general surgeons.
> Q: How many doctors could one find in the [Hakkâri] public hospital in the late 1990s, at best?
> A: We could find five doctors at best.
> Q: At the worst?
> A: No more than one or two. One could always find a gynecologist. They used to come [to Hakkâri] to earn money. They used to spend most of their time in their private clinics.

Due to the lack of specialists and GPs, hospitals in Orumieh in Iran were often the first places Hakkârians would resort to at this time. Indeed, Hakkârians used to cross the border to get treatment in Iraq or Iran throughout the history of the Republic. A famous Turkish journalist reported the poverty of the health workforce in Hakkâri in 2000 and the Orumieh traffic of Hakkârians thus:

> There are four specialists in Hakkâri Public Hospital and three specialists in Yüksekova Public Hospital. As for Şemdinli Public Hospital, there have been no specialists for a long time, and there is only a newly-qualified doctor. There is not even a public hospital in Çukurca ... let alone doctors. Only 11 of 30 health posts are open, and 13 doctors working in these [11] health posts try to ease the specialists' burden. The state cannot send doctors here. Today, the number of patients per doctor [in Hakkâri] is 35, 000.

> Every day 300 Hakkârians pass through the Esendere border gate to go to Orumieh in Iran to get treatment. The first choices of those people going to Orumieh are the state-owned Imam Khomeini and private Azerbaijan hospitals. Fees for all kinds of examinations [. . .] represent a tenth of the fees charged in Turkey.
>
> Although there are 22 specialist cadres assigned to Hakkâri public hospital, only four doctors are actually working and trying to create medical miracles. Those patients who cannot be treated [in the hospital] are transferred either officially to Van or unofficially to Iran. Hakkârians opt for Orumieh, which is 158 kilometers away from [Hakkâri city], over Van, which is 210 kilometers away from [Hakkâri city]. [54]

Likewise, a DPT report prepared by a committee following inspections in Kurdish provinces, having emphasized that there were only three specialists in Hakkâri as against the 25 assigned, suggested that an extra payment be granted to doctors employed in the region in order to attract doctors there and thus remove the necessity for Hakkârians to go to Iran and to other provinces for treatment.[55]

In addition to the shortage of doctors, Hakkârians also faced the problem of finding doctors with a full-time attachment to their institutions. According to a local nurse who had started to work in the hospital in the late 1990s, this situation resulted in various ethical problems. As she recounted, all the regular specialists in Hakkâri Public Hospital had private clinics and directed patients to their clinics by limiting the daily treatment quota in the hospital:

> Q: Were there ethical issues?
> A: Sometimes yes ... They [specialists] used to say, "We will not examine more than 20 patients." Yet the demand was too much. When I compare [those days] with the present, I think that a real injustice was done to the people.

3.3.1.5 From Compulsory Service to Contract System and Back: 2002–2004

One cannot talk about an essential difference of the 2002–4 period from the earlier periods in terms of the numbers and engagement of medical personnel in Hakkâri. Yet, two government health acts at that time resulted in a remarkable increase of medical personnel in the province. These were, firstly, the 2002 annulment of the 1995 suspension of the compulsory service law, and secondly, the 2003 adoption of a contract system (which is still in force) to employ medical personnel in the Kurdish region or in the so-called "regions whose staffing is difficult" (*eleman temininde güçlük çekilen yerler*). For this reason, the years 2002–4 may be identified as a distinct period in the history of the health workforce in Hakkâri.

By June 2002, according to the report prepared by a committee of the Public Health Branch of the Turkish Medical Association (Türk Tabipleri Birliği, TTB), there were 30 GPs in Hakkâri instead of the assigned 170. That meant that health posts were working with a 17.6 percent occupancy rate. In addition, 9 out of 23 health posts were closed, and only two health stations were active. A combined total of 11 specialists were employed in Hakkâri city, Yüksekova and Şemdinli.[56]

In 2002, the compulsory service law enacted by the military regime—which had not been followed in practice since 1995—was reactivated by the Minister of Health (against the opposition of doctors' organizations). This resulted in an increase in the number of specialists and GPs in Hakkâri. And then, the following year, the compulsory service law was completely annulled by the new government.

The incoming AKP government replaced the compulsory service law with a contract system and offered higher wages to specialists, GPs, and other health workers who would work in areas designated by the law as "regions whose staffing is difficult." The contract system prevented a decline that might have occurred due to the annulment of the compulsory service law and even partially encouraged specialists to work in Hakkâri. The number of specialists in Hakkâri increased from 24 in 2003 to 37 in 2005. The contract system did not produce the same positive effect for GPs, but it limited the extent of the fall (from 86 to 68). The major effect of the contract system on the health workforce in Hakkâri concerned other groups of health workers. Through the new system, hundreds of nurses, midwives, and health clerks were appointed to Hakkâri. Thus, while there were 137 nurses, 51 midwives, and 106 health clerks in 2003, these numbers changed to 222, 80, and 194, respectively.[57] My experience in the province confirmed this increase. Excepting the wives of army members and policemen, almost all non-local nurses, midwives, and health clerks I encountered during my fieldwork were contract (or "fixed," *çakılı*) personnel, most of whom had been working in Hakkâri since 2003.[58]

Despite the improvement, however, the overall increase of medical personnel was still insufficient to provide proper healthcare to Hakkârians. The state had to spend a trillion liras in 2004 (equivalent at that time to around 700,000 USD) for the transfer of patients from Hakkâri to Van due to the shortage of medical specialists in the province. While Hakkâri needed 99 specialists in 2004, the number of available specialists actually working there was only 16.[59] The most tragic manifestation of the shortage of GPs and specialists was the deaths of six dialysis patients (the youngest aged 13 and the oldest aged 60) in the first 4 months of 2004 due to the lack of nephrologists.[60]

Doctors' involvement in private practice persisted throughout this period as well, deepening the problems. For instance, the Public Health Branch of the Turkish Medical Organization reported that "The chief doctor of the health post [in Hakkâri city] supports his private clinic more than the health post and answered the question concerning the patient profile of the health post by supposing that it was asking about the patient profile of his private clinic and not that of the health post."[61]

Worse than this negligent attitude was the active exploitation of patients. For instance, according to a former administrator of the hospital, the then head of the Health and Social Services Laborers' Union (Sağlık ve Sosyal Hizmet Emekçileri Sendikası, SES)—and several others—the same doctor used to prescribe third-line antibiotics even for straightforward cases of flu. The intention behind this prescription policy was to make a name for himself among the people, who were unaware of the side effects of antibiotics, as a good doctor healing patients as quickly as possible.

3.3.2 Medical Equipment and Infrastructure in Hakkâri

Apart from the health workforce, a further major aspect of healthcare provision that needs to be addressed in light of the indirect state racism experienced by Hakkârians is the issue of medical equipment and infrastructure. Until the 2008 construction of two modern hospitals equipped with modern devices and machinery, one in Hakkâri city and the other in Yüksekova, which replaced the old ones, the hospitals in the province were no more than large health posts in terms of the number of beds, technology, comfort, and so on.

The first (1968) hospital in Hakkâri was so devoid of necessary medical equipment that for years it could not provide any services beyond simple surgical operations. Focusing on the history of the development of curative institutions in Hakkâri, the following sections describe the poverty of healthcare providers in the province with respect to medical infrastructure and equipment.

3.3.2.1 Curative Institutions in Hakkâri and the Poverty of Medical Equipment and Infrastructure

The first curative institution built in Hakkâri was the five-bed Çölemerik Examination and Treatment House in Hakkâri city, about which little is known.[62] Considering that the opening of Examination and Treatment Houses was decided on in 1924 and that they did not require much investment, one can speculate that the Examination and Treatment House in Hakkâri city was probably opened around then, in the second half of the 1920s.

Examination and Treatment Houses were opened in districts and placed under the responsibility of government doctors in the early Republican period. Government doctors used to reserve some hours of their working time, which was essentially devoted to public health issues and contagious diseases, to examine patients in Examination and Treatment House and provide necessary treatment, free of charge. In small settlements which lacked any hospital, the Examination and Treatment House was the single institution providing curative services, mostly with very poor facilities.

Neither in Hakkâri city nor in any other Hakkâri districts had any hospital been constructed during the Imperial period. Patients with an urgent health problem that could not be treated in the Examination and Treatment House would have to go to Van Maternity and Children's Hospital or Van Memleket Hospital, provided that the roads were not closed by snow and that the patient's health allowed them to endure days of travel under prohibitive conditions. Moreover, unless the patient could report their poverty by a document (*fakirlik mazbatası*) issued by the head of their neighborhood, and the report was accepted by the head doctors of the hospitals, the patient had to pay for treatment. There was neither a national nor private health insurance scheme in those years.

İbrahim Arvas, a member of the Assembly in the single-party period, 1925–50,[63] a centrally appointed deputy of Hakkâri, paid attention in one of his speeches to this situation. The speech reflects the huge pressure placed on him by Hakkârians and the considerable misery of the people. First, it was not very often that Arvas voiced the problems of Hakkâri and Van in the Assembly; and second, it is surprising that as a loyal, non-Kurdist Kurd, he would "remind" deputies of the "specificity" of Hakkâri in a somewhat threatening tone, albeit implicitly:

> Hakkâri has four districts. Along with the Başkale district [of Van], these districts do not have any contact with Van during winter. There are no hospitals in these five districts. I ask the Minister [of Health and Social Assistance] to reserve some resources from the Allocation for the Development of Eastern Provinces for the construction of even a small hospital [in Hakkâri], not a big one. People who get sick go to Iraq because they are not given treatment [in Hakkâri] and neither can they go to Van.[64]

Hakkâri has an additional specificity. I would like to clarify it in your presence. On one side of Hakkâri is Syria; on another side is Iran and on another, Iraq. Thank god that civilization has risen in our Turkey. It is not good that [Hakkâri] remains deserted without doctors and hospitals while civilization prevails [on the other side].[65]

The second institution built to provide curative service in Hakkâri was the health center.[66] The construction of the building was completed in 1955, and it was officially opened in 1962, the delay due to a lack of equipment and doctors. According to Aydın Bilgiç, who was in Hakkâri as a military doctor between 1955 and 1957, the health center was closed during these years and did not host any patients.[67] Thus, he remembers not being able to direct someone suffering from a serious case of typhoid to the health center and instead having to treat him on an unrolled mattress in the entrance of a small hotel.[68]

The statistics concerning the health center's performance during its early years verify its insufficiency. Between 1956 and 1963, not a single surgical operation or even laboratory or x-ray examination was made in Hakkâri Health Center. It was so non-operational that the building was used by reserve army officers as accommodation. Referring to the medicines, "which were rotting for years" in the storehouses of the health center, and to the personnel, "who were paid for nothing," local newspapers demanded the fully-fledged activation of the health center as soon as possible.[69]

When it was finally opened in 1962, the health center served with 30 beds until 1968 when it was transformed into Hakkâri Public Hospital with the addition of a further 20 beds.[70] When the 14 years of the health center are analyzed, one cannot really say that it functioned as a real health center as defined by the ministry (MHSA). Health centers were intended to provide both curative and preventive services in an integrated manner as small, town hospitals, including simple surgical operations. The Hakkâri Health Center, however, still lacked fundamental equipment when it was opened, such as an ambulance, x-ray machines and a generator.[71] Thus, it mainly operated just out-patient services. Sabri Öztürk, who worked in Hakkâri for 2 years during the 1960s as a GP and then became deputy for CHP, described the wretchedness of the health center very strikingly in the Assembly:

> SÖ: I stayed two years in Hakkâri. None of the acute appendicitis cases or transverse arrest cases could be saved. None of the ileus cases could be saved. All died.
> Justice Party (Adalet Partisi, AP) deputies: What did you do there then?
> SÖ: As a GP I used the facilities enabled by the AP, yet I could not save their lives.[72]

Table 8. Performance of Hakkâri Health Center, 1956–1967

	Out-patients	In-patients	Deaths	Bed occupancy (%)
1956	586	0	0	0
1957	370	0	0	0
1958	416	0	0	0
1959	56	0	0	0
1960	263	0	0	0
1961	949	26	0	3
1962	884	143	2	15
1963	866	150	7	11
1964	2,311	173	10	13
1965	1,872	226	3	16
1966	2,788	445	7	27
1967	2,151	412	10	33

Source: Constructed from health statistical yearbooks prepared by the MHSA.[103]

The working capacity and performance of the center between 1956, when it was constructed, and 1968, when it was transformed into a hospital, is shown in Table 8.

Hakkâri Health Center could not provide a healthcare service that was quantitatively and qualitatively fit for purpose, not only in the early 5 years until its official opening in 1962, but later as well. The service provided by the health center was quantitatively inadequate in that, as the single curative institution for a provincial population then of 80,000 people, it was never able to treat more than 3,200 people annually. The service was qualitatively inadequate, too, since the patient profile of the center did not comprise those in most need of serious treatment. This is evident in the low fatality numbers and poor bed occupancy rates (Table 8). That the latter were so low in a context where total bed capacity was already so far from meeting the population requirement is an indicator of the extremely poor quality of healthcare services provided by the center.

With the transformation of the health center into the Hakkâri Public Hospital in 1968 and the start of the appointment of specialists and surgeons to the hospital, a slight improvement occurred in the healthcare service provided through the 1970s. As a result of the medical equipment purchased and the surgeons and specialists appointed, simple surgery, such as hernia operations and appendectomies, could be performed in the 1970s.

The improvement, however, was minimal and slow. The lack of medical personnel and medical equipment continued to place fundamental limits on the hospital's health services throughout the 1970s. For instance, in July 1974, the hospital still lacked, along with regular surgeons, any x-ray machine and personnel able to use one. It also lacked a dental unit and surgery equipment, along with various medicines.[73] The missing x-ray machine was sent to the hospital later that year, in 1974, yet it was only installed in the following April, a delay highlighting the lack of educated personnel in the hospital—with potentially tragic consequences.[74] To cite an example of the consequence of this very basic infrastructure and service delivery issues problem, we read in the *Hakkâri Sesi* of July 1972 that the autoclave machine was out of order, so many people died during surgery.[75]

Table 9. Performance of Hakkâri Public Hospital, 1968–1980

	Out-patients	In-patients	Deaths	Bed occupancy (%)
1968	5,873	625	17	28
1969	3,633	754	12	33
1970	3,010	725	14	30
1971	3,859	708	18	27
1972	7,327	690	26	25
1973	13,760	845	25	34
1974	12,626	930	53	37
1975	n/a	1,047	22	31
1976	n/a	834	20	32
1977	n/a	793	20	21
1978	n/a	773	28	20
1979	n/a	853	32	24
1980	n/a	981	41	23

Source: Constructed from MHSA health statistic yearbooks.[104]

112 | *The Social Policy of the AKP toward the Kurds*

The performance of Hakkâri Public Hospital during the 1970s is shown in Table 9. In parallel with the appointment of rotating doctors, a considerable increase in out-patients occurred during the 1970s, from 2,000–3,000 to over 10,000. There was also an increase in in-patients, albeit at a negligible rate. When considered alongside the number of deaths in the hospital and the consistently low bed occupation rates, the very limited increase of in-patients shows that the

Table 10. Performance of Hakkâri Public Hospital, 1981–2002

	Beds	Out-patients	In-patients	Deaths	Bed occu-pancy (%)	Major surgeries	Medium surgeries	Minor surgeries
1981	50	12,251	1,121	26	30	n/a	n/a	n/a
1983	50	11,468	1,605	41	56	87	144	121
1984	55	14,160	2,154	51	68	167	194	216
1985	55	19,351	2,370	61	83	121	222	196
1986	65	18,915	2,188	49	47	98	133	187
1987	100	25,964	3,253	52	45	106	148	238
1988	100	23,796	3,052	47	42	91	324	201
1989	100	35,002	3,834	23	46	115	272	190
1990	97	34,572	2,971	59	45	257	317	99
1991	100	40,031	3,108	114	50	233	333	116
1992	100	49,779	2,928	57	39	256	360	88
1993	100	20,525	2,855	65	35	323	401	86
1994	100	52,570	3,321	51	36	271	356	194
1995	100	53,694	2,865	35	29	163	220	108
1996	100	19,964	2,358	n/a	29	256	265	144
1997	100	61,642	3,605	20	34	208	333	152
1998	100	80,103	3,596	18	32	140	296	211
1999	100	75,309	4,213	26	36	174	264	190
2000	100	63,614	4,110	26	39	63	307	123
2001	107	27,606	4,502	24	48	18	331	30
2002	104	73,460	n/a	n/a	51	92	505	32

Source: Constructed from MoH/MHSA health statistic yearbooks.[105]

patient profile of the hospital continued to be composed of those not suffering from serious diseases requiring comprehensive treatment and major surgery.

In addition to the shortfall of medical personnel and equipment, problems stemming from the poor coverage and hierarchical structure of the national health insurance system should also be addressed when speaking about the capacity and quality of curative services in Hakkâri. The rural population, shopkeepers, and workers employed in the informal sector, that is, most Hakkârians, were not covered by any health insurance schemes during the 1950s, 1960s, and 1970s. Only civil servants—from 1949, by the Retirement Fund (Emekli Sandığı)—and workers employed in the formal sector—from 1945, by the Social Insurance Institution (Sosyal Sigortalar Kurumu, SSK)—were insured.[76] Moreover, workers insured by the SSK were not allowed to use MoH hospitals, and hence the Hakkâri Public Hospital. Therefore, the overwhelming proportion of Hakkârians could only access the healthcare provided by the poorly equipped and staffed Hakkâri Public Hospital if they had a poverty record accepted by the head of the hospital or else had a payment accepted by the doctors or managed to deceive them by using the health insurance card of a relative working in government service.

Regarding the working performance of Hakkâri Public Hospital during the 1980s and 1990s, again, we cannot observe sufficient progress, certainly not enough to speak of a radical break from the gradually improving but still poor performance of the 1970s. As Table 10 shows, the development in this period was largely focused on the rising number of specialists and practitioners employed in the hospital (albeit very modestly and in a fluctuating manner) and not on the modernization of medical infrastructure. In other words, progress was not so strong as to result in a qualitative change in the patient profile of the hospital.

In the period between 1981 and 2002, the number of in-patients increased from 1,121, which was already very low, to 4,502; recorded deaths in the hospital little changed, at an insignificant level; bed occupation rates were mostly around 30–40 percent, despite the very limited bed capacity; and increases in the numbers of major and medium-risk surgeries were definitely not sufficient for concluding that Hakkâri Public Hospital had started to give decent treatment to seriously ill patients. The single remarkable change in the period is the sixfold increase in the number of out-patients. This confirms that the improvement in the working performance of Hakkâri Public Hospital in the period was more or less limited by a considerable increase in the capacity of the first aid and diagnosis service.

Elsewhere in the province, in Yüksekova, the first institution built to provide curative services was the health center there, which became operative in 1974. However, the service provided by this health center was so poor that it would be more accurate to begin the history of the curative services in Yüksekova with the opening of the 15-bed Yüksekova Public Hospital in 1987. However, even the hospital was not sufficiently staffed and equipped at the end of the 1990s to provide proper health services capable of meeting the needs of seriously ill patients in need of comprehensive in-patient treatment and major surgery. In 1995, for instance, the hospital had 34 beds, used for 362 in-patients with an occupancy rate almost 13 percent. There were only 34 sizable operations performed in the hospital that year (17 major and 17 minor).[77]

In Şemdinli, no curative institution offered in-patient treatment until Şemdinli Public Hospital became active and started to accept patients. The hospital started to function in 1999, albeit very poorly, due to a chronic lack of specialists and medical equipment. It was still unable to offer in-patient treatment until 2005. The bed occupancy rate in Şemdinli Public Hospital in 2003 was 2.1 percent,[78] and the first surgical operation in the hospital, a minor one, was performed in 2006.[79] The state of the hospital in 2002 was described thus:

> The local Director of Health, Dr. Cengiz Alış, says that they try to provide healthcare under very difficult conditions ... The hospital lacks a fully-equipped ambulance, medical equipment, an emergency generator, nurses, midwives, and specialists ...
> "The generator of the hospital is out of order, and there are frequent power cuts due to snow. Because we don't have an emergency generator, we treat even pregnant women under candlelight. That isn't a healthy method of treatment, of course."[80]

Referring to the poor state of Şemdinli Public Hospital in 2003, a contract nurse employed in the Şemdinli health post since 2003 confirmed the words of the local director:

> Q: What was the hospital like six or seven years ago?
> A: There were no doctors and departments or an operating room. I mean, there was nothing. Only ER was available. Internists and general surgeons used to be here, but rotationally and only for one month.
> Q: The hospital was not so busy then?
> A: No, it wasn't. It couldn't provide a proper service. It was like an ER. The facilities weren't active. Nurses, my colleagues, used to stay in them.

They'd use them as their homes. Before us [contract nurses], the hospital used to operate like a health post. At that time, there were no nurses except the wives of soldiers.

Again, a full assessment of curative services in Hakkâri for this period requires that we address the state of the health insurance system. During the 1980s and 1990s, problems stemming from the lack of health insurance coverage and the hierarchical structure of the health insurance system persisted. For instance, as we read from the *Hakkâri Halkın Sesi*, sometimes administrators of Hakkâri Public Hospital would not accept the poverty records submitted by those not covered by a health insurance scheme, who formed the majority of the population (as the rural population was not covered at this time); thus, the poor had to pay for the services provided.[81] The hierarchical structure of the health insurance system, meanwhile, produced discriminations. For example, because workers insured by the SSK were still not allowed to use MoH hospitals in 1987, and hence Hakkâri Public Hospital, some 3,000 workers and their dependents had to go to Van for minor surgery and x-rays.[82]

However, two important developments occurred in health insurance coverage in these years. As of 1985, the Social Security Institution of Craftsmen, Tradesmen, and Other Self-Employed Workers (Esnaf ve Sanatkârlar ve Diğer Bağımsız Çalışanlar Sosyal Sigortalar Kurumu, Bağ-Kur), which had been founded in 1971, started to meet the health expenses of its members.[83] Much more importantly, though, poor households not covered by any health insurance scheme and whose income per member was less than a third of the net minimum wage were given Green Cards in 1992. Even though a Green Card only covered in-patient treatment and not medication, tests, or consultations related to out-patient treatment, it was nevertheless a major advance. Certainly, it freed people from having to convince hospital administrators of their poverty in order to receive in-patient treatment free of charge.[84] In 2000, just over 66,000 Hakkârians (28 percent of the whole population) were Green Card holders and had the right to in-patient treatment in Hakkâri and Yüksekova Public Hospitals free of charge.[85]

3.3.3 Public Health

A children's immunization campaign was on its way. I was very tired. I went to Istanbul to see my family, but I got a call from the Ministry [of Health and

Social Assistance]. When I went there, I noticed it was the Minister who had me called.

"Doctor," he said, "a smallpox epidemic has occurred in India, and the World Health Organization has informed us that it has also spread to Iran. If it spreads to us, they [the WHO] will put the entire country into quarantine and cut all our links to Europe. That would be a disaster for us. All the governors and teams are under your command. Go and do whatever you can do to stop the spread of the epidemic . . ."

We immediately arrived at the Iranian border. It was a big vaccination campaign . . . Home by home; one by one . . . I had a khutba [public religious announcement] delivered in Kurdish when necessary. We made Kurdish announcements. I was authorized to do it. We spoke the language that the citizens speak . . . The women of the region, especially, did not know Turkish, and we had to reach out to them. We achieved many goals, but when a commander in the border region informed me about the Kurdish tribes settled on the two sides of the border, I was horrified. These tribes would earn their living by smuggling. They were sometimes in Turkey and sometimes in Iran . . . All these people had to be vaccinated . . . Secretly I met a prestigious tribe leader and asked him to inform the leaders of all these tribes that I wanted to get them vaccinated by my team in a place that would be determined by consensus. The answer coming from these tribes reflected their great mistrust: "Will the doctor gather us in a place with the pretext of vaccination and then hand us over to the gendarmerie?"

I negotiated this issue with the governor and the military authorities. Then I decided on a location close to the region and declared to the leaders of these tribes that this place was demilitarized and that I was the guarantor of their security. They checked the region for a while, and then they got in touch with me when they realized that the region really had been demilitarized . . . I warned all the authorities not to intervene in this issue.

Thousands of people . . . They came . . . Women, men, children, elders . . . They came from the lands of Iran to Turkey in a way that you only see in films . . . We got all of them vaccinated without exception. The state withdrew from the border during the vaccination . . . We stopped the epidemic at the border.[86]

Thus, Dr. Neşet Adnan Zentürk recounts his mission in the early 1960s to prevent the spread of a dangerous smallpox epidemic at the Turkish-Iran border, including in Hakkâri. Tellingly, this success story in public health services depended on the complete suspension of the ordinary realities of the area. Following the "exception confirms the rule" principle, it is clear that the success sheds light on why public health in Hakkâri was a failure throughout Kemalist Turkey.

Listing item by item the conditions that enabled this exceptional achievement allows us to see the usual insufficiencies of Hakkâri that resulted in the general failure. Medical teams, normally missing in Hakkâri, were sent in sufficient numbers. A systematic and comprehensive vaccination program, normally missing in Hakkâri, was carried out. The official ban on the Kurdish language was suspended, and Kurdish was used systematically and officially to communicate with the people. The cross-border tribes' distrust of the whole state apparatus—resulting from the usual mix of sovereign violence and indirect state racism—was recognized, negotiated, and settled. The national border dividing the ordinary habitus of tribes was annulled and demilitarized (temporarily). In short, had the vaccination campaign led by Zentürk not suspended the ordinary realities of Hakkâri, it could not have stopped the spread of the smallpox epidemic to Turkey.

This list surely does not uncover all the shortcomings behind the failure of public health services in Hakkâri, such as infrastructure problems and poor nutrition, but it still clearly shows the strong link between the poverty of public health in Hakkâri in Kemalist Turkey and the everyday life of Hakkâri characterized by sovereign violence and indirect state racism.

3.3.3.1 Poverty of Public Health in Hakkâri: Results

In order to indicate the extent of the poverty of public health services in *Hakkâri*, two criteria often used in public health scholarship applied to test the quality of services in a specific location may be employed: infant mortality rate (number of deaths among children under one-year-old per 1000 live births); and child (under-five) mortality rate (number of deaths among children under five-year-old per 1000 live births).

The statistics for infant and child mortality rates in Hakkâri are not available, especially for the pre-2000 period, but they can be constructed using the DİE yearly health statistics. Unfortunately, one still encounters a serious problem, for the numbers of infant deaths and total live births reported are totally unreliable. As acknowledged by the DİE in the 1970s, in rural areas of the East, village roads were closed by snow for months, and this—coupled with insufficient staff and the villagers' distrust of outsiders, especially state professionals—made the proper collection of statistical data concerning births and deaths, especially infant deaths, a very difficult task.

118 | *The Social Policy of the AKP toward the Kurds*

At the end of the research conducted in the villages of the Eastern Region in 1972, the experts of the Medical Statistics Department of the MHSA and members of the DİE realized that the birth rates in villages where midwives were present were reported as being around 40–45 percent, which decreased to 25–30 percent for other villages simply because the midwives did not have access

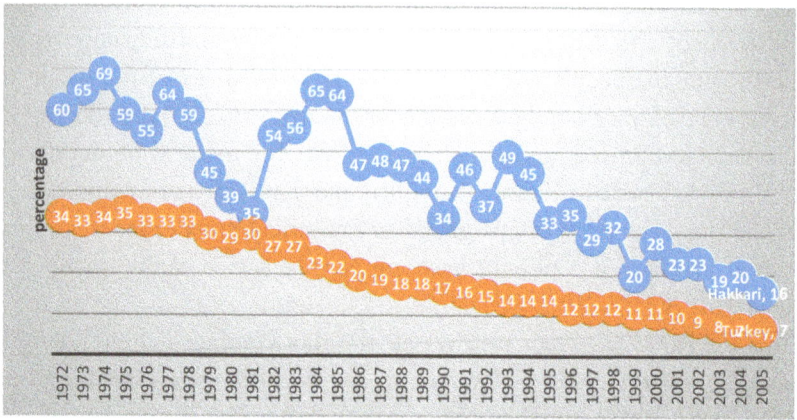

Figure 7a. The Ratio of 0-4 Age Group Mortalities to All Mortalities (Hakkari and Nationwide, Urban Settlements).
Source: Compiled from Mortality Statistics of Urban Settlements prepared by DİE mortality figures (TURKSTAT Library; TÜİK Kütüphanesi website).

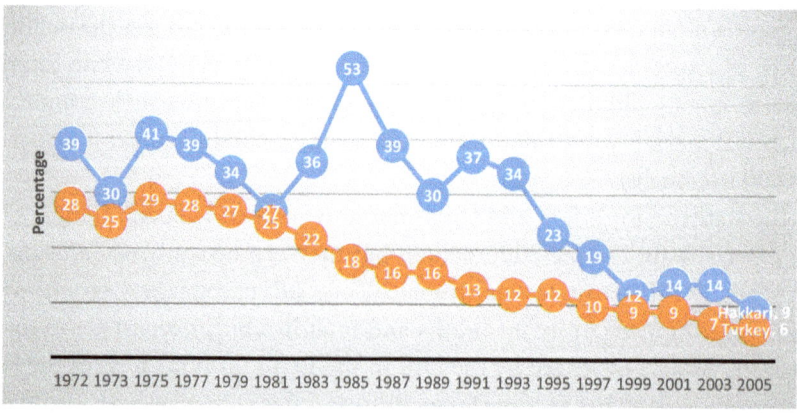

Figure 7b. The Ratio of 0-1 Age Group Mortalities to All Mortalities (Hakkari and Nationwide, Urban Settlements).
Source: Compiled from Mortality Statistics of Urban Settlements prepared by DİE mortality figures (TURKSTAT Library; TÜİK Kütüphanesi website).

to them.⁸⁷ There were similar issues with the death statistics. Mortality rates were reported to be much higher in villages with a midwife than in villages without.⁸⁸

Indeed, most children in Hakkâri used to be delivered with the help of traditional midwives: generally older women who had experienced numerous births. Among the 2002 births reported by midwives in 1967, for example, 1,122 infants were delivered without any help from certificated health staff.⁸⁹ According to Lale Yalçın-Heckmann, who carried out a field study in a Hakkâri village between 1980 and 1982, official, formally educated midwives located in big villages were called to help only when a serious complication or an unpredicted problem occurred.⁹⁰

In addition to material hardships, people's unwillingness to register babies' birth and deaths made the proper gathering of birth and death statistics almost impossible. According to Yalçın-Heckmann, many newborn babies delivered without any help from official midwives—especially female babies—would not be registered by their parents for a long time.⁹¹

In order to overcome the impossibility of obtaining anything like accurate knowledge about births and infant and child mortalities in the 0–4 age group in the province as a whole, I employed the mortality statistics given in the DİE statistical yearbooks for urban settlements. Using the annual, age-based classification of officially recorded mortalities—based on the death certificates issued by doctors—I calculated the share of mortalities occurring in the 0–1 and 0–4 age groups among all officially recorded mortalities in the urban settlements of Hakkâri province. I made the same calculation for urban settlements of Turkey as a whole and compared these two (Figures 7a and 7b).

For the period analyzed, the number of officially recorded mortalities annually in urban settlements in Hakkâri was never less than 28 or more than 200 and typically around 120–30. These extremely low figures in comparison to the population mean that only a fraction of all mortalities in the urban areas of Hakkâri could have been recorded. Yet, assuming that it is more difficult to conceal infant and child mortalities from the official authorities in urban contexts than it is in rural contexts, the comparative rates for the province and the whole country can be used.

As can be seen from the two sets of statistics (Figures 7a and 7b), both infant mortality and child mortality rates in Hakkâri were considerably higher than the Turkish average in the pre-AKP period. And the actual gap between Hakkâri and Turkey rates was most probably greater than recorded due to the lack of sufficient personnel in Hakkâri and the unwillingness of Hakkârians to register babies' births and deaths. As is also evident, the gap had gradually declined over the previous 30 years. This would have been a consequence of the Expanded Program of Immunization (*Genişletilmiş Bağışıklama Programı*), introduced in 1981 and further accelerated by a nationwide vaccination campaign in 1985 and a polio eradication program in 1989.[92] However, 0–4 age-group mortalities still formed no less than 60 percent of all mortalities in Hakkâri until the mid-1980s, most of which were from the 0–1 age group, which continued to form one-fifth of all mortalities until the end of the 1990s.

3.3.3.2 Poverty of Public Health in Hakkâri: Reasons

The high rates of infant and child mortality indicate the poverty of public health services. As it is mentioned in the "Hakkâri" article in the Yurt Encyclopedia, which remains an invaluable source of information on the province, the usual high rates of infant and child mortalities in Hakkâri was the result of undernutrition and malnutrition, low immunization levels, unfavorable environmental conditions, the lack of healthcare provision, and the low cultural and educational level of the people.[93] To proceed with a closer examination of the social, economic, and political causes of infant and child mortality rates that were much higher than national averages—and which I therefore characterize in terms of

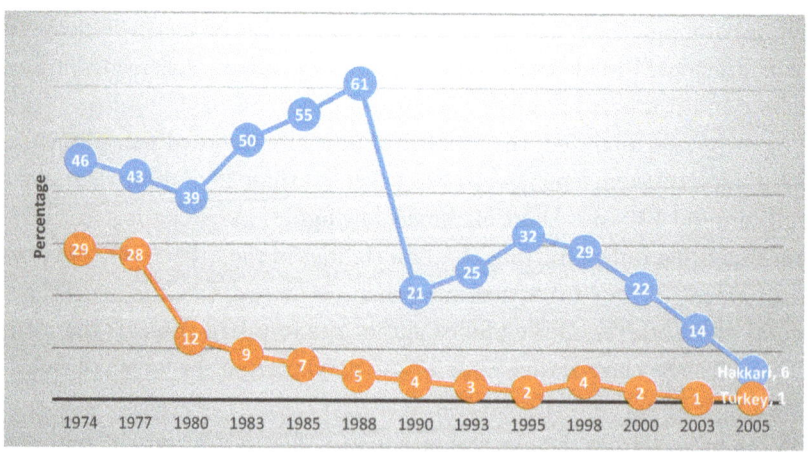

Figure 8. The Ratio of Mortalities from Pneumonia, Enteritis and Other Diarrheal Diseases, and Perinatal Mortalities Combined to All Mortalities in Hakkâri, 1975–2005 (Urban Settlements).

Source: Compiled from Mortality Statistics of Urban Settlements prepared by DİE mortality figures (TURKSTAT Library; TÜİK Kütüphanesi website).

(evidence for) indirect state racism—an analysis of the causes of the mortalities in Hakkâri is instructive.

Checking the annual mortality statistics for urban settlements, which classify mortalities in each province by their 50 main causes, we find the five major causes of mortality in Hakkâri between 1977 and 2005 to be, in order: heart disease, pneumonia, birth-related issues, cancer, and enteritis and other diarrheal diseases (at 25, 15, 11, 7, and 7 percent, respectively). The most striking feature of these numbers is that among the leading causes of mortalities in Hakkâri were pneumonia, enteritis and other diarrheal diseases, and birth-related and perinatal illness, which were easily preventable by the late 1990s. These diseases together made up around half of all mortalities in Hakkâri until the late 1980s and more than a fifth of all mortalities until the late 1990s (Figure 8).

Following the advice of Nancy Scheper-Hughes and Margaret M. Lock that the " individual body should be seen as the most immediate, the proximate terrain where social truths and social contradictions are played out,"[94] one may ask what the information presented in Figure 8 tells us about the "social truths" of Hakkâri. To begin with the two leading causes of death, pneumonia and perinatal illness, these direct us to the poverty of maternal and infant health services and preventive services. The inadequacy of these services had objective and subjective reasons. Leaving aside objective factors, such as the lack of good or any health services, harsh winters, and remote rural settlements, which have been discussed (above), an important subjective factor can be identified as Hakkârians' unwillingness to cooperate with the health staff providing maternal and infant health services and preventive services. Complaints about the health services have already been mentioned in this chapter, including the dissatisfaction recorded in the 1998 UNDP report, but there was also a suspicion of the state which, as has also been noted, was thought not to properly value their (Hakkârian, Kurdish) lives and rather represented a repressive apparatus.

The stance taken by Hakkârians against the family planning works carried out in the province after 1965 offers a good example of this distrust.[95] In "Designing a Family Planning Program for Hakkâri Province," a thesis submitted to the Institute of Population Studies of the Hacettepe University (the foremost in its field in Turkey), it was argued that:

> According to the data for 1972, there are 17,190 married women in Hakkâri province. It can be predicted that 15,000 of these women are still in the reproductive age group. According to the administrators of the General Directorate of Family Planning of the MHSA, in 1970, mobile teams were able to insert

intrauterine contraceptive devices (IUCDs) into only 75 of the married women who were still in the reproductive age group. In 1971, 1972, and 1973, no women were given IUCDs, and also in these years, the delivery of condoms and contraceptives did not occur. In fact, to take a look at the goal set for Hakkâri by the General Directorate of Family Planning, each month one needs to insert IUCDs into 51 women in the reproductive age group.[96]

Table 11. TT Vaccination Coverage for Hakkâri and Turkey (%), 1996–1999

	1996		1997		1998		1999	
	TT1	TT2	TT1	TT2	TT1	TT2	TT1	TT2
Hakkâri	5	3	4	2	3	2	3	1
Turkey	35	32	35	36	35	35	36	36

Source: Constructed from MoH Health Statistical Yearbooks.[106]
Note: The vaccination program involved two doses (TT1 and TT2).

Regardless of gender and other issues, there is manifestly a high level of distrust being recorded here. In fact, the thesis author observed so much suspicion that the most appropriate tactic for the first year of his proposed five-year family planning program was to do nothing about family planning at all, and instead just focus on gaining people's trust via public health work:

> The first year is the most critical stage when it comes to gaining the trust of the people. Even a small act of misconduct or a false word from team members may lead people to develop prejudices toward the future works of the team. This may put at risk all the work that is to be carried out and all the efforts to draw people in and hence the success of the program.
>
> In the first year, concepts like contraception, family planning, and limiting numbers of children would be forgotten, and only public health issues would be addressed. This is because, due to ethnic issues, the local people may regard family planning as a conspiracy aiming to lessen their population and thus strength.[97]

A GP who worked in a health post in Hakkâri city between 1983 and 1988 also confirmed this interpretation. She explained that although she was trained and capable of inserting IUCDs, she could only provide IUCDs for very few women when she was in Hakkâri. According to her, there had been strong resistance to

Table 12. Measles Vaccination Coverage for Hakkâri and Turkey (%), 1997–2002

	Hakkâri	Turkey
1997	7	76
1998	18	78
1999	15	80
2000	29	81
2001	39	84
2002	45	82

Source: Constructed from MoH Health Statistical Yearbooks.[107]

IUCDs, which the women suspected that the state intended to use to somehow control them.

The same distrust persisted in the 1990s when women avoided cooperating with maternal and infant health workers. Clear evidence of this reluctance can be seen in the low tetanus toxoid (TT) vaccination coverage in women of reproductive age. In 1994, the MoH started a country-wide Maternal and Neonatal Tetanus (MNT) Elimination Program and carried out a TT campaign in Eastern Anatolia where the risk of MNT was high due to the high numbers of nonhygienic home deliveries. Women believed that the vaccines would sterilize them, not only in Hakkâri but also in other Kurdish provinces, and refused the vaccination in massive numbers.

The resistance to health staff visiting villages and neighborhoods to vaccinate infants and ensure their immunization against basic diseases like measles and polio was also a manifestation of distrust toward the state. I was told by a Hakkârian nurse who worked for a polio immunization program at the end of 1990s that villagers from a village in Yüksekova did not let the immunization team into the village, arguing that they planned to sterilize the children. Looking at the coverage of measles vaccinations,[98] we see the poor immunization performance of the medical establishment.

The cases of enteritis and other diarrheal diseases, grouped as another of the leading causes of mortality in Hakkâri until the late 1990s, shed light on a different aspect of the poverty of public health services in Hakkâri. When I conducted my research, deaths from typhoid, cholera, and infantile diarrhea had not yet been consigned to history in Hakkâri. The last identified case of typhoid fever was seen in March 2007, most probably because sewage seeped through cracks and into the city's water supply.[99] This is not so surprising given that none of the districts of Hakkâri, including Hakkâri city, have ever had an adequate sewage system. There was no sewage system in Hakkâri province at all until 1986, when construction of one was begun in Hakkâri city. The informal development of new neighborhoods in the mid-1990s following the village evacuations deepened the problem. In 2009, only 40 percent of Hakkâri city had a sewage system. Yüksekova, a district with 70,000 people, had no sewage system in 2014. In the small provincial districts of Şemdinli and Çukurca, the sewage systems have failed to meet actual needs. According to statistics prepared by the Turkish Statistical Institute (Türkiye İstatistik Kurumu, TÜİK) in 2010, only just over half the population of these districts was served by a sewage system (54 percent in Şemdinli, 55 percent in Çukurca).[100]

3.4 Conclusion

Reviewing the healthcare provisioning in Hakkâri during the pre-AKP period establishes the nature of state-citizen relations during the Kemalist period. Using anecdotes, local newspapers, observations, interviews, official reports, and statistical tables, this chapter has shown how healthcare provision in Hakkâri in the pre-AKP period was always far—too far—from meeting the needs, even the vital ones, of Hakkârians. This was due specifically to the lack of sufficient medical personnel and medical infrastructure and more generally to the low levels of urban and rural infrastructure and lack of cooperation and trust between the state and the local people.

The chronic nature of these healthcare provision insufficiencies in the Kurdish Southeast may be denoted by the concept of "indirect state racism." This idea refers to the distinction made between more and less worthy lives, where the distinction is made indirectly via the distribution of public resources among groups of people that is not in proportion to actual needs or protective basic rights but is rather determined according to cost and benefit to the economy as a whole or the proximity and distance of the groups to established social and national norms.

Overall, Hakkâri healthcare provision in the pre-AKP period, just as for all public services in the province and the region in that period, was always too problem-ridden and insufficient to be defined with the language of "omissions." One cannot fail to notice the political stance underpinning the lack of change in Hakkâri. There was no established will to expend sufficient effort and reserve sufficient resources to increase the quality of public services in this province whose needs and demands were never placed at the top of governments' to-do lists. Government priorities were instead largely shaped by the imperative of fast development and not by the requirements of balanced regional development.

Notes

1 Michel Foucault, *Society Must Be Defended: Lectures at the Colláege De France, 1975–76*, ed. Mauro Bertani and Alessandro Fontana, trans. David Macey (New York: Picador, 2003), 256.
2 Ibid., 22.
3 Ibid., 255.
4 D. J. K. Peukert, *Inside Nazi Germany: Conformity Opposition and Racism in Everyday Life* (London: Batsford, 1987), 208–36.
5 Foucault, *Society Must Be Defended*, 256.
6 For a Turkish elaboration of state racism, see Zeynep Gambetti, "Yönetimsellikten Irkçılığa," *Dipnot*, no. 6 (2011).
7 Paul Farmer, *Pathologies of Power: Health, Human Rights, and the New War on the Poor* (Berkeley and London: University of California Press, 2005).
8 Immanuel Maurice Wallerstein, *The Modern World System 1: Capitalist Agriculture and the Origins of the European World-Economy in the Sixteenth Century* (Berkeley and London: University of California Press, 2011).
9 See Edhem Eldem, Daniel Goffman, and Bruce Alan Masters, *The Ottoman City between East and West: Aleppo, Izmir, and Istanbul* (Cambridge: Cambridge University Press, 1999); Şevket Pamuk, *The Ottoman Empire and European Capitalism, 1820–1913: Trade, Investment, and Production* (Cambridge and New York: Cambridge University Press, 1987).
10 İlhan Tekeli, *Türkiye'de Bölgesel Eşitsizlik ve Bölge Planlama Yazıları* (Istanbul: Tarih Vakfı, 2008), 46–52.
11 Veli Yadırgı, *The Political Economy of the Kurds of Turkey: From the Ottoman Empire to the Turkish Republic* (Cambridge: Cambridge University Press, 2017), 265.
12 Servet Mutlu, *Doğu Sorununun Kökenleri: Ekonomik Açıdan* (Istanbul: Ötüken, 2002), 188–91.
13 Tekeli, *Türkiye'de Bölgesel Eşitsizlik ve Bölge Planlama Yazıları*, 66.
14 Sırrı Erinç, *Doğu Anadolu Coğrafyası* (Istanbul: Sucuoğlu Matbaası, 1953), 58.
15 See Devlet İstatistik Enstitüsü (State Statistical Institute), *Tarımsal Yapı Ve Üretim 1990* (Ankara: DİE, 1993); *Tarımsal Yapı: Üretim, Fiyat, Değer, 1995* (Ankara: DİE, 1997).
16 Michel Foucault, *Security, Territory, Population: Lectures at the CollèGe De France, 1977–78*, ed. Michel Senellart (Basingstoke and New York: Palgrave Macmillan, 2007), 18.

17 Servet Mutlu, "Economic Bases of Ethnic Separatism in Turkey: An Evaluation of Claims and Counterclaims," *Middle Eastern Studies* 37, no. 4 (2001): 110.
18 Ibid.
19 Mutlu, *Doğu Sorununun Kökenleri: Ekonomik Açıdan*, 379–413.
20 Sait Aşgın, *Cumhuriyet Döneminde Doğu Anadolu'ya Yapılan Kamu Harcamaları, 1946–1960* (Ankara: Atatürk Kültür, Dil ve Tarih Yüksek Kurumu, Atatürk Araştırma Merkezi, 2000).
21 Although there are Kurdish districts in *Erzurum* and *Kars*, these provinces are not classified as Kurdish, either demographically or politically.
22 Meltem Ahıska, *Occidentalism in Turkey: Questions of Modernity and National Identity in Turkish Radio Broadcasting* (London: I. B. Tauris, 2010), 16.
23 Ibid., 14–17.
24 "Human Development Report: Turkey 1998," UNDP, accessed February 15, 2022, http://www.tr.undp.org/content/turkey/tr/home/library/national-hdrs/nhdr-1998.html.
25 "Human Development Report: Turkey 2001," UNDP, accessed January 13, 2022, http://www.tr.undp.org/content/dam/turkey/docs/Publications/nhdrs/NHDR2 001.pdf.
26 "Human Development Report: Turkey 1998," UNDP.
27 For healthcare provision in Turkey between 1920 and 1960, see Asena Günal, "Health and Citizenship in Republican Turkey: An Analysis of the Socialization of Health Services in Republican Historical Context" (Ph.D. diss, Boğaziçi University, 2008), 143–98.
28 We learn from a petition written by a local party organization of the DP to the Prime Minister's Office in December 15, 1955, for example, that although Çukurca was given the administrative status of district in 1953, no government doctors were appointed there. See *BCA BMGMK* [Catalogue Number: 030 01/117 740 6].
29 Günal, "Health and Citizenship in Republican Turkey," 258. Günal argues that the worries of the military officers concerning the Kurdish issue was a factor that led the military officers to initiate the socialization of health services in the Kurdish provinces. Ibid., 202.
30 Ibid., 262.
31 Republic of Turkey, *Cumhuriyet Senatosu Tutanak Dergisi*, term 1, session 33, volume. 63, January 31, 1971.
32 *Hakkâri Sesi*, February 6, 1973.
33 *Hakkâri Sesi*, August 19, 1975.
34 *Hakkâri Sesi*, December 17, 1975.
35 Hakkari Valiliği (Governorship of Hakkari), *Cumhuriyetin 50. Yılında Hakkari: 1973 İl Yıllığı* (İstanbul: Pera Basımevi, 1974), 126.
36 *Hakkâri Sesi*, February 6, 1973.
37 Ibid.

38 Fahamettin Altun, *Hakkari İl Yıllığı, 1967* (Ankara: Gürsoy Matbaacılık Sanayi, 1972), 95.
39 *Hakkâri Sesi*, March 29, 1977.
40 *Hakkâri Sesi*, March 4, 1977.
41 *Hakkâri Sesi*, August 1, 1974.
42 *Hakkâri Sesi*, October 21, 1972.
43 Devlet Planlama Teşkilatı (State Planning Organization), *Kalkınmada Öncelikli İller İnceleme Raporu* (Ankara: DPT, 1981), 9.
44 Ibid., 48.
45 *Milliyet*, October 22, 1981.
46 *Kalkınmada Öncelikli Yöreler Raporu 1985* (Ankara: DPT, 1985), 3; Devlet Planlama Teşkilatı (State Planning Organization), *Kalkınmada Öncelikli Yöreler Ve Türkiye İçin Seçilmiş Göstergeler 1991* (Ankara: Devlet Planlama Teşkilatı, Kalkınmada Öncelikli Yöreler ve Bölgesel Kalkınma Genel Müdürlüğü, 1991), 61–62.
47 *Hakkâri Halkın Sesi*, January 2, 1984.
48 *Hakkâri Halkın Sesi*, January 9, 1986.
49 *Hakkâri Halkın Sesi*, July 11, 1985.
50 *Hakkâri Halkın Sesi*, May 13, 1986.
51 *Milliyet*, June 23, 1998.
52 See *T.C Resmi Gazete*, no. 22240, March 27, 1995; *T.C Resmi Gazete*, no. 22415, September 25, 1995; *T.C Resmi Gazete*, no. 24078, June 13, 2000.
53 Sağlık Bakanlığı (Ministry of Health), *Sağlık İstatistikleri 2002* (Ankara: Sağlık Bakanlığı Araştırma, Planlama ve Koordinasyon Kurulu Başkanlığı, 2003), 32; *Sağlık İstatistikleri 1996* (Ankara: Sağlık Bakanlığı Araştırma, Planlama ve Koordinasyon Kurulu Başkanlığı, 1997), 32.
54 *Milliyet*, September 17, 2000.
55 Devlet Planlama Teşkilatı (State Planning Organization), *İl İncelemeleri (Batman, Bingöl, Bitlis, Diyarbakır, Elazığ, Hakkari, Mardin, Muş, Siirt, Şırnak, Tunceli, Van) Ön Raporu* (Ankara: DPT, 2000), 36.
56 "Doğuda ve Kırda Sağlık," Türk Tabipler Birliği (Turkish Medical Association), accessed August 10, 2013, http://www.ttb.org.tr/halk_sagligi/ges/GES2002.pdf.
57 Türkiye İstatistik Kurumu (Turkish Statistical Institute), *Bölgesel Göstergeler TRB 2: Van, Muş, Bitlis, Hakkari 2009* (Ankara: TÜİK, 2010), 55.
58 They are known as fixed personnel because the contract does not allow appointment elsewhere.
59 *Milliyet*, June 13, 2004.
60 Ibid.
61 Turkish Medical Chamber, "Doğuda ve Kırda Sağlık."
62 Birinci Genel Müfettişlik, *Güney Doğu/Birinci Genel Müfettişlik Bölgesi* (İstanbul: Cumhuriyet Matbaası, 1939), 361.

63 İbrahim Arvas, *Tarihi Hakikatler: İbrahim Arvas'ın Hatıratı* (Ankara: Yargıçoğlu Matbaası, 1964).
64 Republic of Turkey, *Millet Meclisi Tutanak Dergisi*, term 8, session 54, vol. 24, February 23, 1950.
65 Ibid.
66 Health centers were first opened in 1940s during the single-party period, although they were not extended to whole country until the 1950s (by the DP governments). A typical health center had 10–20 beds and was staffed by one or two doctors and other health workers. Its primary duty was to provide preventive services, though it was also obliged to provide curative services as well. See Erdem Aydın, *Türkiye'de Sağlık Teşkilatlanması Tarihi* (Ankara: Naturel, 2002), 46–66.
67 Aydın Bilgiç, *Yaslı Gittim Şen Geldim: 1955–1957 Hakkari Anıları* (Ankara: Özsan Matbaacılık, 1999), 52.
68 Ibid., 53.
69 *Hakkâri*, January 19, 1962.
70 With the start of the socialization of the health system in early 1960s, the distinction between curative institutions and public health institutions was boldly underlined, and health centers in Anatolian and Kurdish towns were gradually turned into hospitals with small renovations. The public health work of the health centers was taken over by the health posts.
71 *Hakkâri*, August 13, 1962.
72 Republic of Turkey, *Millet Meclisi Tutanak Dergisi*, term 5, session 115, vol. 4, February 24, 1978.
73 *Hakkâri Sesi*, July 9, 1974.
74 *Hakkâri Sesi*, April 12, 1975.
75 *Hakkâri Sesi*, July 12, 1972.
76 Nadir Özbek, *Cumhuriyet Türkiyesi'nde Sosyal Güvenlik Ve Sosyal Politikalar* (Istanbul: Emeklilik Gözetim Merkezi: Tarih Vakfı, 2006), 251–314.
77 Sağlık Bakanlığı (Ministry of Health), *Yataklı Tedavi Kurumları İstatistik Yıllığı 1995* (Ankara: Sağlık Bakanlığı Tedavi Hizmetleri Genel Müdürlüğü, 2001), 179.
78 *Yataklı Tedavi Kurumları İstatistik Yıllığı 2003* (Ankara: Sağlık Bakanlığı Tedavi Hizmetleri Genel Müdürlüğü, 2004), n.p.
79 *Yataklı Tedavi Kurumları İstatistik Yıllığı 2006* (Ankara: Sağlık Bakanlığı Tedavi Hizmetleri Genel Müdürlüğü, 2007), 87.
80 *Hakkâri Ekspress*, February 1, 2002.
81 *Hakkâri Halkın Sesi*, January 3, 1986.
82 *Hakkâri Halkın Sesi*, February 13, 1987.
83 See Özbek, *Cumhuriyet Türkiyesi'nde Sosyal Güvenlik ve Sosyal Politikalar*, 315–24.
84 Günal, "Health and Citizenship in Republican Turkey," 431.
85 *Milliyet*, August 20, 2000.

86 "Bir Salgını Önlemek," Ardan Zentürk, April 1, 2022, http://www.sdplatform.com/Dergi/224/Bir-salgini-onlemek.aspx.
87 Devlet İstatistik Enstitüsü (State Statistical Institute), *Sosyalizasyon Bölgelerinden Derlenen Doğum İstatistikleri 1972* (Ankara: DİE, 1977), 3.
88 *Sosyalizasyon Bölgelerinden Derlenen Ölüm İstatistikleri, 1973–74–75* (Ankara: DİE, 1978), 3.
89 Sağlık ve Sosyal Yardım Bakanlığı (Ministry of Health and Social Assistance), *Sağlık İstatistik Yıllığı 1964–67* (Ankara: Güneş Matbaacılık, 1971), 316.
90 Lale Yalçın-Heckmann, *Tribe and Kinship among the Kurds* (Frankfurt am Main: P. Lang, 1991), 86.
91 Ibid., 82.
92 Elif N. Özmert, "Dünya'da ve Türkiye'de Aşılama Takvimindeki Gelişmeler," *Çocuk Sağlığı ve Hastalıkları Dergisi* 51, no. 3 (2008): 168–175.
93 "Hakkari," 3242.
94 Nancy Schepher-Hughes and Margaret M. Lock, "The Mindful Body: A Prolegomenon to Future Work in Medical Anthropology," *Medical Anthropology Quarterly* 1, no. 1 (1987): 31.
95 The family planning program initiated in 1965 was not peculiar to Kurdish provinces but rather a manifestation of a transition to an anti-natalist policy (following fast population growth) from the pro-natalist policy (employed since the beginning of the Republic to compensate for the massive population loss undergone during the Ottoman collapse, WWI and foundation period).
96 Tolga Hakan, "Bir Aile Planlaması Program Denemesi Hakkari İli İçin" (MA thesis, Hacettepe Üniversitesi, 1976), 30.
97 Ibid., 37.
98 GPs who worked in *Hakkâri* in the 1980s and 1990s reported that most pneumonia-related deaths in Hakkâri occurred as a complication of measles.
99 Rahmi Özdemir and Emine Kayataş, "Hakkari İlinde Tifo Salgını-Mart 2007: Etkilenen Pediatrik Olguların Değerlendirilmesi," *Journal of Dr. Behcet Uz Children's Hospital* 2, no. 3 (2012): 139.
100 Türkiye İstatistik Kurumu (Turkish Statistical Institute), *Seçilmiş Göstergelerle Hakkari 2012* (Ankara: TÜİK, 2013), 136.
101 At https://khgmistatistikdb.saglik.gov.tr/TR-43867/istatistik-yillari.html. The Ministry of Health and Social Assistance (MHSA) was restructured and renamed the Ministry of Health (MoH) in 1989.
102 *Bölgesel Göstergeler TRB 2*, 55.
103 At https://khgmistatistikdb.saglik.gov.tr/TR-43867/istatistik-yillari.html.
104 At https://khgmistatistikdb.saglik.gov.tr/TR-43867/istatistik-yillari.html.
105 At https://khgmistatistikdb.saglik.gov.tr/TR-43867/istatistik-yillari.html.
106 At https://khgmistatistikdb.saglik.gov.tr/TR-43867/istatistik-yillari.html.
107 At https://khgmistatistikdb.saglik.gov.tr/TR-43867/istatistik-yillari.html.

4

Turkish Nationalism, the Kurdish Question, and Hakkâri: Discourses and Practices, 2003–2014

This chapter provides an analysis of how the AKP dealt with the Kurdish issue in the period 2003–14, paying particular attention to Hakkârians' experience with the AKP-led governments. The analysis consists of two parts. In the first part, it is shown that, despite fluctuations, the AKP had a coherent Kurdish strategy, which was part of a wider political transformation that can be considered a "passive revolution" against the Kemalist establishment. In the second part, government practices in Hakkâri are analyzed, revealing both the tangible improvement of healthcare provision in Hakkâri during this early AKP period, via statistical indicators of healthcare providers, but also the persistence of sovereign violence, now in a new, more individualizing fashion made possible by the increased surveillance capacity of the state.

The AKP's passive revolution against the Kemalist establishment involved a socially and culturally inclusive reformism that curbed the more extreme aspects of Turkish state-nationalism; it renounced some of collective punishment techniques of rule, recognized Kurdish cultural rights on an individual basis, and developed social policy and public investment tools. But it made no concession to the Turkish nationalist principle of "one, indivisible nation" and continued to criminalize forms of politicized Kurdishness.

Similarly, the AKP's social policy and public investment tools were developed in this context of a reformed Turkish nationalism—and thus, arguably, aimed less to end the decades-long "elitist-Kemalist" neglect of Kurds than to make a political claim to that, to (re)institute Turkish control of the region. Given the extent of the historical failure of the Republic there, the new approach can even be seen as a type of soft assimilationism, one that took the attempt at Turkification not further but deeper (winning "hearts and minds" and denying political recognition claims).

Overall, therefore, this did constitute a major shift in governance. It can be characterized as reflecting a strategic transition in the practice of Turkish dominance over Kurds, from one without hegemony to one with hegemony. The former was essentially exclusionary, oriented toward disallowing Kurdishness, while the latter was selectively inclusionary, allowing Kurdishness but with restrictive conditions (i.e., under the hegemonic control of the Turkish nation-state). The chapter thus concludes by pointing to the limits of this strategy, with a focus on how the persistence of sovereign violence integral to the new strategy had effects that countervailed the message sent by the improvement of healthcare provision. It undermined the very idea it professed to bear, that Hakkârians' lives really were worthy of care in the eyes of the state, and thus was ultimately self-defeating.

4.1 The AKP: From Conservative Democracy to Authoritarian Conservatism

The AKP was founded in 2001 by a splinter group from the Islamist Virtue Party (Fazilet Partisi, FP). The group was led by Recep Tayyip Erdoğan, former mayor of Istanbul Metropolitan Municipality, and emerged with distinctive ideological motives that distinguished the AKP from its Islamist predecessors. Unlike the Islamist FP, the AKP was careful not to be defined by Islamism and not to oppose the EU and Western modernity; it was rather "conservative democrat."[1] Another difference of the AKP from the Islamist FP was its stance toward the free market and neo-liberalism. While the Islamist FP emphasized the role of the state in the economy in a national-developmentalist fashion, the AKP adopted a neoliberal language, emphasizing the importance of integration into global markets and defending the retreat of the state from the economy.[2]

In the general election of 2002, the AKP swept to power. It won a simple majority of the seats in the assembly, partly because it adopted a modernist, "soft" Islam and because of the personal charisma of its leader, Erdoğan, but also and in large measure due to the great resentment of the masses toward the parties of successive coalition governments that were held responsible for political paralysis and the exorbitant inflation and economic mismanagement in the second half of the 1990s that culminated in 2001 with a full-blown financial crisis requiring an International Monetary Fund (IMF) emergency bailout. Following this success, the AKP went on to win all of the subsequent general elections, never securing less than 40 percent of the vote, which was unprecedented in the history of Turkish electoral democracy.

One can divide the first decade of AKP rule into two main periods. In the first period, between 2003 and 2007, the AKP did not hold power in the full sense of the term. With the IMF program already implemented by the outgoing coalition, the AKP had little room for maneuver in the economic field. Politically, the AKP enthusiastically continued the ongoing EU membership process until 2006, both because EU norms were in accord with those defended in the party program and because its commitment to the EU process was a source of legitimacy. This legitimacy was vital for the party in the early years of its power when it was accused of concealing its real intentions and having a hidden agenda by Kemalists, who remained in positions of power (particularly in the state, e.g., the judiciary and army, and the mainstream media).[3]

The period beginning with 2007 witnessed the gradual elimination of dual power and the establishment of the AKP as the single ruling authority. The lessening of financial constraints by the strict implementation of the IMF program, the government's decision in 2008 not to resume the standby agreement with the IMF, and also high growth rates achieved between 2002 and 2007, granted the government some autonomy in the economic sphere.[4] This resulted in a certain increase in the resources reserved for social assistance and public expenditures, which partially explains the persistence of the AKP's electoral success.[5] The AKP's capacity to act autonomously increased in the political sphere from 2007, the year in which it achieved its second general election victory and managed to get its candidate chosen as President of the Republic, despite the resistance of the Kemalist Constitutional Court (Anayasa Mahkemesi) and the Turkish Armed Forces (Türk Silahlı Kuvvetleri, TSK).

With the strong anti-Turkey stance of the conservative right in the EU and diminishing support for EU enlargement, especially in France and Germany following the 2007–8 financial and economic crisis, in addition to the complications introduced by Cyprus' accession,[6] the international impetus behind the AKP's reformism began to fade. Given the increase in its capacity to act as an autonomous power, the AKP moved toward alternative paths: its reformism lost momentum, and the party increasingly retreated to its Islamist and conservative origins. The former was identified as Sunni, while the latter, of course, included Turkish nationalism.

The primary assertion emanating from the AKP sociopolitical base, that conservative Sunni Muslims form the core of the nation, was adopted in a majoritarian style.[7] Meanwhile, political power has been used to promote a new group of loyal capitalists.[8] The "Anatolian tigers" (new businesses) that had led Turkey's drive toward newly industrialized country (NIC) status were co-opted into the developing regime as a clientalist class (tending toward a system of crony patronage and large-scale corruption). It was observed that the Turkish Industry and Business Association (Türk Sanayicileri ve İş Adamları Derneği, TÜSİAD) consisting of "the secular elites of large-scale businesses that had been favored in the previous era were being pushed out."[9]

Objections to an increasingly authoritarian orientation of the AKP and Erdoğan, which many compared to despotism of Sultan Abdul Hamid II and dubbed neo-Ottomanism,[10] started to become delegitimized as non-national and marginal (against the general will), and violently suppressed. The Gezi uprising in 2013, prompted by opposition to the government's decision to construct a shopping center in Gezi Park in Istanbul's Taksim square and spreading across the country, was the peak point of this tension.[11] Thereafter, in a deeply divided country, the suppression of the anti-authoritarian demands of the secular public gave rise to a (re-) securitization of the state that extended to all oppositions—including the Kurdish movement. The collapse of the negotiations with the PKK in 2015, extraordinary measures taken after 2016 coup d'état attempt led by Gülenists, and finally transition to the "Turkish type" presidential system in 2017 were the final milestones in the evolution of the conservative democracy into an authoritarian, one-man rule.

4.2 The AKP and the Kurdish Question

On the afternoon of December 29, 2011, I had been studying for hours in the archive of the Çapa Medical Faculty when a message arrived on my mobile phone. It came from an unregistered number and invited everyone to Taksim Square to protest against a massacre committed by the armed forces in Uludere (Roboski), a former district of Hakkâri and current district of Şırnak. I thought that the message was an invitation to the commemoration of the victims of the brutal military operations carried out by the state in Şırnak in 1992 and continued my archival work, assuming that this was an ordinary invitation to one of the many similar demonstrations taking place in Taksim Square. A few hours later, when I turned on the television, I learned with shock that aircraft had bombed a group of villagers from Uludere crossing the border the previous night. Thirty-five people engaged in the usual illegal border trade but apparently or supposedly mistaken for PKK guerillas were thus brutally killed.

I do not begin the section on the AKP's Kurdish policy with this brief anecdote in order to underline the continuity between the pre-AKP period and the AKP period with regard to the approach toward Kurds. The reverse is true: the AKP's way of handling the Kurdish question had led me to think that collective punishment was no longer the basic ruling instrument in the Kurdish issue; hence my supposition that the massacre mentioned in the message had taken place 20 years ago, and not in 2011. Learning the truth prompted a critical rethinking of what had led me to misunderstand the message and to attribute the Roboski massacre to the past.

That review gave me a new understanding that reconceived the AKP's Kurdish policy as a shift; although gradual, fluctuating, and never linear, this shift had moved the state from a strategy of Turkish dominance over Kurds without hegemony to one with hegemony. As argued in Chapter 2, the usual Turkish policy of the Kemalist Republic in the Kurdish region had been to rely on collective techniques of punishment of Kurds for the establishment of sovereignty. Despite the assimilationist rhetoric, weak infrastructural power of the state, especially in Hakkâri and border provinces, did not allow it to put the rhetoric into practice in any effective way. The Kurdish policy of the AKP between 2003 and 2014 was an unprecedented reformist one.

In the first period of it rule, the AKP addressed Kurds as equal members of the nation (*millet*), essentially a Muslim one, and whose ethnic and social rights had been systematically violated by secular, Westernizing Kemalist elites alienated from the nation as a whole, including Turkish Muslims. This was fundamental to the AKP's approach to the PKK insurgency. The more the violated ethnic and social rights of Kurds were restored, the AKP reasoned, the less the ground for exploitation of Kurds by the PKK, and the more peaceful the state-Kurds relations would be. In other words, the Kurdish policy of the AKP in 2003–14 was part of a wider agenda of refashioning the nation on an anti-Kemalist, anti-elitist, and essentially Muslim basis with a claim to end social and cultural exclusion. The AKP constituency, therefore—and a major reason why it enjoyed electoral victories that also shifted, from stunning to routine (later enforced)—encompassed not just the religious masses, but also the rural masses, the poorly educated and casual workers of the subaltern underclass of Kemalist Turkey, the ordinary folk everywhere. In this electoral representation, or sum, Kurds were not just another group but a key one, making up 15–20 percent of the population and historically victim to the sovereign violence and indirect racism of the state.

The novel aspect of the Kurdish policy of the AKP was most visible in the negotiations between the PKK and the Turkish state, which can be traced back to 2007 and definitely ended in 2015. In three rounds, the first one in 2007–9, the second in 2010–11, and the last third in 2013–15, the conditions of a peaceful resolution of the Kurdish issue and disarmament of the PKK were negotiated with the participation of the leading figures of the AKP, National Intelligence Service (Milli İstihbarat Teşkilatı, MİT), Abdullah Öcalan, other leading figures of the PKK, deputies of the pro-Kurdish party, and some NGOs.[12] In these negotiations paving the way for and part constituting the Kurdish Opening, the leader of the Kurdish unrest (both the individual and the organization) was openly recognized as a political actor for the first time in the history of the Republic. These negotiations laid the necessary ground for many reforms enacted in this period.

Though liberatory in many respects, the Kurdish policy of this time had many limitations. These account for how the AKP could easily evolve away from its reformist stance negotiating with the PKK over Kurdish rights toward a total counter-insurgency strategy resembling the past. For the AKP's challenge to Kemalist Turkey *only* bore the character of a *passive* revolution.[13] It was a passive revolution not just because it contained the subaltern and Islamic opposition to social exclusion and reconciled it with capitalism but also because it sought to satisfy Kurdish demands in such a way as to weaken and dissipate the Kurdish national consciousness and movement without the basic concessions necessary to properly address the Kurdish grievance. The invariable elements of the undulating Kurdish policies comprising this passive revolution led by the AKP against the Kemalist establishment can be formulated as follows:

- Devaluing politics of identity by making a distinction between the politics of identity and politics of service to assert the latter against the former in a partly neoliberal and partly developmentalist fashion;
- Increasing the use of social policy and public investment;
- Minimizing the open/public offensive references to the Turkish character of nation but without ever questioning the Turkish foundations of the nation-state (official language, historical narrative, unitarian administrative structure);

- Emphasizing Islam and the Ottoman heritage as the common bond tying the members of the nation together;
- Openly recognizing Kurdishness as an ethnic difference worth recognition but depoliticizing it as a folkloric diversity;
- Criminalizing Kurdishness as the basis of a right to a separate polity; and
- Attributing the responsibility of the Kurdish massacres of the past to the Kemalist elites without fulfilling the legal, political, and ethical requirements incumbent on this recognition.

4.3 The AKP's Turkish Nationalism

This consideration of the AKP's Turkish nationalism distinguishes it in terms of power, as a productive power and as a coercive power.

4.3.1 The AKP's Turkish Nationalism as a Productive Power

The AKP's nationalism as a productive power can be divided into its approach to Kurds and the Kurdish issue from a biopolitical perspective—here, *Kurds as Living-Beings, the Kurdish Question as an Economic Burden, and Kurdish Parties as Troublemakers*—and to the broader issue of national identity in a reformist fashion—here, the *AKP and the Turkishness of the Nation*.

4.3.1.1 Kurds as Living-Beings, the Kurdish Question as an Economic Burden, and Kurdish Parties as Troublemakers

The Kurdish policy of the AKP between 2003 and 2014 had many variables. These included the ideological background of the AKP, the EU membership process, the shifting strategies of the PKK and other Kurdish actors, and political competition among the main Turkish parties as well as with the main Kurdish party. Among these factors, the one that was not conditional but rather essential to the larger political and ideological orientation of the AKP was the distinction made between a "politics of service" and "politics of identity."

Prime Minister Erdoğan, the position held by the AKP leader from March 2003 to August 2014 (which thus also characterizes this period), argued that his party stood for a politics of service. He meant all policies that treated citizens as service-beneficiaries addressed through their material "needs"—such as those concerned with the construction of roads, airports, and hospitals, improvement of social services, and provision of social assistance. The concept of "politics of identity" in Erdoğan's political vocabulary referred to the unfruitful discussions and empty rhetoric around identities. Erdoğan sometimes used "politics of ideology" instead of "politics of identity" in a manner reflecting the AKP's anti-intellectualist stance inherited from the conservative center-right tradition of Turkish politics.[14] The politics of identity/ideology was, according to Erdoğan, enacted by the ultra-Turkish nationalist MHP (then electoral opponent of the AKP), the Western-minded and secular CHP (inheritors of the Kemalist tradition, now the main opposition), and the repeatedly banned and reformed pro-Kurdish party (now HDP, during most of this period the DTP and then BDP).

As is evident in their naming, the distinction between these two types of politics—of "service" as opposed to "identity/ideology"—reflects the depoliticizing language of managerialism.[15] This is related to an engagement with neoliberal, conservative, and pragmatic understandings of politics—which can be traced back to Erdoğan's municipal experience in Istanbul (as the former mayor made popular by effective service delivery), the center-right tradition of Turkish politics as self-defined (in opposition to the pedagogical politics of the center-left strand of Kemalism), and also the biopolitics of developmentalism (which has its roots in the national-developmentalist orientation of the Islamist parties preceding the AKP).[16] Of these, the distinction pertained mostly to the biopolitics of developmentalism.

The distinction made between the politics of identity and the politics of service to assert the latter over the former should be seen first and foremost as part of a nation-building, discursive strategy. This strategy aimed to overcome the fragmentary effects of identities (Turk-Kurd) and ideologies (left-right) by devaluing such politics (of identity/ideology) and embracing all as bare life. Thus, the nation was refashioned as a community of service-beneficiaries who were—ought to be, should become—satisfied with the ever-increasing quality of life built on economic growth and modern development.

The expression of this biopolitical orientation in the Kurdish issue was a form of state-nationalism seeking to contain Kurdish unrest by addressing Kurds first and foremost as living-beings, as service-beneficiaries with needs hitherto ignored but as deserving of satisfaction as the needs of, in Erdoğan's words, "first-class citizens of Turkey." This state-nationalism was evident in the spectacular increase of public investment in Kurdish provinces. Nominal public investment in the Kurdish provinces increased tenfold between 2003 and 2013, three times the rate of increase in the rest of the country (Table 13).

The increase in the total populations of Turkey and the Kurdish provinces during this time—up by about an eighth (from around 68 to 77 and 6 to 6.7m,

Table 13. Progressive Rates of Increase in Nominal Public Investment in the Kurdish Provinces and the Rest of the Country in 2003–13 (index: 2003=100)

	Kurdish Provinces	Rest of the Country
2003	100	100
2004	101	98
2005	209	147
2006	204	155
2007	201	172
2008	217	186
2009	347	204
2010	448	242
2011	647	244
2012	694	290
2013	1,004	333

Source: Constructed from the DPT and Ministry of Development data.[53]
Note: Calculated from budget program allocations; public investment not calculable on provincial basis not included; Kurdish provinces: Diyarbakır, Ağrı, Muş, Hakkâri, Şırnak, Van, Batman, Siirt, Bingöl, Bitlis, Mardin, and Tunceli.

respectively) between 2000 and 2013—was fairly insignificant compared to the nominal public investment increases generally and its concentration on the Kurdish provinces, in particular. The rate of inflation for this period (December 2013–January 2003), a little over 150 percent overall, was also considerably less than the increase in investment in the Kurdish provinces.[17] Most of this raised input occurred between 2009 and 2013, when the growth of the Kurdish movement forced the AKP to intensify its efforts and use benevolent strategies along with violent ones in attempting to undermine the mass support and electoral success of the HDP in the region and nationally (Section 1.1). It should be noted that security investment calculable on provincial basis is included in the total public investment calculable on provincial basis—in which context it is notable that security investment calculable on provincial basis accounted for less than 10 percent of the public investment calculable on provincial basis in the Kurdish provinces during 2003–13.

One can detect another instance of embracing Kurds via redistributive policies in the social assistance provided by the central government. Through a regression analysis of a dataset generated by a nationwide representative sampling survey carried out in 2011 by the prominent Turkish polling and public research company KONDA, Erdem Yörük shows for the period 2003–11 that "social assistance programs in Turkey" were "disproportionately directed towards the Kurdish minority and to the Kurdish region on an ethnic basis."[18]

From this biopolitical point of view, the Kurdish question appeared first and foremost as an economic burden dragging the country down and slowing the imperial take-off of Turkey. This was most obviously articulated in the brochure entitled "The Democratic Opening Process with Questions and Answers: The Project of National Unity and Brotherhood," released by the AKP in January 2010 to convince the Turkish masses that the reform process of its Kurdish (now Democratic) Opening would not result in the disintegration of the country.

This brochure consists of 30 questions that an ordinary Turkish individual (i.e., one indoctrinated with Turkish nationalism) might ask about the reform process, together with their answers. It was the single, publicly available document in which the AKP institutionally delineated its strategy in any detail, its promises, and its limits in respect of the Kurdish issue. The first question asked in the brochure was, "What is the democratic opening process, and what purpose does it serve?" The implication already contained in the opening question, therefore, is that democratization in the Kurdish issue was instrumental (to serve a purpose). It was not regarded as an end itself or an outcome of an introspective and self-critical gesture, as the answer revealed:

> In the contemporary world, democracy has become the main ground of advancement and development in all fields, especially that of economic development. Turkey has built its strong economy and respectable foreign policy on the steps taken toward democracy in the last seven years. Today discourses, such as "Let's have a strong economy at the cost of the restriction of liberties"; "Let's be active in foreign politics at the cost of postponing contemporary democratic reforms", and: "Let's live in a secure country at the cost of concessions on democracy," have no chance of success ... The more Turkey becomes democratized and improves its democratic standards, the stronger it will be in the international community ... The Project of National Unity and Brotherhood aims at the advancement, development, and growth of our country and the rise of its national and international prestige, as well as the increase of the welfare and peace of our nation ... .[19]

Thus, the true goal was advancement, development, and growth. These words betray the deeper ambition. The discourses promoting the economy over liberty are only stated as having "no chance of success" (*başarı şansı kalmamıştır*), an excessively weak and pragmatist formulation. In fact, the Kurdish question does not once appear in the brochure as a primarily ethical problem pertaining to the recognition of an ethnic difference historically embedded in the nation-state but until then brutally denied.

Referring to public investment in the Kurdish region, Erdoğan quite often compared and contrasted the AKP politics of service—or "real nationalism"—with the pro-Kurdish party politics of identity, with the latter leading to nothing but the worsening of living conditions among the Kurdish people. According to the AKP, the pro-Kurdish party had just exploited the ethnic identity of Kurds and never really been interested in their quality of life. Erdoğan expressed this in biopolitical terms when addressing the Kurdish party (then BDP): "You're looking for Kurds. We're looking for human beings."[20]

One can distinguish two discursive strategies used to present the Kurdish movement as economically detrimental to the Kurds. One of these dates back to the 1990s, when calculations concerning the economic cost of the military struggle against the PKK began to be made.[21] In this discourse, the PKK had caused a waste of resources that could have been reserved for the Kurdish people and had even been fed by their poverty. Therefore, the argument continues, the PKK did not want the enrichment of the people of the region, quite the reverse. Erdoğan's frequent comparisons between the poor developmental performance of Diyarbakır, a stronghold of the PKK, and the much better developmental performance of Gaziantep, where the Kurdish movement had not had similar mass support, constituted a typical and much-pronounced example of this view.[22]

The second discursive strategy used by the AKP was to criticize the services provided by the municipalities governed by the pro-Kurdish party (or parties, the distinct and different iterations of the main party). In this discourse, the poverty of the municipal services provided in municipalities governed by the pro-Kurdish parties was taken as illustrative of the political mentality that exploited the Kurdishness of the people but did not pay any attention to their living conditions and well-being. The following quotation is a typical example of this discourse:

> The BDP makes ideological politics and has nothing to do with service provision. Let's look at Hakkâri. In the middle of the city, sewage flows. As for Diyarbakır, I cannot see any municipal services there. It's like this because they make politics of ideology, not politics of service.[23]

To sum up, the AKP's Kurdish policy in 2003–14 was strongly informed by an emphasis on the biopolitical care of bare lives and life-fostering technologies addressing Kurds primarily as living-beings and service-beneficiaries. This is visible both in the messages sent to Kurds via the spectacular increase in public investment and social assistance and also in the political language that devalued the identity-centered politics of the Kurdish movement.

4.3.1.2 The AKP and the Turkishness of the Nation

The AKP's distinction between the politics of service and identity may seem to have entailed an all-embracing attitude to the Kurdish issue. It put forth an identity-blind policy and seemed to rely on an understanding of nation not defined by any ethnic identity. More precisely, the biopolitical interest in bodies and indifference to identities—looking for human beings rather than Kurds—may be expected to have produced a more welcoming stance toward Kurdish identity. Erdoğan often repeated that he was opposed to both Turkish and Kurdish nationalism:

> Nobody ought to oppose us ... in the name of Kurdishness or of Turkishness. We are a government that has trampled on all sorts of nationalisms. We do not accept vain nationalism. Do you know what there is in our understanding of nationalism? There is patriotism, humanism, taking the side of the poor, waifs and strays, making this beautiful country one of the top ten countries of the world.[24]

At first sight, this sort of nationalism, which the AKP sometimes called "positive nationalism," may be thought to have worked against the earlier disciplinary aspects of official-Kemalist Turkish nationalism that imposed Turkishness as the norm until the 1990s. Yet this would not be correct, for, in addition to the distinction made between politics of identity and politics of service, another slogan was much repeated and practiced by the AKP during and after this period: "One nation, one state, one flag, one land."

Prime Minister Erdoğan would repeat this slogan in all his speeches. A definition of the "one nation" and the source of other "ones" was supplied in 2013 thus:

> We say "one nation" ... What is a nation? The nation is not only composed of Turks. In the nation are Turks, Kurds, Laz, Circassians, Georgians, Arabs, Roma, and Bosnians. [The nation] is the sum of all ... In the opening of the first assembly, Ghazi Mustafa Kemal said, "The people present here are

Islamic communities including Turk, Kurd, Laz, Circassian, Georgian, and Abkhazian." [. . .] It is these that make up the nation.[25]

In this passage, one of hundreds of similar speeches, Erdoğan returns the basis of the oneness of the nation, flag, land, and state to an Islamic brotherhood and not to a common ethnic origin. In the manifest discourse of the AKP, it was not the common ethnic origin but rather the common culture, largely determined by Islamic belonging and Ottoman heritage, which formed the nation.[26] Nationalism promoted by the AKP had never been, then, immune to the politics of identity that the AKP itself so often criticized. The more religious (Sunni Islam) a citizen is, the more they belong to the nation as imagined by the AKP.[27]

One may assert that this understanding of nation, which does not place a special emphasis on ethnicity, should still be given credit because it embodies a clear break from the Turkish ethnonationalism of Kemalism and at least does not discriminate against citizens based on their ethnic identities. This, however, mistakenly directs us to close our eyes to the inevitable "representation" problem manifesting in the reduction of multiplicities to one: in the conflict between the "particular" and "universal" addressed by Ernesto Laclau.[28] Once the oneness of the nation is posited, that oneness has to be represented. The function of representation can only be assumed by a particular element of the multiplicity that is reduced to one.

Thus, we can state simply that Kemalist Turkish nationalism persisted in the AKP's silent acceptance of Turkishness as the privileged particular embodying the oneness of the state and its territory (less silent after the final collapse of the Peace Process negotiations in 2015, which foreshadowed its Turkish nationalist pivot and eventually an alliance with the MHP).[29] The Turkish character of the AKP's nationalism, especially before 2015, was materialized mainly not in what it did, but rather in what it *avoided* doing, not in its slogans but rather its silence.

A pertinent example here follows Althusser's remark on the "material existence" of ideologies.[30] In every city in Turkey, there is a prominent statue of Atatürk in the central square erected as part of the Kemalization—so also Turkification—of civic space. Visiting these statues, singing national marches in front of them, and leaving garlands at their feet are constituent elements of ceremonies organized on the anniversary of important dates in the national struggle. There is a large Atatürk statue right in the center of Hakkâri city as well.

Until 2011, the front face of the statue featured the following text quoting Mustafa Kemal's famous motto, "How happy is the one who calls himself a Turk." In 2011, in the midst of the Kurdish Opening, so-called, the statue was refurbished by the governorship. When this was completed, the slogan was no longer there. It was replaced by another slogan from Atatürk: "Peace at Home, Peace in the World." The change was a clear message to the people of Hakkâri that the state would no longer impose Turkishness as a norm to be achieved and Kurdishness as a burden to be disposed of. Yet the very form through which this message was transmitted was no less illustrative of the AKP's Kurdish policy.

The change was made on the pretext of the refurbishment of the statue. The statue itself was not changed, a representation of Atatürk, and nor was the more subtle adjustment declared. In short, the change was not made in a politically courageous way. It was certainly not a publicly self-critical act of the state and expressing apology embodying a clear break from the past. In this regard, then, despite the fact that Kemalists emphasized Turkishness and the AKP emphasized Islamic brotherhood and the Ottoman heritage as the bond uniting the nation, it is continuity rather than rupture that better defines the relation between conceptualizations of "nation" during the two periods.

To present the continuity between the two nationalisms in more theoretical terms, we can employ a distinction between pragmatist/realist and normative *moments* of Turkish nationalism. By the pragmatist moment of Turkish nationalism, I mean the real-political aspect of Turkish nationalism that takes as a

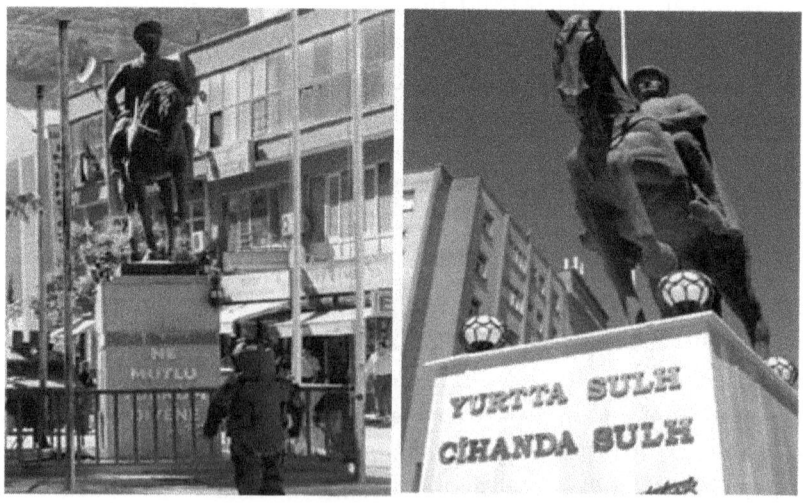

Figure 9. From "How Happy is the One Who Calls Himself a Turk" to "Peace at Home, Peace in the World."
Source: Yüksekova News Portal (Yüksekova Haber Portalı website).

given—though not as an ideal—the circumstances in which it acts. The normative moment of Turkish nationalism refers to its transformative aspect, which tries to *change* the nation through ideals and norms attached to the nation. Following on this distinction, the pragmatist basis of the Kemalist nation, Islamic brotherhood, emerges as the normative basis of the AKP's nation, and the normative basis of the Kemalist nation, Turkishness, is the pragmatist basis of the AKP's nation.

As mentioned above and in Chapter 2, it was Kemalists who first defined the nation according to an Islamic brotherhood, albeit covertly. Although it was not openly declared, being Muslim was the required and minimum condition of eligibility for the nation of Kemalists. It should be added that taking religious belonging as the constitutive criterion of the nation was not a matter of choice for the secular and Western-minded Kemalists. Rather, it was a necessity given that due to massacres, population exchanges, and migrations, "Anatolia, which had been 80 percent Muslim before the wars," by 1923 was "approximately 98 percent Muslim."[31] Islam was the single common feature of the different ethnicities comprising the population. Excepting for the speeches delivered during the National Struggle of 1919–22, including the one Erdoğan cited above—that it was the people as Islamic communities that made up the nation—Kemalists remained notably silent when it came to this Islamic character of the new national state, the Western-styled Republic.

While Islam was the unavowed basis of the nation, Turkishness was claimed as the national norm by Kemalists, especially after the Sheikh Said rebellion of 1925. All ethnic differences in the nation were regarded as remnants of the Ottoman Empire, and the Turkification of the nation and elimination of the "remnants" were sought. Different instruments were employed to this end, such as the national education system, settlement, and resettlement policies, Turkification of place names, banning of non-Turkish languages from official use and sometimes even from daily use.[32]

Thus, the *limits* of the transformative capacity of Kemalist Turkish nationalism were defined by the Islamic basis of the nation. Turkish nationalism, for instance, never went so far as to abandon Islam and to defend a return to the pre-Islamic, shamanistic Turkic beliefs and practices of Central Asia. Kemalist Turkish nationalism did not acquire an exclusionary stance toward non-Turkish Muslim ethnicities so long as they did not resist Turkification. They were welcomed to Turkishness via the famous motto of the Republic stating that "How happy is the one who calls himself a Turk." Non-Muslim ethnicities, recognized as minority groups in the Lausanne Treaty, were, however, devoid of the protective shield of Islam against the Turkish nationalism of Kemalism and frequently fell victim to the state's discriminatory policies.

In order to better understand the disciplinary aspect of the AKP's nationalism, one must take the heritage of Kemalist Turkish nationalism into consideration. At the end of dozens of years of assimilation policies, the gap between the pragmatist and normative bases of Kemalist nationalism closed as the homogenization project was applied, but with the exception of the Kurds. Other than Kurds and their Kurdishness, the Turkish state had managed to institute Turkishness as the overriding identity of the great majority of people and to reduce ethnic belonging to the level of folkloric diversity, posing no political challenge to Turkish sovereignty. Sociologically speaking, the nation had already acquired its Turkish character when the AKP came to power in 2002.[33]

Rather than denying or problematizing it, the AKP pragmatically and silently built on the Turkishness of the nation it inherited in the 2000s, just as Kemalists had built on Islam in the 1920s. In 2003–14, Erdoğan rarely referred to the Turkishness of the nation and even sometimes openly condemned Turkish nationalism as a fundamentalism; yet Turkishness as the unavowed basis of the nation has always set the limit to the transformative capacity of the normative aspect of the AKP nationalism, which sought (and still seeks) to shape the nation according to its notion of Islamic brotherhood and Ottoman heritage. More precisely, the AKP's Islamic and Ottomanist revision of Kemalist Turkish nationalism has never gone so far as to fundamentally destabilize the "one nation" narrative. Erdoğan did not recognize Kurds as a separate national community existing alongside the Turkish nation.

The silence of the AKP on the Turkishness of the nation and its rhetoric on Islamic brotherhood and Ottoman heritage should not lead us to conclude that Turkish nationalism has not been an integral part of the AKP's nationalism, however.[34] Indeed, a consideration of the AKP reforms concerning the Kurdish issue between 2003 and 2014 offers a good perspective to elaborate on and deepen the argument for the limits of AKP reformism and the disciplinary aspect of the AKP's nationalism.

In *The Silent Revolution*, a book on the reform performance of the AKP released by the Undersecretariat of Public Order and Security, the main reforms listed included the following:

- Bans and limitations on . . . the languages to be used in associations' activities were abolished;

- Legal limitations against broadcasting in different languages and dialects were eliminated;
- Barriers against ... citizens' naming their children with names of their choice [were eliminated];
- Compensation for damages of terror victims [was introduced];
- Convicts and detainees in prisons [were allowed] to speak to their kinsmen in their native language;
- The "Institute of Living Languages in Turkey" composed of Departments of Kurdish Language and Culture, Assyrian Language and Culture and Arab Language and Culture was established;
- It was made possible to restore former names of settlement areas;
- It was ensured that political parties could make speeches in different languages and dialects spoken by ... citizens during their election campaigns;
- Important works in the Kurdish language and literature, such as *Mem-u Zin* [a classic Kurdish love story] were translated and published.
- Through the "Law Amending Primary Education Law and Some Laws," a gradual system was initiated in education ... this legal amendment paved the way for choosing Kurdish as an elective course;
- TRT started broadcasting a Kurdish news site called "TRT XEBER";
- [Defendants were granted] the right to defend themselves in a language that ... [they] have stated, in order to express ... [themselves] in a better manner.[35]

Despite some reforms made by the preceding governments in the 1990s—notably, the abolition of the death penalty and lifting of the state of emergency—those made by the AKP in the Kurdish issue in 2003–14 were of unprecedented breadth. And, as mentioned (above), the negotiations with the PKK and its imprisoned leader over the peaceful resolution of the Kurdish issue constituted a real rupture in the firmly established state discourse framing the Kurdish issue as an issue of terrorism. Yet, none of these falsify the argument concerning the AKP's Turkish nationalism.

To be clear, the intention here in emphasizing the continuity between Kemalists and the AKP with regard to the persistence of Turkish nationalism is not to deny the partial emancipatory space opened by the interchange of Islam and Turkishness (i.e., moving Turkishness from a norm to pragmatist basis and Islam from pragmatist basis to norm). In the Islamic ontological premises of the normative aspect of the AKP nationalism, ethnic differences as such do not embody a degeneration or a threat to be eliminated.[36] Otherwise, the series of

148 | *The Social Policy of the AKP toward the Kurds*

AKP reforms lifting bans on Kurdish identity—as well as the "democratic opening" process—would probably not have been possible.

However, being ideologically flexible so as to accommodate ethnic differences is one thing, but assuming a political stance actively working for the recognition of ethnic differences is quite another. It is evident that the AKP reformism in 2003–14 regarding the Kurdish issue did not extend as far as an appreciation of the collective rights for Kurds as an ethnopolitical community, much less their legal recognition and promotion.[37] All the reforms listed above grant individual rights to Kurds as individuals of a single Turkish nation. The AKP reformism was blind to Kurds as a collective entity. This is not only an abstraction that we can derive from the reform list of the AKP; it was so deeply a part of the AKP's stance toward Kurds that the party did not refrain from openly declaring it in the "Democratic Opening Process with Questions and Answers" document.

In that brochure, it was stated that "neither a discussion around our unitary structure nor a concession on the principle of 'one state, one nation, one land, one flag' is on the agenda." Furthermore, it was added that "Turkish is the language of instruction and will remain so . . . no preparatory work is underway to render different languages spoken in Turkey as languages of instruction." So a bilingual education system—a key Kurdish demand—was ruled out from the start. The message is clear enough. The oneness of the nation, that is, its Turkishness, was never an issue for discussion and negotiation. The AKP's passive revolution was always an essentially reformist project, not a radical one.

4.3.2 The AKP's Turkish Nationalism as a Coercive Power

The less violent, more benevolent Kurdish policy of Turkish state-nationalism led by the AKP in 2003–14 did not cancel out practices and rhetoric pertaining to the moment of sovereignty of Turkish nationalism. A total of 1,902 PKK guerillas were eliminated in these years (Table 14). In addition to the 1,902 guerillas who lost their lives in military operations, hundreds of civilians, including dozens of children, were killed by security forces during street demonstrations.[38]

Table 14. PKK Guerillas Killed Yearly in Military Operations, 2003–2016

2003	2004	2005	2006	2007	2008	2009	2010	2011	2012	2013	2014	2015	2016
102	103	149	145	223	177	103	155	232	426	47	30	292	662

Source: Constructed from data available at *Şehîden Me Rûmeta Me Ne.*[54]

It would not really be accurate, however, to conclude that it was the military operations or murder of political opponents that characterized sovereign violence employed against the cadres of the Kurdish movement in 2003–14. Rather, this comprised the arrest and detention of the cadres and sympathizers of the PKK-linked civil Kurdish movement, the Association of Communities in Kurdistan (Koma Civakên Kurdistan, KCK). The police operations deployed with judicial support to take down the KCK between 2009 and 2012 tell us much about the nature and methods of sovereign violence under the AKP during this time.

Before the capture of Öcalan in 1999, the PKK was fighting for national liberation and adopted a Marxist-Leninist ideology. Öcalan used his trials to present what became known as the "defense texts" and the marker of the ideological and organizational transformation of the PKK. In these texts, Öcalan presented the state as "the 'Original Sin' of humanity" to argue that "liberation cannot be achieved by means of state-building, but rather through the deepening of democracy."[39] Inspired by the writings of Murray Bookchin, the PKK leader formulated a project of radical democracy. According to Öcalan, "this project builds on the self-government of local communities and is organized in the form of open councils, town councils, local parliaments and larger congresses"; in a bottom-up structuring, "The citizens themselves are agents of . . . self-government, not state-based authorities."[40] The KCK was the umbrella organization of the self-governing local communities that the PKK-affiliated Kurdish movement in Turkey had been slowly constructing since 2005.

It was said many times by Öcalan and the PKK leaders that the KCK was not based on a program committed to taking over state power.[41] Nevertheless, the emphasis on self-government was perceived as a threat by the AKP government. According to Yalçın Akdoğan, then the chief supervisor to Erdoğan and claimed to be one of the masterminds of the KCK operations, it undermined the sovereignty of the state as a form of "parallel state":

> The organization tries to undertake the functions . . . of a state, like "taxation," "establishment of courts and practicing judicial function," [and] "institution of security and defense" . . . Trying to institute its authority in the region, the organization exacts tribute from the people, waylays and abducts the people, takes statements from the people and judges them, and tries to institute field domination via Self-Defense Units.[42]

Akdoğan's words show that the AKP read the attempts of the Kurdish movement to reorganize itself around the principles of self-government as a refashioning of separatism. In other words, one of the motives behind the KCK operations was to reinforce and fortify the state sovereignty that was thought to be under attack from the self-governmental attempts of the KCK.

Although the KCK operations embodied a sovereign practice of police detention and legal charges, they were completely different from the earlier sovereign practices in the Kurdish region, which had been characterized by techniques of collective punishment. Systematic torture and forced disappearances were not part of the KCK operations as a rule. The strong biopolitical emphasis on the care of bare lives made via the distinction between the politics of service and identity was one of the factors limiting the use of draconian methods of the 1990s. The claim to restore the violated human rights of Kurds and end the extra-legal counter-insurgency methods used by the Kemalist state against which the passive revolution was launched was another factor behind renouncing the techniques of collective punishment. Also, the advancement of the disciplinary capacity of the state to individualize suspects determined the form that the KCK operations took.

After the village evacuations of the 1990s, the majority of Kurds were living in urban areas. These neighborhoods were constantly monitored through dozens of police cameras known as "MOBESE," and Kurds, too, had started to use modern communication channels, which were open to police control and surveillance. Therefore, the KCK operations were police operations that relied on an advanced disciplinary capacity to identify individuals and networks through recording telephone conversations, identifying IP addresses, checking electronic mail, photographs, and videos shot by MOBESE cameras, and other audio-visual techniques.[43]

The KCK case files were filled with transcriptions of telephone conversations between suspects and photos of suspects detained, shouting slogans in a demonstration, talking with other suspects, or entering the building of a pro-Kurdish institution. This why many Hakkârians jailed during the KCK operations and later released in 2012–14 stopped using cell phones and why the first targets of young protesters during street clashes with the police would be the MOBESE cameras, which they attacked with stones, bombs, and guns.

Accusing the KCK of being a parallel state trying to establish its sovereignty by taxing and judging people by its own mechanisms, anti-terror police teams took thousands of Kurdish activists into custody between April 2009 and 2012, including elected mayors and members of the BDP, academics, lawyers, journalists, and trade unionists. According to numbers given by the BDP, between April 2009 and October 2011, 7,748 people were taken into custody and 3,895 of those detained were jailed.[44] The KCK operations aimed at depriving the Kurdish movement of the cadres who could carry out the political activity of constructing the grounds of self-government.

4.4 The AKP's Turkish Nationalism and Hakkâri

State-nationalism carried out by the AKP in the Kurdish region can be clearly followed in the policies put into practice in Hakkâri. As a province where the hegemony of the Kurdish movement is obvious, in Hakkâri, in 2003–14, the AKP employed an effective combination of benevolent and coercive instruments, on the one hand to embrace Kurds as service-beneficiaries with needs hitherto ignored but deserving to be satisfied as needs of "first-class citizens of Turkey," and on the other to punish them as members of an ethnopolitical community with claims to self-rule.

4.4.1 The AKP's Turkish Nationalism in Hakkâri as a Benevolent Power: Embracing Kurds as Bodies

The AKP adopted a more generous stance toward the Kurdish provinces with respect to public investment than previous governments, but the rate of increase in Hakkâri was even more striking. While nominal public investment increased tenfold in the Kurdish provinces in 2003–13, over three times the figure for the rest of the country, the figure for Hakkâri was over double that for the region as a whole, with a 22-fold rise (Table 15).

This remarkable difference was one of the most striking manifestations of the AKP shift in approach to a consent- and compromise-seeking Turkish dominance. Addressing Kurds as service-beneficiaries was central to the move, as is evident in the major tangible improvement made to healthcare provision in the Kurdish provinces. And this was especially the case in Hakkâri, with its two new, modern public hospitals in Hakkâri city and Yüksekova opened in 2008 and the general upgrading of personnel and improvements to the medical equipment and infrastructure. The province obviously benefited also from the law on contract personnel issued in 2003 to staff health institutions primarily in the Kurdish region, and the law on compulsory service issued in 2005 to appoint newly qualified specialists and GPs, again primarily to the Kurdish provinces.

Apart from these policies that aimed directly at improving healthcare provision in Kurdish provinces, including Hakkâri, certain nationwide policies

Table 15. Progressive Rates of Increase in Nominal Public Investment in Hakkâri, Kurdish Provinces, and the Rest of the Country (index: 2003=100), 2003–2013

	Hakkâri	Kurdish Provinces	Rest of the Country
2003	100	100	100
2004	185	101	98
2005	228	209	147
2006	757	204	155
2007	257	201	172
2008	214	217	186
2009	700	347	204
2010	1,100	448	242
2011	1,157	647	244
2012	1,728	694	290
2013	2,214	1,004	333

Source: Constructed from DPT and Ministry of Development data.[55]
Note: Calculated from budget program allocations; public investment unclassified into provinces not included; Kurdish provinces: Diyarbakır, Ağrı, Muş, Hakkâri, Şırnak, Van, Batman, Siirt, Bingöl, Bitlis, Mardin, and Tunceli.

also contributed considerably to the improvement of healthcare provision in the Southeast. With the gradual replacement of the fragmented and hierarchical health insurance system by a General Health Insurance Scheme (Genel Sağlık Sigortası, GSS) from 2003, the distinctions between different health schemes were eliminated. That meant that from 2003–4, Green Card holders, who formed almost half of the population in Kurdish provinces and Hakkâri, now had guaranteed free access to consultations, tests, and medications related to out-patient treatment and the right to go to the better staffed and equipped state university (teaching) hospitals. Also, conditional cash transfers in 2003 and the transition to a family practice (local GP) system in 2010 ensured regular check-ups of babies, children and pregnant women and a considerable increase of vaccination rates (see below).

The considerable improvement in hospital medical equipment was one of the most important transformations in the medical establishment in Hakkâri. Prior to 2007, according to the response to a request under the Freedom of Information Act, Hakkâri Public Hospital lacked such items as a multifunctional surgery table, tomograph, color Doppler ultrasound, MRI scanner, mobile x-ray machine, endoscopic camera system, and gastroscopy and colonoscopy sets, without which many operations simply could not be performed. Only then did it become possible to avoid having to transfer patients to Van, Ankara, and Istanbul, as indicated by the rise in operations carried out at the hospital (Table 16).

Table 16. Surgical Operations Performed in Hakkâri Public Hospital (by category), between 1995 and 2013

	Major Operations	Medium Operations	Minor Operations
1995	163	220	108
1996	256	265	144
1997	208	333	152
1998	140	296	211
1999	174	264	190
2000	63	307	123
2001	18	331	30
2002	92	505	32
2003	152	471	43
2004	277	515	128
2005	219	504	107
2006	93	296	124
2007	299	1,763	1,427
2008	2,152	1,680	1,208
2009	2,517	1,623	1,490
2010	3,731	2,087	2,047
2011	3,320	2,478	2,538
2012	4,133	5,570	3,119
2013	2,472	4,337	4,567

Sources: Constructed from MoH (General Directorate of Public Hospitals) Health Statistical Yearbooks[56] and Hakkâri Public Hospital data.

With the construction of a new hospital building in 2008, there was a huge leap in the numbers of surgical operations performed in Hakkâri Public Hospital—from a total of 629 in 2002, the year when the AKP came to power to 11–13 thousand by 2012–13, the end of the period covered (or, from an average of less than two a day to 30–35). Both medium and minor surgical operations increased tenfold between 2002 and 2012. Most critically, there was a massive increase in the number of major operations performed, from under 100 in 2002 to over 40 times that number a decade later, indicating that the hospital was at last serving as a real hospital, with risky surgeries carried out and complicated cases managed.

In addition to the surgery performance, other indicators of the advancement of the health services in Hakkâri in these years include bed occupancy, registered deaths, and patient numbers (Table 17). In the hospital, bed occupation rates can be taken as a reliable indicator of service improvements. Previously, although there were never more than a few dozen hospital beds—100 by the 1990s—only a quarter or third of them would typically be in use; seriously ill patients had to be transferred to better-equipped and staffed hospitals. During the early AKP period, as treatment began to be given to seriously ill patients locally, bed occupation rates increased up to over 85 percent, in spite of the increased bed capacity (over 70 percent higher).

The increase in the number of deaths occurring in Hakkâri Public Hospital in 2003–14 likewise confirms the improvement of health services in Hakkâri. Given that most people did not have access to state treatment and anyway the state's provincial medical facilities had no intensive care unit and little or no treatment could be given to seriously ill patients in the pre-AKP period, the numbers of deaths occurring in Hakkâri's medical facilities amounted to only a minute proportion of all deaths occurring in the province. Thus, the opening of intensive care units and the treatment of seriously ill patients in Hakkâri Public Hospital resulted in an increase in the number of deaths recorded there.[45] In other words, somewhat paradoxically at first sight, the increase in the number of patients dying in Hakkâri Public Hospital confirms the advancement of the hospital.

A much more explicit expression of the improvement of health services in Hakkâri is the simple increase in the number of users of the main hospital in the province. The appointment of specialists under the law on compulsory service and the purchase of medical equipment had a direct impact on the number of hospital in-patients and out-patients. Between 2002 and 2012, the number of out-patients and in-patients increased by around six and four-and-a-half times, respectively.

Table 17. Performance of Hakkâri Public Hospital, 1995–2013

	Beds	Bed Occupancy (%)	In-patients	Out-patients	Deaths
1995	100	29	2,865	53,694	35
1996	100	23.8	2,358	19,964	n/a
1997	100	33.8	3,605	61,642	20
1998	100	31.9	3,596	80,103	18
1999	100	36.1	4,213	75,309	26
2000	100	39.3	5,010	63,614	26
2001	107	47.8	4,502	27,606	24
2002	104	50.9	4,526	73,460	18
2003	102	43.6	3,751	78,255	16
2004	100	43	n/a	127,332	n/a
2005	118	41.3	3,717	161,188	24
2006	96	58.2	4,970	201,194	45
2007	125	75.7	8,722	268,880	11
2008	173	64.4	9,871	235,021	43
2009	173	96.3	13,778	344,281	69
2010	173	83.4	14,900	374,325	85
2011	173	86.5	15,483	408,327	84
2012	173	74.4	20,318	391,570	124
2013	173	77.2	28,677	338,833	135

Sources: Constructed from MoH (General Directorate of Public Hospitals) Health Statistical Yearbooks[57] and Hakkâri Public Hospital data.

Hakkâri Public Hospital acquired the capacity to provide health services in a wide range of medical branches, including neurosurgery, cardiovascular, thoracic, and, plastic surgery, gastroenterology, nephrology, and psychiatry, none of which existed in any hospitals in the province before the AKP health reforms. Now, in sharp contrast to the situation in the 1970s, 1980s and 1990s, the most-needed medical specialists, like general surgeons, gynecologists, pediatricians, internists, ophthalmologists, orthopedists, and urologists, were posted and working there. However, it must be noted, medical specialists were still insufficient to meet the actual need, and it was not exceptional for gynecologists, internists, pediatricians, ophthalmologists, dermatologists to see more than 70–80 and sometimes even more than 100 patients a day, which practically means reserving only a couple of minutes for each patient (see Appendix 3).[46]

The improvement of the medical establishment in Hakkâri at this time was not limited to the improvement of curative services. The basic indicators for preventive medicine also signify a striking improvement in preventive services and in maternal and child health services in the province, facilitated in part by the modernization of medical infrastructure (Figures 10a and 10b) but also and especially by conditional cash transfers.

Conditional cash transfers were introduced in Turkey for the first time in 2001 (against the harsh consequences of the financial crisis) by the Social Assistance and Solidarity Foundation (Sosyal Yardımlaşma ve Dayanışma Vakfı) as part of the Social Risk Mitigation Project (Sosyal Riski Azaltma Projesi) with credit provided by the World Bank. The system was initially implemented in six provinces as a pilot scheme and then gradually expanded to the whole country after 2003.[47]

Combined with the systemic transition to family practice (neighborhood GPs), the conditional cash transfers enabled relatively quick and easy access to services. This led Hakkârians to adopt preventive healthcare measures, with high rates of delivery in hospital, vaccination coverage, and follow-ups for infants and children (up to 6 years old), and pregnant woman.

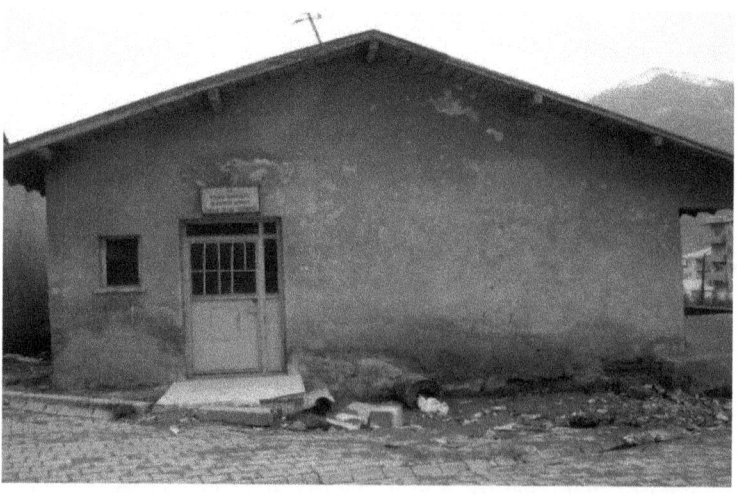

Figure 10a. Old Central Health Post in Şemdinli (opposite the Şemdinli Public Hospital).

Turkish Nationalism, the Kurdish Question, and Hakkâri

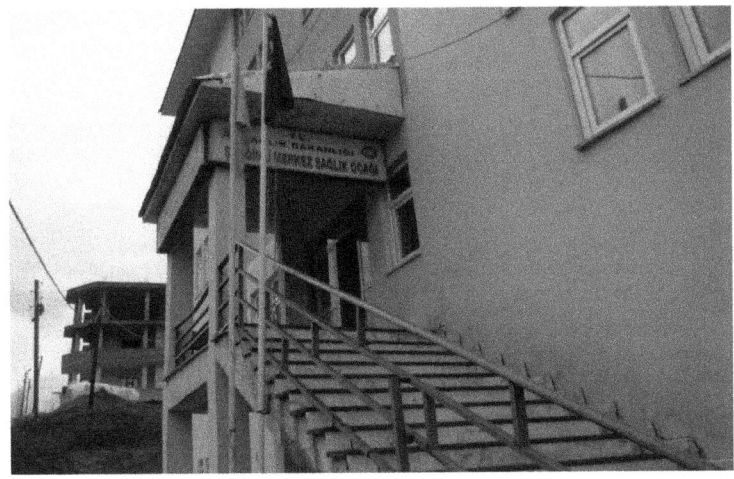

Figure 10b. New Central Health Post in Şemdinli.
Note. The first three floors of the building include operational units and rooms of the health post, local health bureaucracy, and Green Card unit; the fourth and fifth floors are reserved for the accommodation of the GP and health staff employed at the health post.

Beginning in 2004, the year when the conditional cash transfer program started to be effectively implemented, there was a leap in the number of follow-ups (especially for infants and pregnant women) while the percentage of home deliveries plummeted from nine in every ten births to less than two (Table 18).

Vaccination rates in Hakkâri likewise confirm the massive improvement in preventive services and in maternal and child health services. Previously, routine immunization programs would fail for two main reasons. First, families would not usually allow immunization teams to vaccinate children or women. Especially, vaccines given to children and tetanus vaccines given to women of child-bearing age (15–49 years old) were declined by Hakkârians due to the largely accepted rumors of a secret sterilization program by the Turkish state. Second, the clashes between the PKK and the state also many times decreased the efficiency of routine immunization programs. A GP who worked at a health post in Yüksekova between 1995 and 1996, the peak years of the war, recalled that they would not undertake any fieldwork in the area under their responsibility. They only used to vaccinate those babies and children brought by their parents to the health post.

It is not surprising, therefore, to see that the main vaccinations—against tuberculosis (BCG), diphtheria, tetanus, whooping cough, and polio (DTaP+OPV), hepatitis B (HBV), and measles—were very poorly performed until 2004. The

Table 18. Maternal and Child Health Services in Hakkâri, 1996–2014

Year	Follow-ups (n)						Home deliveries (%)	
	per Infant		per Child		per Pregnant woman			
	Hakkâri	Turkey	Hakkâri	Turkey	Hakkâri	Turkey	Hakkâri	Turkey
1996	0.9	3.7	0.1	1.1	0.9	2.0	85.4	29.6
1997	1.3	3.6	0.1	1.1	1.8	1.9	84.2	23.3
1998	0.5	3.4	0.1	1.0	0.5	1.8	72.4	21.1
1999	0.2	3.4	0.1	1.0	0.1	1.8	77.4	17.7
2000	0.2	3.2	0.1	1.0	0.1	1.7	89.2	16.0
2001	0.3	3.5	0.2	1.1	0.2	1.9	90.7	14.5
2002	0.9	3.4	0.5	0.8	0.3	1.7	92.3	12.4
2003	0.9	3.3	0.5	2.0	0.3	1.8	86.9	10.2
2004	3.0	4.3	1.9	1.3	1.1	2.2	56.5	10.8
2005	3.7	4.8	2.1	n/a	1.9	n/a	n/a	n/a
2006	3.8	5.2	2.1	1.2	1.7	2.7	41.9	12.4
2007	n/a	6.0	n/a	1.6	n/a	3.1	20.3	10.7
2008	5.6	6.4	n/a	1.6	4.2	3.3	30.4	8.7
2009	6.6	6.8	n/a	1.6	4.8	3.6	21.7	9.0
2010	5.8	7.1	n/a	1.6	4.0	4.2	17.2	8.0
2011	n/a	8.1	n/a	2.0	2.1	4.3	n/a	6.0
2012	5.8	8.6	1.1	2.2	3.3	4.1	n/a	3.0
2013	6.6	8.8	1.8	2.2	4.2	4.4	n/a	2.6
2014	6.6	8.2	1.7	2.2	n/a	4.8	n/a	2.0

Sources: Constructed by the author based on data obtained from Hakkâri Provincial Directorate of Health and the MoH and on data available at the MoH (General Directorate of Public Hospitals) Health Statistical Yearbooks.[58]

conditional cash transfers employed in 2004 had a noticeable positive impact on this situation, and Hakkârians' resistance to the immunization program was largely overcome (Table 19). In today's Hakkâri, almost all those who need to be vaccinated are vaccinated without any remarkable resistance, as the table below confirms clearly.

The contribution made by the shift to the family practice system to preventive medicine and maternal and child health services in Hakkâri was twofold.

Table 19. Immunization Rates in Hakkâri and Turkey, 1996–2012

Year	BCG Hakkâri	BCG Turkey	DTaP+OPV 3 Hakkâri	DTaP+OPV 3 Turkey	Measles Hakkâri	Measles Turkey	HBV 3 2001–	MMR 2006– Hakkâri	Pentaxim 2008–	PCV 3 2008–
1996	12	69	31	84	60	85				
1997	12	73	8	79	7	76				
1998	11	76	10	80	18	78				
1999	12	78	11	79	15	80				
2000	18	77	22	80	29	81				
2001	34	82	40	83	39	84	13			
2002	35	77	44	78	45	82	15			
2003	33	76	50	68	51	75	24			
2004	56	79	75	85	68	81	39			
2005	83	88	88	84	Replaced by MMR		75			
2006	76	88	87	90			84	80		
2007	66	94	73	96			68	n/a		
2008	105	96	Replaced by Pentaxim				87	92	74	n/a
2009	94	96					93	101*	98	92
2010	83	97					90	92	87	90
2011	90	95					95	104*	95	95
2012	94	96					95	98	94	94

Sources: Constructed by the author based on data obtained from Hakkâri Provincial Directorate of Health and on data available at the MoH (General Directorate of Public Hospitals) Health Statistical Yearbooks.[59]

* Rates of over 100 percent may occur when the number of people vaccinated within the working area of a health post/family health center exceeds the number of people in locally registered population who need to be vaccinated. In 2011, for example, there was an influx of people into Hakkâri from Van due to an earthquake, so the migrant infants were immunized in the Hakkâri family health centers and recorded thus.

First, family doctors were paid based on a negative performance system. The final salary that a family doctor received comprised of a remainder after deductions; these were automatically calculated according to the numbers of unperformed follow-ups and ungiven vaccinations as against those assigned. Thus, family doctors were financially motivated to convince mothers to have their children vaccinated. Second, the negative performance system parameters were fixed so that the family doctors received relatively high salaries, with one result being that new Hakkârian graduates of medical faculties tended to return to their hometown to work. The majority of family doctors working in Hakkâri city were thus Hakkârians, able to speak with their patients in their mother tongue and familiar with their psychology. This development played a major role in reinforcing patients' relationships with the family health centers and linking them thus to the state provisioning of healthcare at the local level.

4.4.2 The AKP's Turkish Nationalism in Hakkâri as a Coercive Power: Excluding Kurds as Members of an Ethnopolitical Community

The state as enacted by the AKP in Hakkâri in 2003–14 was not only a "servant state";[48] it was also a Turkish nation-state, and sovereign. That is to say, if the striking improvement in healthcare provision was one face of the AKP's Turkish nationalism in Hakkâri, the intense sovereign violence employed to suppress ethnopolitical claims was another. Almost a hundred Hakkârian PKK guerillas were killed in military operations between 2003 and 2014 (Table 20). Dozens of civilians in Hakkâri were also killed by security forces during street demonstrations.

Yet, as stated above, it was not the murder of political opponents that characterized the sovereign violence employed by the AKP against the cadres and supporters of the Kurdish movement during this period but the arrest and detention of political activists, especially between 2009 and 2012, when the KCK operations were carried out. Given the strong connections of the Kurdish movement with the Kurdish people as a whole, the arrest and detention of activists did not take the shape of a sterile isolation of small pockets of agitants committed to a

Table 20. Hakkârian PKK Guerillas Killed, 2003–2014

2003	2004	2005	2006	2007	2008	2009	2010	2011	2012	2013	2014	TOTAL
4	1	5	5	10	9	9	4	15	25	9	2	96

Source: Constructed from data at *Şehîden Me Rûmeta Me Ne.*[60]

violent and deadly warfare; rather, it resulted in the arrest and detention of thousands of Hakkârians.

During the KCK operations, as stated, politicians, old and new, and members and administrators of the legal party (BDP) and NGOs affiliated with the Kurdish movement were taken into custody and jailed. As operations carried out to reinforce Turkish sovereignty against the self-governmental attempts of the Kurdish movement by separating PKK affiliates from the masses, KCK operations were centrally coordinated operations whose political character went far beyond their juridical aspect. According to İsmail Akbulut, the then head of the provincial branch of the Human Rights Association (İnsan Hakları Derneği, İHD), who was arrested in the KCK operations in Hakkâri and imprisoned for months, it was not the evidence per se that determined who was jailed and who was released:

> A: I was only jailed because I took the corpses of some killed PKK guerillas from the rural area with the permission of the official authorities and handed them to their families. That was the single accusation leveled against me.
> Q: How did the legal process proceed?
> A: They took me to the police headquarters after I was taken into custody. Members of anti-terror police units told me I was going to be jailed. "How do you know?" I asked, "Are you the judge?" "It's been decided," they said. They said, "You and you and you are going to be jailed, and you and you and you are going to be released." When we were taken to the prosecution office, the police were proved right. What can you believe in? The law?

Despite the rumors circulating about the total numbers taken into custody and arrested in Hakkâri during the KCK operations, reliable statistics were not made available. When I asked İsmail Akbulut whether they had prepared a report on the KCK operations in Hakkâri, he told me that the association's computer had been seized by police.

Following this answer, I decided to try to get information from the Hakkâri Police Department using the Freedom of Information Act. I petitioned the Hakkâri Police Department for information about the number of people taken into custody over the last 5 years in relation to terror crimes. No response was forthcoming. I then called the Hakkâri Police Department to ask why my question had not been answered despite the legal obligation. I was informed that they do not answer "such" questions and was advised to bring an official paper from the Rector of the University of Hakkâri and meet with the Hakkâri Police Chief to discuss the subject. I realized that further insistence might be risky for me and did not follow the advice.

The only remaining alternative was to calculate the numbers myself using the İHD annual reports on violations of human rights. In these reports, prepared based on detention cases reported in the local and national media, political detention cases in Turkey are recorded with the place and date of detention and number of detained. According to the detention entries for Hakkâri for the 4 years, 2009 through 2012, when the KCK operations took place, the numbers of those taken into custody in the province due to PKK/KCK affiliations were 376, 470, 794, and 434, respectively, making a total of 2,074 people.[49] In addition to those taken into custody, many who learned and guessed that they would be arrested escaped to Iraqi Kurdistan. For instance, the former head of the Şemdinli branch of İHD fled there and stayed for 2 years before it was safe to return.

Given that in Hakkâri extended family patterns are not exceptional, kinship relations are strong, and the average size of households is around seven,[50] the operations are likely to have directly affected the lives of not less than 20–30,000 people, which equates to a direct blow to the lives of approaching a tenth of the population. This surely has to do with the strong mass connections of the movement in Hakkâri.

The Kurdish movement is so hegemonic a power in Hakkâri that attempts to make clear-cut distinctions between institutions and people with this or that level of contact with the PKK-KCK and those with no such contact is quite problematic. This can also be seen in the criminalization of the traditional mechanism of *rîspî* (lit.: white-bearded). *Rîspî* refers to the intermediary role played by old, respectable men between sides in a dispute—negotiations with elders, one might say, which are usual in nations with strong, traditional, communal traditions. Although a traditional way of settling disputes in Hakkâri, *rîspî* was criminalized during the KCK operations in Hakkâri.

By way of an example of a case involving the legal party, Mehmet Sıddık Yıldırım, former head of the provincial branch of the BDP, was accused thus:

> It has been understood that Mehmet Sıddık Yıldırım has assumed duties in the so-called Justice Commission brought into being by the KCK . . . ; he tries to settle legal disputes between the people of the region based on the non-legal authority of the armed terrorist organization PKK over the people . . . ; he invited people to the party (provincial branch of the BDP) to take their statements as "defendant", "victim" and "witness"; he allegedly assumed the position of judge in the Justice Commission during the settlement of legal problems,

such as pecuniary causes, causing offense, and female abduction; he processes applications, takes decisions, and follows the implementation (enforcement) of these decisions, ...[51]

In fact, what was criminalized as a parallel court alternative to the courts of the state was not a process carried out secretly, behind closed doors. Once, when I went to the provincial organization of the BDP to conduct an interview with its head, I saw a group of people waiting in the party building. I found out that they were there to ask for the help of the party in settling a dispute. What the BDP did was no more than to refashion the old *rîspî* system led by leading figures of tribes and religious leaders and reinstitute it under the guidance of the party administrators. Therefore, the Yıldırım defense against the accusation can be taken as a precise description of the reality on the ground:

> Hakkâri has some specific traditions and customs. It is not a true approach to attribute our efforts at reconciling disputing parties . . . to the KCK contract. The history of this sort of effort dates back to hundreds of years. The people with disputes used to go to the leaders of the tribes for settlement . . . Because issues like female abduction are shameful, no side in a dispute wants to bring such issues to the courts. Citizens trust the BDP . . . and apply to the BDP for the settlement of such disputes. This has nothing to do with the KCK contract. Sometimes, security forces cannot settle the dispute between two families. For instance, regarding a dispute mentioned in Tape Record 46, due to which a person was murdered, I was called by the Governor to settle this dispute. Our efforts were expended so as not to let a new death occur.[52]

4.5 The Limits of the AKP's Turkish Nationalism in Hakkâri

A Hakkârian dentist affiliated with the Kurdish movement once stated that "The WHO defines 'health' as a state of complete physical, mental and social wellbeing, but we add to this definition that health is also a state of political wellbeing." He described the following case:

> Recently, a woman came to my clinic with her sister. She was complaining of an ache on the right side of her head. Before she came to me, she'd visited a brain surgeon. The brain surgeon had told them that he hadn't seen anything to treat. Then they'd visited a neurologist who couldn't see anything to treat, either. Then they'd visited an otolaryngologist. He hadn't seen anything

to treat, either, and directed them to me. When I was examining the patient, her sister was saying in Kurdish to the women around, "We went to see her son. She saw that he wasn't in a good way. After she saw him like that, she had such a headache." I talked with her and learnt that one of her sons had fallen, martyred as a guerilla, and two others are in prison. If I were this woman, I'd have had a headache as well.

Many doctors similarly reported women complaining of pains that were never relieved and whose particular situation was unclear. According to some of the Hakkârian doctors, this kind of unrelieved, general pain should be seen as symptomatic of post-traumatic stress disorder (PTSD) resulting from the continuing effects of the war. Regardless of the medical diagnosis and how one analyzes the relationship in Hakkâri between the prevalence of this sort of pain and the human cost of the war, one thing is evident: the persisting traumatic effects of fears, risks, tortures, and human losses caused by the intense use of sovereign violence in Hakkâri in the pre-AKP period (via draconian collective punishment), which the AKP could not address properly but rather added to by causing new traumas during their first decade in power (via police operations) substantially weakened and undermined, if not completely voided, the inclusive message sent through the improvement of healthcare provision that Kurdish lives mattered in the eyes of the state.

This was the main point communicated by eight Hakkârian women from the women's branch of the provincial organization of the BDP. Our interview was in the party building. Obviously, they would be heavily politicized, but in a situation of decades of war and suffering and given that the BDP was then supported by more than three-quarters of Hakkârians, the views they expressed should, as a whole, not be so different from those of other people in the area. One should mostly expect just relatively well-formulated and passionate versions of the local perceptions and prevailing mood in general.

So, I asked my main question straight out, why they did not vote for the AKP despite the striking improvement in healthcare provision in Hakkâri:

> Q- Erdoğan … built a hospital in Hakkâri and sent doctors here, but Hakkârians don't give their votes to him. Why don't you vote for Erdoğan?

The participant who answered my question first described herself as a forty-year-old housewife:

> My two children are in the mountains, and my brother-in-law is in prison now. But what good is the hospital to me? Even if you gave all Hakkâri to me, it wouldn't be enough.

The woman explained that because her two children were constantly harassed by the police and threatened with arrest, they had to join the PKK guerillas in the mountains in the end, proving, to her, indeed, that "Kurds have no friends but mountains." Then Ayşe [pseudonym], a 22-year-old woman employed in Binevş Women's Municipal Counseling Center whose brother was in prison, started speaking. She was extremely angry:

> Hey, look! We'd never sell our votes for a hospital . . . Why would I give my vote to him if I'm not free? Why would I give my vote to him if my brothers, fathers, mothers go to the mountains due to this psychology? Why would I give my vote to him if I'm not happy? Is a hospital enough to make me happy?

Referring to the mother whose two children were in the mountains, she continued:

> The mother said that she's forty years old. You're coming from the West. Please tell me whether a mother there aged forty looks like this. How old does she look? [Referring to the mother.] She looks as if she's sixty years old. Why? She's suffered too much at the hands of the state. We've all suffered at the hands of the state. I don't care whether it provides a service or not.

Indeed, I had been surprised when the mother said that she was 40 years old because, as Ayşe said, she really did seem no less than 60. Ayşe's reference to the woman's appearance highlighted how the incongruity between her age and physical appearance did not have to do much with perception but was a simple fact. To ask this physically collapsed woman the question in Erdoğan's mind, why Hakkârians ungratefully failed to appreciate that the state had changed and started to value Kurds' lives through reforms, hospital construction, and the appointment of doctors, was therefore quite meaningless, absurd even, an insult. The answer I received from her, therefore, did not go beyond the rhetorical response, "What good is the hospital to me?"

Another participant, a housewife in her mid-30s, drew attention to the "paradox" of the simultaneous use of sovereign violence and provision of healthcare:

> Yes, the hospital has been built, but do you know how many corpses of soldiers and sons of the people, guerillas, have been taken there so far? Did he build the hospital to serve the people or for the corpses?

This expression of the inherent contradiction of the AKP approach for local people prompted a dialogue involving another participant. This woman, a former teacher in her early forties, who later said she had been expelled from the profession for political reasons, added, "Yet the corpses of his soldiers arrive at the hospital whole, while ours arrive in pieces." Referring to the woman sitting beside her, who was around 65 years old, the co-president of the provincial organization of the BDP joined the discussion:

> The son of this mother was martyred as a guerilla. Those killing him did not stop at killing him and detached his head from his body. She wanted to see her son last time when he was buried. How could we show him to his mother? But we had to show him, she insisted.

The woman referred to was looking at the ceiling of the room, and tears were falling from her eyes.

I felt ashamed and fell silent as I realized that I was asking questions about the quality of state healthcare provision to women whose sons had recently been brutally killed, had run off and joined the PKK after police threats, whose brother-in-law was in prison. I apologized. I was told not to feel sad: "We got to let off some steam."

Clearly, the persistence of sovereign violence in Hakkâri for decades, including the period of 2003–14, has created a physically and psychologically injured population group, such that talking with them even about the state's healthcare provision, let alone about its quality and improvement, is quite beyond the point and actually a little offensive. Given the very high level of Hakkârians' ethno-politicization, the mood of these women should rather be taken as illustrative of the mood of large numbers of Hakkârians and lead us to question the limits of the governmental strategy dividing Kurds into their bare and politically qualified lives in order to embrace the former and punish the latter. Even hoping for this betrays a fundamental misconception of the depth and nature of the problem.

It was precisely these limits of governance that I was invited to recognize throughout the conversation with the BDP women, especially in the context of the women with children in the mountains:

> *Former teacher:* I'd like to put a question to you: even if we have plenty of doctors, very good doctors, do you think that they can give treatment to these mothers?

Me:	No, that job is not one they can perform.
Mother:	A doctor cannot treat me. No doctor can help me. There are photos of my children and brother-in-law on the wall in the home. Every time I open the door . . . [She pauses.]. Are you married, do you have children?
Me:	Yes.
Mother:	You can imagine the grief of losing a child. You wouldn't trade your child for the world. When he has a temperature, you cannot sleep till morning. My children have been in the mountains for three years. I cannot sleep a moment, thinking about whether they're hungry, thirsty, dead, or alive. Enough is enough. We're already exhausted. Go and tour Hakkâri, you'll see someone like me in every home. It's just too much.
Former teacher:	Is a hospital enough to treat our pain?

4.6 Conclusion

The state-nationalism that the AKP practiced between 2003 and 2014 was a version of Turkish nationalism aiming to contain Kurdish unrest through the simultaneous use of both coercive and benevolent instruments of power. It embraced Kurds as individual citizens of the single nation bearing a Turkish and Islamic character, and as bodies, as service-beneficiaries worthy of care, while at the same time criminalizing Kurdishness as the basis of a right to separate polity.

The biopolitical distinction made between a "politics of service" and of "identity" or "ideology," asserting the former against the latter, and the oft-cited "one nation, one state, one flag, one land," were two mottos of the Turkish nationalism enacted by the AKP in 2003–14. The first was most strikingly materialized in the tangible improvement of healthcare provision in terms of medical infrastructure and the health workforce, while the latter manifested as the transference, thus persistence, of sovereign violence, from collective punishment techniques to an individualized targeting that aimed at anyone and everyone linked to the KCK.

The simultaneous use of benevolent and coercive instruments in this way aimed to shift the expressions of power in normative ways. Kurds were to be brought within the nation-state hegemony, and that hegemony was to be transformed in a way that would facilitate this inclusion. The intention was to refashion the nation in a more Islamic, less ethnically marked way, but still on a Turkish basis, and as a community of service-beneficiaries satisfied with the ever-increasing quality of life built on economic growth and development. In the context of the history of the Kemalist Republic, the AKP approach was path-breaking in many ways. At the very least, it involved a huge reform of policy. But it failed.

The AKP was able to provide service provisioning for the treatment of bodies, one might say, but it could not capture hearts and minds. Politically, in terms of the bottom line of electoral support, Kurds in the Southeast were attracted by the possibilities of the new governance, but as time progressed and the structural flaws of the AKP approach became evident, so did limitations. In Hakkâri, it could not overcome the people's firmly established conviction that their lives still counted for little in the eyes of the state. This failure to incorporate the mass of Hakkârians into the new national narrative can be seen in the widespread, endemic persistence of patient dissatisfaction, which is the subject of the next chapter.

Notes

1 See Ergun Özbudun, "From Political Islam to Conservative Democracy: The Case of the Justice and Development Party in Turkey," *South European Society and Politics* 11, no. 3–4 (2006): 20–35; Yalçın Akdoğan, "The Meaning of Conservative Democratic Political Identity," in *The Emergence of a New Turkey: Democracy and the Ak Party*, ed. M. Hakan Yavuz (Salt Lake City: University of Utah Press, 2006), 49–65.

2 See Cihan Tuğal, *Passive Revolution: Absorbing the Islamic Challenge to Capitalism*; Simten Coşar and Aylin Özman, "Centre-Right Politics in Turkey after the November 2002 General Election: Neo-Liberalism with a Muslim Face," *Contemporary Politics* 10, no. 1 (2004): 57–74.

3 Erhan Doğan, "The Historical and Discoursive Roots of the Justice and Development Party's EU Stance," *Turkish Studies* 6, no. 3 (2005): 421–37.

4 For an analysis of the economic performance of the AKP, see Şevket Pamuk, *Türkiye'nin 200 Yıllık İktisadi Tarihi* (Istanbul: Türkiye İş Bankası Kültür Yayınları, 2014), 285–97.

5 Ziya Öniş, "The Triumph of Conservative Globalism: The Political Economy of the Akp Era," *Turkish Studies* 13, no. 2 (2012): 141–42.

6 Nilgün Arısan Eralp and Atila Eralp, "What Went Wrong in the Turkey-EU Relationship?" in *Another Empire? A Decade of Turkey's Foreign Policy under the Justice and Development Party*, ed. Kerem Öktem, Ayşe Kadıoğlu, and Mehmet Karlı (Istanbul: Istanbul Bilgi Üniversitesi Yayınları, 2009), 163–83.

7 Ergun Özbudun, "Akp at the Crossroads: Erdoğan's Majoritarian Drift," *South European Society and Politics* 19, no. 2 (2014): 155–67.

8 See Ayşe Buğra and Osman Savaşkan, "Politics and Class: The Turkish Business Environment in the Neoliberal Age," *New Perspectives on Turkey* 46 (2012): 27–63.

9 Şevket Pamuk, *Uneven Centuries: Economic Development of Turkey since 1820* (Princeton, NJ: Princeton University Press, 2018), 289.
10 See Hakan Yavuz, *Nostalgia for the Empire: The Politics of Neo-Ottomanism* (New York: Oxford University Press, 2020), 144–78.
11 Erdem Yörük and Murat Yüksel, "Class and Politics in Turkey's Gezi Protests," *New Left Review* 89, no. 1 (2014): 120–22.
12 Mesut Yeğen, "The Kurdish Peace Process in Turkey: Genesis, Evolution and Prospects," in *Global Turkey in Europe III*, ed. Senem Aydın-Düzgit, Daniela Huber, Meltem Müftüler-Baç, E. Fuat Keyman, Michael Schwarz and Nathalie Tocci (Istanbul: Stiftung Mercator, 2015).
13 Tuğal, *Passive Revolution*.
14 Tanıl Bora, "Türk Sağı: Siyasal Düşünce Tarihi Açısından Bir Çerçeve Denemesi," in *Türk Sağı: Mitler, Fetişler, Düşman İmgeleri*, ed. İnci Özkan Keresteciöğlu and Güven Gürkan Öztan (Istanbul: İletişim, 2012), 14–18.
15 See John Clarke and Janet Newman, *The Managerial State: Power, Politics and Ideology in the Remaking of Social Welfare* (London and Thousand Oaks, CA: SAGE Publications, 1997).
16 Ömer Turan, "Kudretli Devlet, Manevi Kalkınma, Ağır Sanayii: Türk Sağı Ve Kalkınma," in *Türk Sağı: Mitler, Fetişler, Düşman İmgeleri*, ed. İnci Özkan Keresteciöğlu and Güven Gürkan Öztan (Istanbul: İletişim, 2012), 459–508.
17 153.67 percent; calculated with the Central Bank of the Republic of Turkey the inflation calculator. See https://www3.tcmb.gov.tr/inflationcalc2/inflationcalc.php.
18 Erdem Yörük, "Welfare Provision as Political Containment the Politics of Social Assistance and the Kurdish Conflict in Turkey," *Politics & Society* 40, no. 4 (2012): 535.
19 "Soruları ve Cevaplarıyla Demokratik Açılım Süreci: Milli Birlik ve Kardeşlik Broşürü," AK Party, January 2010, https://serdargunes.files.wordpress.com/2015/08/acilim220110.pdf. The brochure was removed from the official website of the AKP after the peace process ended.
20 "Recep Tayyip Erdoğan'ın 1 Haziran 2011 tarihli Diyarbakır mitinginde yaptığı konuşma," Recep Tayyip Erdoğan, last modified November 27, 2017, https://tr.wikisource.org/wiki/Recep_Tayyip_Erdo%C4%9Fan%27%C4%B1n_1_Haziran_2011_tarihli_Diyarbak%C4%B1r_mitinginde_yapt%C4%B1%C4%9F%C4%B1_konu%C5%9Fma.
21 See Servet Mutlu, "The Economic Cost of Civil Conflict in Turkey," *Middle Eastern Studies* 47, no. 1 (January 2011).
22 "Diyarbakır bir Gaziantep Olamadıysa . . .," TRT Haber, last modified January 19, 2013, https://www.trthaber.com/haber/gundem/diyarbakir-bir-gaziantep-olamadiysa-71534.html>.

23 "Erdoğan: 'BDP ideoloji siyaseti yapıyor'," Doğruhaber, last modified March 10, 2014, https://dogruhaber.com.tr/haber/120489-erdogan-bdp-ideoloji-siyaseti-yapiyor/.
24 *Hürriyet*, February 18, 2013.
25 "Erdoğan'dan 'bayrak' tepkisi," Anadolu Ajansı, December 1, 2013, https://www.ntv.com.tr/turkiye/erdogandan-bayrak-tepkisi,4lhAdJc1x0q0vzOrI_3BfA.
26 Cenk Saraçoğlu, "İslami-Muhafazakar Milliyetçiliğin Millet Tasarımı: AKP Döneminde Kürt Politikası," *Praksis* 26 (2011): 45–47.
27 Jenny White, *Muslim Nationalism and the New Turks* (Princeton, NJ: Princeton University Press, 2013), 53.
28 See Ernesto Laclau, *Emancipation(S)* (New York: Verso, 1996), 20–35.
29 For example, in the last draft submitted by the AKP to the parliamentary Constitutional Reconciliation Commission (founded in October 2011 to produce a common draft for the new constitution), the AKP did not refrain from defining the nation as a "Turkish nation." See http://t24.com.tr/haber/iste-tbmm-anayasa-uzlasma-komisyonu-tutanaklarinin-tam-metni,245108.
30 Louis Althusser, *On the Reproduction of Capitalism: Ideology and Ideological State Apparatuses* (London: Verso, 2014), 156.
31 Zürcher, *Turkey*, 172.
32 *T.C Resmi Gazete*, no. 18199, October 22, 1983. In 1983, the military council had enacted the "The Law Concerning Publications and Broadcasts in Languages Other Than Turkish," which stated that "Disclosure, dissemination and publication of ideas in any language other than the first official languages of the states recognized by the Turkish State is prohibited."
33 According to a KONDA survey carried out in July 2010, 76.7 percent of Turkish citizens defined themselves as Turkish, 14.7 percent as Kurdish, and 8.5 percent by other ethnic identities (Konda, *Kürt Meselesi'nde Algı ve Beklentiler* [Istanbul: İletişim, 2011], 87).
34 For an article avoiding a definition of AKP nationalism as Turkish nationalist due to a lack of open reference to Turkishness, see Cenk Saraçoğlu, "Türkiye Sağı, Akp Ve Kürt Meselesi," in *Türk Sağı: Mitler, Fetişler, Düşman İmgeleri*, ed. İnci Özkan Kerestecioğlu and Güven Gürkan Öztan (Cağaloğlu, Istanbul: İletişim, 2012), 243–79.
35 Republic of Turkey Prime Ministry Undersecretariat of Public Order and Security, *The Silent Revolution: Turkey's Democratic Change and Transformation Inventory 2002–2012* (Ankara: Undersecreteriat of Public Order and Security Publications, 2013), 169–257.
36 Erdoğan frequently repeated the thirteenth verse of the Al-Hujurat sura of the Holy Quran to argue that, for the AKP, it was not ethnic belonging but rather religiosity

that really mattered. The translation of the Holy Quran made by Ahmad Zaki Hammad contains the following verse:
O humankind! Indeed, We have created all of you from a single male and female. Moreover, We have made you peoples and tribes, so that you may come to know one another. And, indeed, the noblest of you, in the sight of God, is the most God-fearing of you. Indeed, God is all-knowing, all-aware.
The Gracious Quran: A Modern-Phrased Interpretation in English, trans. Ahmad Zaki Hammad (Lisle, IL: Lucent Interpretations, 2009), 904.
37 Cuma Çiçek, "Elimination or Integration of Pro-Kurdish Politics: Limits of the AKP's Democratic Initiative," *Turkish Studies* 12, no. 1 (2011): 20–24.
38 See "1988–2014 Yılları Arası Çatışmalı Süreçte Katledilen Çocuklar Raporu," İnsan Hakları Derneği Diyarbakır Şubesi (Diyarbakır Branch of Human Rights Association), accessed November 25, 2014, https://ihddiyarbakir.org/
39 Ahmet Hamdi Akkaya and Joost Jongerden, "Reassembling the Political: The Pkk and the Project of Radical Democracy," *European Journal of Turkish Studies* 14 (2012): 5.
40 Abdullah Öcalan, *War and Peace in Kurdistan* (Cologne: International Initiative Freedom for Öcalan-Peace in Kurdistan, 2008), 32.
41 See PKK, *Partiya Karkerên Kurdistan Pkk Yeniden İnşa Kongre Belgeleri* (İstanbul: Çetin Yayınları, 2005).
42 *Yeni Şafak*, October 7, 2011.
43 See "Human Rights, the Rule of Law, and the Protection of Human Rights Defenders: Report on the Diyarbakır KCK Case," İHOP, accessed December 17, 2021, http://www.ihop.org.tr/wp-content/uploads/2011/04/20110414_KCK_ENG.pdf.
44 "30 Ayda KCK'den 7748 gözaltı, 3895 tutuklama," Bia Haber Merkezi, accessed March 13, 2022, https://bianet.org/bianet/siyaset/133216-30-ayda-kck-den-7748-gozalti-3895-tutuklama.
45 The first intensive care unit in Hakkâri Public Hospital was opened in August 2009.
46 When I conducted interviews with doctors in 2009–10, the specialists were all preoccupied with preparing tender specifications concerning the purchase of medical devices they need to examine their patients and complained of having to lose time with a task that was the duty of the administration but whose personnel were insufficiently experienced and informed to do.
47 Since 2006, it has been provided by the Social Assistance and Solidarity Fund (Sosyal Yardım ve Dayanışma Fonu). "Türkiye'de Uygulanan Şartlı Nakit Transferi Programının Fayda Sahipleri Üzerindeki Etkisinin Nitel ve Nicel Olarak Ölçülmesi Projesi Final Raporu," *Aile ve Sosyal Politikalar Bakanlığı* (The Ministry of Family and Social Policies), accessed January 26, 2022, http://www.sck.gov.tr/wp-content/uploads/2020/02/SNT-Program%C4%B1n%C4%B1n-Etkisinin-%C3%96l%C3%A7%C3%BClmesi-Raporu.pdf.

48 Bülent Küçük ve Ceren Özselçuk, "'Mesafeli' Devletten 'Hizmetkâr' Devlete: AKP'nin Kısmi Tanıma Siyaseti," *Toplum ve Bilim* 132 (2015): 162–190.
49 "Yıllık Raporlar," *İnsan Hakları Derneği* (Human Rights Association), accessed March 5, 2022, https://www.ihd.org.tr/td_d_slug_2/.
50 "Nüfus ve Konut Araştırması 2011," *Türkiye İstatistik Kurumu* (TurkStat), accessed January 20, 2022, https://data.tuik.gov.tr/Bulten/Index?p=Nufus-ve-Konut-Arastirmasi-2011-15843.
51 KCK trial held in Van Heavy Penal Court. Indictment File No. 2012/171, Interrogation File No. 2012/1231.
52 Ibid.
53 At https://katalog.sbb.gov.tr/Record/44192.
54 At https://hpgsehit.com/index.php/ehit-kuenyeleri.
55 At https://katalog.sbb.gov.tr/Record/44192.
56 At https://khgmistatistikdb.saglik.gov.tr/TR-43867/istatistik-yillari.html.
57 At https://khgmistatistikdb.saglik.gov.tr/TR-43867/istatistik-yillari.html.
58 At https://khgmistatistikdb.saglik.gov.tr/TR-43867/istatistik-yillari.html.
59 Ibid.
60 https://hpgsehit.com/index.php/ehit-kuenyeleri.

5

The Persistence of Patient Dissatisfaction as a Mass Phenomenon

While the state health service in the province of Hakkâri had previously been very poor and it could be no surprise if local people were dissatisfied with it, one might expect local public opinion to change with the improvements. Even if the Turkish-Islamic hegemony of the AKP nation-state had failed to win over Kurds, one might still have anticipated that Hakkârians would recognize the improvements to service provisioning and thus no longer express dissatisfaction. But the dissatisfaction continued. Why was this? Why did patient dissatisfaction with state health services persist as a mass phenomenon in an area where all indicators concerning the medical infrastructure, health workforce, and immunization performance of the local health organization showed a striking development in the capacity to meet the needs of residents and the end of the chronic dearth of state healthcare provision there?

Normally, one would expect a solid majority of citizens in Hakkâri to have compared the past and present healthcare provision in the province and appreciate the progress made, especially since Hakkârians had lacked any healthcare provision at all worthy of mention until the early 2000s, let alone anything like a competent, reasonably funded professional service. Yet, a considerable proportion of Hakkârians did still complain about the shortcomings, as though nothing had substantially changed.

In the anthropology of policy and state[1] and critical engagement with governmentality as an approach,[2] scholars have already revealed not only that service-beneficiaries may respond to policy instruments in a way that is not predicted by policymakers but that, moreover, this is not an exceptional state of affairs. As Gritt B. Nielsen argues, "ethnographic explorations into people's everyday lives often show that their subjectivities and their use of technologies are rarely as clear-cut and neat as is presented in a political rationality."[3] After all, no place or space is actually a clean slate onto which policymakers can simply write anything at will.

The persistence of patient dissatisfaction in Hakkâri in 2003–14 despite the tangible progress in the quality of healthcare provision there relates to the fact that issues pertaining to race/ethnicity and culture affect patient satisfaction in various complicated and unforeseeable ways. Manifestly, even after the resolution of issues with the access of a minority group to service provision, the dissatisfaction of these groups may still persist due to the politico-cultural gap between the group and the provider, the agents and actors involved.[4] Such was the case in Hakkâri.

Making sense of patient dissatisfaction in an ethnopolitically polarized context may require us to go beyond a purely logical way of reasoning—beyond, that is, operating with solely "objective" (quantitative) indicators. We need to situate the research object in its historical context, here, that of state-citizen relations in Hakkâri and the ethnopolitical subordination of Kurds in Turkey. The persistence of patient dissatisfaction in Hakkâri during the period under consideration confirms the conclusion drawn by John D. O'Neil in his work on patient satisfaction among Inuit people in Canada:

> In situations in which a dominant ethnic group provides healthcare to a subordinate group . . . the importance of relating wider issues of political economy, racism, and exploitation to individual medical encounters and patient satisfaction is apparent.[5]

The evidence from areas as diverse as Inuit Canada and Kurdish Turkey indicates that the macro-political contexts of biomedical encounters, especially those characterized by racial, ethnic, and cultural hegemony, can very well affect patient satisfaction in various complicated and unforeseen ways.[6]

The literature on ethnic/racial disparities in healthcare places a strong emphasis on the role of healthcare providers' cultural competence in the satisfaction of the needs of minorities with health services.[7] Healthcare providers' cultural competence refers to their capacity to "work effectively in cross-cultural situations."[8] The dissatisfaction examined here, by contrast, is not one that begins and ends with healthcare providers; rather, it is a particular manifestation of a more general dissatisfaction with state institutions that is linked to a fundamental crisis in state-citizen relations pertaining to belonging and identity.

Thus, this chapter is guided by a sensitivity to patient dissatisfaction in societies where state authority-local relations are characterized by alienation due to ethnic and racial subordination. In ethnically and racially divided and unequal societies, as Horowitz argues, "issues that elsewhere would be relegated to the category of routine administration assume a central place on the political agenda"[9] and that political issues, likewise, affect routine administration. Therefore, as Fanon reveals,[10] the greater the alienation between ruler and ruled, the more difficult it is to isolate patient dissatisfaction from general discontent among the ruled and classify the factors behind patient dissatisfaction, to divide them neatly into medical, non-political factors, on the one hand, and non-medical, political factors, on the other. Patient dissatisfaction in a divided society cannot be conceived independently of a totalizing distrust, a distrust of the intentions, skills, practice, and the infrastructure of state-run healthcare providers. This is nothing more or less than a particular reflection of the strong political distrust of the whole state apparatus perceived as an alien entity.[11]

This chapter, therefore, does not focus on the cultural competence of healthcare providers or the role of (dis)trust in patient dissatisfaction in the doctor-patient encounter per se but seeks to prioritize the entirety of ethnopolitical power relations informing the attitudes of the subordinate as recipient to the dominant as provider in the healthcare context. Two main ethnopolitical factors that largely account for the persistence of patient dissatisfaction in Hakkâri as a mass phenomenon in 2003–14 are identified.

The first, as previously introduced, was the deeply entrenched conviction on the part of large masses of Hakkârians that their lives were not so worthy of care in the eyes of the Turkish state. This entailed a pessimistic way of seeing in which negative aspects of healthcare provision—shortcomings, malfunctions, mistakes, etc.—became more visible than and magnified over positive aspects—increased health staff numbers, medical infrastructure modernization, etc. This conviction reflected the burden of the history of state-citizen relations in Hakkâri characterized by sovereign violence/collective punishment and indirect state racism.

The second factor concerned the full and equal citizen status assumed by large masses of Hakkârians. The criterion used in Hakkâri in 2003–14 to assess the quality of healthcare provision tended not to be the relative progress of healthcare provision there over time, a criterion that can be employed by the citizen in the making in developmentalist or pedagogical narratives of nationalism. Rather, there was a strong inclination to measure local healthcare provision by comparing it to the that in other provinces, mainly developed Turkish ones, or by its capacity to meet the absolute standard of the right to qualified healthcare provision promised in law and by the constitution to all Turkish citizens. The widespread desire to assume full and equal citizen status, a counter-move against the dehumanization and degradation imposed through sovereign violence and indirect state racism, was an important factor at play in this respect.

The following sections expand these arguments, drawing on ethnographic evidence and a detailed analysis of the persisting patient dissatisfaction in Hakkâri as a mass phenomenon. First, that needs to be explicitly shown.

5.1 Dissatisfaction with Healthcare Provision in Hakkâri: A Mass Phenomenon

In spite of the undeniable improvement of healthcare provision in Hakkâri with regard to the medical infrastructure and health workforce, the first things Hakkârians would talk about concerning healthcare provision in the early 2010s would typically *not* be the replacement of the old, decayed public hospitals in Hakkâri city and Yüksekova with modern ones, a huge improvement in facilities, the appointment of hundreds of specialists and GPs and thousands of nurses and midwives, introducing medical operations in Hakkâri that could not be performed in Hakkâri in the past, and, if necessary, the facility to make emergency transfers of patients to Van by air ambulance helicopter. Instead, one most probably heard complaints concerning the lack of doctors and the inadequacy of the facilities of the hospitals. Then, if one responded to these complaints by pointing out, say, the construction of the new hospital building, one would be refuted with more criticism: "The building is good, but it's empty inside," or "It's like a statue, it's no use."

In response to objections to local people's claims about the lack of doctors and reminders that sometimes a single specialist would serve the whole province in the past and now dozens of newly qualified specialists and other doctors were in Hakkâri doing their compulsory public service, complaints would shift again: "They're inexperienced doctors, they're medical interns," and "They do their internship on our bodies and then leave." Given the tangible, remarkable even, improvements in the service, there could be no doubt that one was witnessing a complex case of persisting and profound dissatisfaction that went beyond healthcare provision. Thus, I conducted a questionnaire-based research survey in Hakkâri city to establish this on a solid quantitative grounding as a basis for discussing trends and counter-trends in patient satisfaction in Hakkâri.

5.1.1 Methodology

The questionnaire consisted of 15 questions with responses made according to a five-point Likert scale. Questions were limited to the subject of Hakkâri Public Hospital, assuming that the level of patient satisfaction with the hospital, the biggest healthcare provider in the province, should provide a reliable basis of a discussion of the overall patient satisfaction with the medical establishment there.

Respondent selection was determined by the goal of developing a sample so as to facilitate discussion on the basic trends and patterns of patient dissatisfaction in Hakkâri. Therefore, selection criteria were applied for the sampling:

1. Considering the social, cultural, and political homogeneity of districts, research was confined to residents of Hakkâri city (the urban center);
2. Considering that patient responses could be biased by their immediate experiences were the questionnaire to be implemented inside the hospital, I worked with patients going to family health centers, which, as institutions providing healthcare free of charge, accepted patients from all segments of society; and
3. Considering the socioeconomic and political nuances distinguishing the various neighborhoods of the city, the research was conducted in five different family health centers in five different neighborhoods.

The study was conducted during the month of May 2013. I spent 2 days at each family health center. All visitors of the family health centers were asked to participate in the research without any pre-selection. They filled in the questionnaires while waiting in line or after being seen by the doctor or the nurse. Most respondents filled in the questionnaires unaided. A few, mostly illiterate, older women who did not know Turkish well were not able to fill in the questionnaire by themselves. I filled their questionnaires by interviewing them, with the support of research assistants as necessary.

A total of 427 respondents completed the questionnaire, of whom 58 were not counted as they were not permanent residents of Hakkâri city (some questionnaires were completed by temporary residents—civil servants or students of the university—or people living outside of the city). Thus, the sample comprised 369 respondents.

Since respondents were exclusively users of family health centers, the results did not represent a random sampling of the local population and thus did not authorize any generalization with complete confidence of representativeness and its margin of error. It nevertheless provided good quantitative grounds from which to develop discussion as the sample size was high enough to show major tendencies and broadly reflect the demographic composition of the population of the city (see below), while the respondents were regular users of the healthcare provisions in the city but not preselected.

5.1.2 Respondents

The research study was restricted to the permanent residents of the city. When asked about their background, how they had ended up in Hakkâri city, the answers collected were thus: 175 respondents defined themselves as locals (i.e., as native to the city), and of the remainder, 143 were village evacuees, 30 had moved voluntarily to the city from outlying villages in the local area (Hakkâri district), and 21 had moved there from other districts in the province. In absence of research on the places of origin of the permanent residents of Hakkâri city, I can confirm based on my personal experiences and impressions from the field that these constitute a reasonable representation.

In addition to place of origin, the other demographics that were checked and controlled for were gender, age, education, employment, monthly income, and social security coverage. Regarding gender, the 181 male and 188 female gender split was similar to the city as a whole. Regarding age, 30 of the 369 respondents were 15–18 years old, 183 were 18–29, 104 were 30–44, 40 were 45–59, and 11 were over 60 years old (one respondent did not give his age) (Table 21).

The slight overrepresentation of women largely resulted from the fact that maternal and child healthcare is one of the main services provided by family health centers. The overrepresentation of the 15–29 age group respondents to the cost of some underrepresentation of respondents over 45 and especially those over 60 most probably had two causes. First, high school students in Hakkâri, as with their counterparts across Turkey, paid frequent visits to family health centers to obtain sick reports enabling them to skip school courses and thus gain time to study for the university entry exam or sit school makeup exams, instead. Second, the poor health of older people would prevent them from traveling to family

Table 21. Gender and Age Composition of the Sample and Hakkâri City (%)

	Sample	City*
Male	49.05	53.41
Female	50.95	46.59
15–29	57.88	51.51
30–44	28.26	28.82
45–59	10.86	12.80
60–	2.98	6.85

Source: (City figures) TÜİK, *2013*.[52]
* City age percentages for the over 14s.

health centers, and when they did require intervention, it would most often be for a serious condition needed specialist treatment in a hospital.

With regard to education level, 60 of the 369 respondents were illiterate, while 13 were literate but had not completed primary school; 141 respondents had only completed primary and junior high school, and of the remaining 154 people, 99 were high school graduates, 50 had bachelors' degrees, and five were postgraduates (one respondent did not give information on education) (Table 22). With less than half of respondents having gone beyond a basic, junior level of schooling, the general education level of the sample was low—which was fairly well representative of the local (city) population. The overrepresentation of the illiterate and uneducated grouping stems from the fact that women are more inclined to use family health centers than men (for the maternal and child health services), and the education of girls has lagged far behind that of boys until recent times, in Turkey generally but especially in the Kurdish region.

Regarding employment, 38 respondents were civil servants, 29 were unskilled workers/laborers, 19 were shopkeepers, and four had other professions; 28 respondents were self-employed, and 25 were unemployed; 117 respondents were housewives,[12] 103 were students, and two were retired (four respondents gave no information on employment). With regard to monthly income, 228 respondents declared that their monthly household income was less than 1,000 TL (c. 550 USD),[13] 82 declared it was 1,000–2,000 TL, 33 declared 2,000–3,000 TL, and 19 declared more than 3,000 TL (seven respondents did not declare their monthly household income). With regard to social security coverage, 172 respondents declared that they were Green Card holders, with the same number saying

Table 22. Educational Background of the Sample and Hakkâri City (%)

	Sample	City *(over 14)*
Illiterate/no former education	19.83	15.70
Primary/junior high school	38.31	41.48
High school	26.90	26.66
University graduate	13.58	12.94
Postgraduate	1.35	0.66
Unknown	–	2.53

Source: (City figures) TÜİK, *2013*.

that they were insured as premium payers; 23 respondents said they were not covered by any scheme (two respondents did not give their social security status).

Overall, the sample was workable as it broadly reflected the local population. It reflected the socioeconomic composition of the city, as is evident in the information given about health insurance status. In the health insurance scheme GSS introduced by the AKP, citizens employed in the formal sector and their dependents had full access to state (MoH) health services, as well as partial access to private hospitals, through the premiums paid to the Social Security Institution (Sosyal Güvenlik Kurumu, SGK). The premiums of the unemployed and those employed in the informal sector but deemed by the state unable to pay premiums were paid by the state, fully or in part, depending on the level of poverty.

Therefore, there were two main groups of people with respect to the GSS: those employed in the formal sector who could pay the premium and those who were unemployed or else working informally (low-paid, temporary, causal workers) and unable (or unwilling) to pay premiums. One could also speak of a third category of people uncovered by the GSS because they could not pay the premiums they were expected to, including self-employed people (in the formal sector) and those poor people who had to contribute a certain part of their premiums but could or did not.

To distinguish between these groups—those covered and uncovered by the GSS—respondents were asked if they were Green Card holders. In fact, Green Cards had previously been delivered to people registered as unemployed who could not afford to pay for health services and had been annulled before the transition to the GSS (toward the end of 2011). However, the overwhelming majority (approximately 80 percent)[14] of former Green Card holders in Hakkâri had been identified as so poor that, in the new system, their premiums needed to be paid by the state, so practically, nothing had changed for former Green Card holders other than the bureaucratic title of the new status ascribed to them by the GSS. Naturally, these people were less concerned with the bureaucratic change of titles than the fact that they were not expected to pay for treatment, but also the new status had neither a non-bureaucratic, concrete title to replace "Green Card Holder" nor its own physical card or similar to use as a name for the status. Thus, the reference continued in everyday language, and people still self-identified as "Green Card holders" when asked.

A little under half—46.61 percent—of respondents defined themselves as "Green Card holder," with the same proportion declaring that they were insured as premium payers; 6.23 percent were not covered by any social security scheme. At first sight, these percentages do not seem to match the reality on the ground at the time. According to the official records for May 2013, not much more than a third—around 36 percent—of Hakkârians were too poor to pay premiums, while well over half—57 percent—of Hakkârians were insured as premium payers (4 percent were poor but deemed able to pay a part of the premium, and 3 percent were uncovered).[15] Green Card holders and those not covered by any scheme seem to be overrepresented in the sample and people insured as premium payers underrepresented.

An important point with respect to this divergence is that the respondents designated by the GSS as dependents—that is, the respondents below 18 and housewives whose coverage status depended on parents and husbands, respectively—were most often not completely sure about their current health insurance status. In fact, although approximately 20 percent of former Green Card holders in Hakkâri were now insured as premium payers, many dependents who were former Green Card holders and were now insured as premium payers probably responded though they were still Green Card holders. Indeed, the composition of the sample with respect to health insurance status does not overlap with the reality on the ground in May 2013, but it does largely do so with the reality on the ground in December 2011, the last month when the Green Card scheme was still valid. According to the monthly bulletin released by the SGK in December 2011 that detailed health coverage in Hakkâri on the eve of the transition to the GSS in January 2012, Green Card holders formed 46 percent and those insured as premium payers formed 52 percent of the population of the province, with two percent of people uncovered.[16]

182 | *The Social Policy of the AKP toward the Kurds*

The reliability of the sample can also be tested by excluding dependents since they were often unsure about their health insurance status. Then, the composition of the sample with respect to health insurance status becomes 35 percent Green Card holders and 57 percent premium payers, with 7 percent uncovered. These percentages largely matched the reality on the ground in May 2013.

5.1.3 Results

The results of the questionnaire research concerning the level of patient satisfaction in Hakkâri city are shown in Figures 11a and 11b. As can be seen, only two-fifths of the respondents could clearly state that they had no complaints about the hospital. Given the dimensions of the improvement of healthcare provision in the city, this scale of negative response is too large to ignore.

The findings of the official statistical agency's life satisfaction survey of 2013 essentially confirmed these findings, with a single exception resulting from the trade-off between those "satisfied" and those "neither satisfied nor unsatisfied." According to the TÜİK results, Hakkâri was even the province where the least people were satisfied with healthcare provision in the whole of Turkey. While the average rate of satisfaction with healthcare provision in Turkey for 2013 was almost three-quarters (75 percent), the proportion of those satisfied in Hakkâri was only just over half (55 percent), with eight percent neither satisfied nor unsatisfied, and almost two in five (38 percent) dissatisfied.[17] In sum, the experience of the medical establishment of almost half (46 percent) of Hakkârians was officially reported as unsatisfactory (Figure 12).

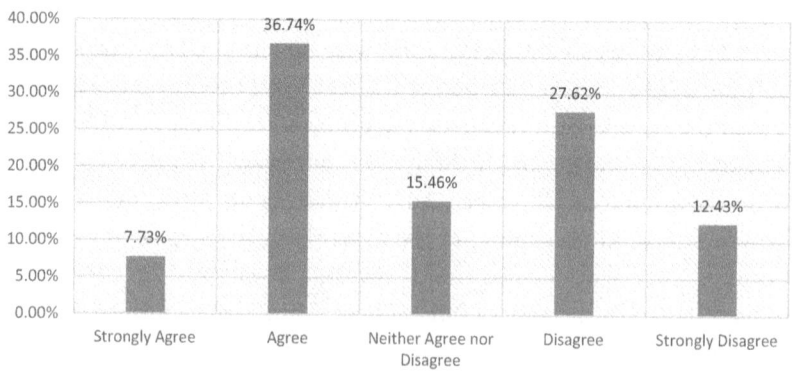

Figure 11a. Responses to the Statement on Hakkâri Public Hospital: "I'm Fairly Satisfied with the Healthcare Provision at Hakkâri Public Hospital."

The Persistence of Patient Dissatisfaction as a Mass Phenomenon | 183

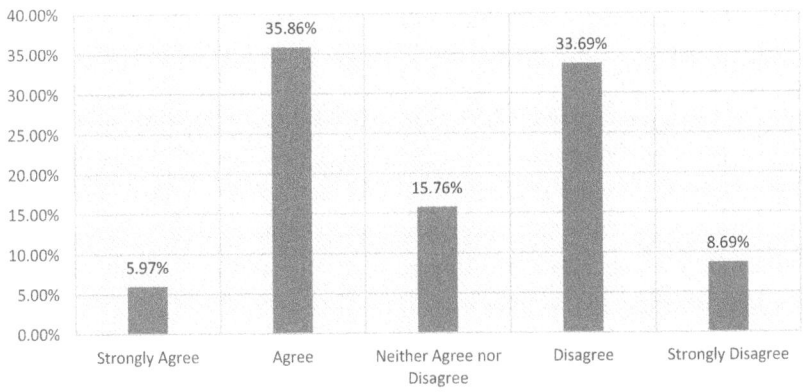

Figure 11b. Responses to the Statement on Hakkâri Public Hospital: "I Do not Have Any Significant Complaints about Hakkâri Public Hospital."

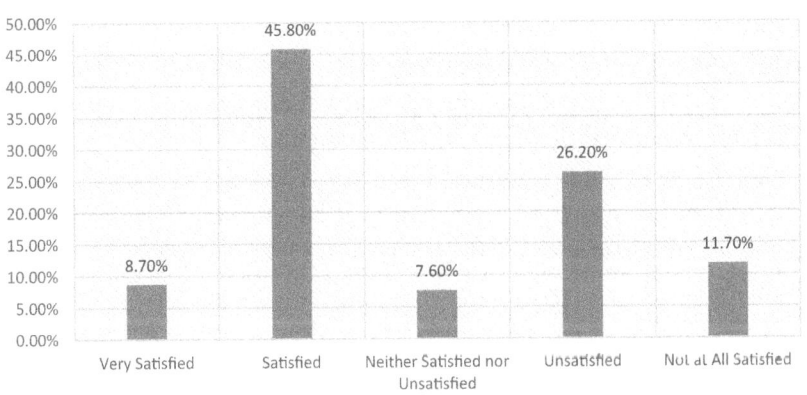

Figure 12. The Level of Satisfaction of Hakkârians with Healthcare Provision. *Source*: TÜİK, 2013.

5.2 An Analysis of Dissatisfaction with Healthcare Provision in Hakkâri

Clearly, the level of discontent with the healthcare provisioning in Hakkâri was such that this can only be considered as a mass phenomenon, not a marginal one. The following sections provide an analysis of this mass phenomenon with regards to the health workforce and medical infrastructure, first as an issue of distrust, then as an issue of equal citizenship.

5.2.1 Dissatisfaction with Healthcare Provision as an Issue of Distrust

Reviewing the issue of trust, issues that may be distinguished include the long history of problematic relations, their specific expression and experience among the health service providers and recipients (doctors, nurses, and patients), and the relationship among these (focusing on patient dissatisfaction). These are interpreted here in the conclusion of a lingering, insidious distrust characterized as a specter that haunts.

5.2.1.1 The Burden of History or the Problem of Trust

A scandal occurred in the biweekly summer school organized in 2011 for the future professors of the University of Hakkâri, most of whom were then research assistants at other Turkish universities where they were writing their postgraduate theses. Organizing the summer school, the rector aimed to familiarize the research assistants with the city and local area since they were legally obliged to return there to fulfill their compulsory service at the end of their postgraduate study—the rector hoped that the research assistants would be more likely to return to the province if they felt a closer connection with the place. His concern was valid. The most popular topic of conversation among the research assistants during the summer school concerned how to avoid returning to Hakkâri without having to pay (the state offered a financial opt-out from the system for those able to afford it).

On the last day of the summer school, a closing dinner was organized in the courtyard of the Çölemerik Vocational School. The Dean of the Faculty of Engineering attended and was expected to deliver a short speech. When he took the microphone, his anger was already noticeable: "You always complain!" he accused the assembled research assistants. "You even avoid filling in the questionnaire," referring to a questionnaire designed to measure participant satisfaction with the summer school.

"If we had not recruited you," the dean continued, "You all would have gone astray." Everybody was shocked, for the meaning of the Turkish phrase for going astray used here (*kötü yola düşerdiniz*) is very clear: it refers to the desperate situation of someone condemned to resort to prostitution (women) or criminal acts (men) to make a living.

The dean, most probably drunk at the moment of his speech, employed this scandalous phrase on the not unreasonable conviction that only the least talented graduates, those not hired anywhere else, would accept work in Hakkâri.

Following long years of sovereign violence and socioeconomic suffering laid upon a history of minimal development and acute poverty, Hakkâri has become an emblem of inferiority. In fact, it was identified in everyday Turkish culture as the worst place in the whole of the country. While making comparisons between the best and the worst, for example, it is conventionally the Hakkâri data that would be chosen by the Turkish politicians and policymakers to stand for the worst. Expressions, such as "While the [assessment item] is [. . .] in Ankara, it is [. . ..] in Hakkâri," were in standard use, along with sentences beginning with phrases like "Even in Hakkâri" (e.g., government politicians would prove how hardworking they were by highlighting their investments "even in Hakkâri"). The most popular among these phrases was to "exile someone to Hakkâri," which referred to the Turkish state tradition of forcing leftist or corrupt civil servants to resign by appointing them to Hakkâri.

The employment of Hakkâri as emblematic for inferiority in Turkey attests to the extent of the issue at hand and why it was not just the actual quality of health services in 2003–14 that Hakkârians used in their assessments of that quality. The history of state-citizen relations in Hakkâri—involving collective punishment and indirect state racism—also played a key role in this. The stance of many Hakkârians toward the state had been structured by their conviction of worthlessness in the eyes of the state based on their own personal experience. A conversation I had with the head of a branch of the Provincial Directorate of Health illustrates this.

In the course of our conversation, I shared with the official my observations about Hakkârians' dissatisfaction with healthcare provision. He did not agree with them and stated that "The numbers do not say so," in a manner not concealing his discontent with my critical perspective. He was referring to the patient satisfaction surveys periodically made by the quality management unit of Hakkâri Public Hospital. In these surveys, he continued, patients seemed quite satisfied with the health services offered there.

Upon his objection to my observation, I went to the quality management unit of Hakkâri Public Hospital. The unit, like all quality management units in other public hospitals of Turkey, measured the level of patient satisfaction on a monthly basis, using standard, centrally designed questionnaires prepared by the MoH. There were three standard questionnaires, one for in-patients, one for out-patients, and the third for ER patients, each of which was answered by 15 patients each month. When the coordinators of the unit allowed me to check the monthly results, I saw that the level of patient satisfaction with Hakkâri Public Hospital was surprisingly high. The results were largely similar each month; the survey on out-patient satisfaction from March 2013 is given by way of example (Table 23).

Unfortunately, rather than refuting the findings reported above, these results signified the incapacity of the questionnaires to measure patient satisfaction in Hakkâri due to the blindness of the questionnaires to the specificity of the place, the local situation. The questions asked concentrated exclusively on patient satisfaction as it pertained to the relatively objective factors in the immediate experience with the healthcare provider (cleaning, waiting time, respect of privacy, etc.). Thus, they were designed as if the history of patients' experience with the medical establishment and the state and the way of seeing entailed by that history had no significant impact on patient satisfaction with the medical establishment now.

Asserting the blindness of the questionnaires to the potentially negative impacts of the wider context of state-citizen relations is not to refer to a deliberate ethnic (Turkish) blindness to the complicated relationship between the

Table 23. The Level of Out-Patient Satisfaction with Hakkâri Public Hospital, March 2013

	Yes 3	Partially 2	No 1
I did not spend much time on patient admission procedures.		2.7	
I chose the doctor who examined me.		2.9	
The waiting lounge was comfortable.		2.7	
The doctor who examined me reserved time for me and informed me about my illness.		2.7	
The doctor who examined me was kind and respectful.		3	
The health staff were kind and respectful.		3	
All the health staff respected my privacy		2.9	
The tests/analyses did not take much time.		2.4	
I would recommend this hospital to other people.		2.7	
If I need to go to hospital again, I will choose this hospital.		2.8	
Out-patient clinics (treatment room, waiting lounge, toilets) were generally clean.		2.9	
The service provided by the hospital was generally good.		2.9	

Source: Quality Management Unit (Kalite Yönetimi Birimi), Hakkâri Public Hospital.

Kurdish question and patient dissatisfaction. Rather, the issue pertains to the general insufficiency of the standard patient satisfaction questionnaires to measure patient satisfaction in contexts informed by ethnic, racial, and colonial hegemony. Annette Jo Browne argues for this in her ethnographic research on how health services given to Canadian Aboriginal women are characterized by colonial and ethnic relations of power:

> A particular methodological implication warrants mention ... This relates to the current use of patient satisfaction surveys/questionnaires in quality assurance programs ... Patient satisfaction questionnaires, based on the assumption that healthcare interactions involve neutral players and are inherently apolitical, tap into surface-level information. This results in a fairly narrow understanding of how patients experience healthcare, and overlooks the complexities and contexts that influence patients' experiences, interpretations and expectations.[18]

Suffering from this "narrow understanding," the questionnaires deployed in Hakkâri failed to take into account that the stance of many Hakkârians toward the state has been structured by their conviction based on their first-hand knowledge that their Kurdish lives counted for little in the eyes of the Turkish state. As expressed by a DPT expert in 1978, "The conviction among the citizens in Hakkâri that the state doesn't give them the necessary support is so widespread that it's even accepted by the civil servants in the province."[19]

To see how widespread this conviction is among Hakkârians, one only needs to look at the everyday language of Hakkârians. Despite the absolute and relative increase of benevolent elements in the Kurdish strategy carried out in Hakkâri during 2003–14, the word "specialist" (*uzman*), for example, was not still generally used for and understood as referring to a medical specialist who was an expert in a specific branch of medicine; instead, it meant specialist sergeant in the military. The mentalities conditioned by violent policies and indirect state racism of Kemalist Turkey, which the AKP-style Turkish nationalism further reproduced, continued to inform the way many Hakkârians made sense of state policies and services.

The characterization of the questionnaires as not locally sensitive and taking into account the perceptions of locals about the lack of value of their lives in the eyes of the state can be expressed thus: they asked whether doctors reserved sufficient time for patients and approached them in a respectful manner but not whether patients trusted their medical capabilities and experience. The reason why this question was not asked in the questionnaire is not hard to understand. It was not asked in public hospitals in the West, in big cities like Ankara and

Istanbul either, where the questionnaires were prepared—because it did not occur to administrators to include such a question. Where the question writer is not informed by the negative burden of the history of the state-citizen relations, why should the doctor-patient encounter be imagined as an issue of trust? The absence of such a question in the questionnaire thus left a fundamental issue pertaining to patient satisfaction in Hakkâri unaddressed, which was especially important given the local feeling (as widely expressed in comments like "The state does not send us experienced doctors" and "The doctors appointed are the newly-qualified ones").

If the issue of distrust had been included in the questionnaires, it would have been seen that there was a very serious problem. According to the results of the questionnaire carried out for this research, only two in every five respondents trusted the diagnosis made by the doctors in Hakkâri Public Hospital, and few of them expressed great confidence; almost a third had no such trust (Figure 13).

The low level of Hakkârians' trust in the medical capabilities of doctors at the central hospital was not the single issue unaddressed and unmeasured by the official quality assessment questionnaires. Seeming to suggest that the only potential problems with medical tests and analyses were long queues and the efficiency of the laboratory processes, the standardized questionnaires also failed to take into account patient mistrust of the *results* of medical tests and analyses. In fact, only 45 percent of my respondents trusted the results of tests and x-ray, ultrasound, and MR imaging, with a third positively *dis*trusting them (Figure 14).

If they really did not trust the medical capabilities of doctors and results of medical tests and analysis, one can ask why patients responding to the hospital

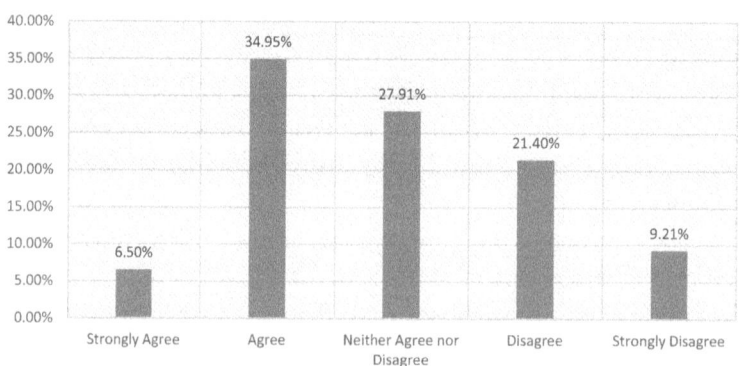

Figure 13. Responses to the Statement "I Trust the Diagnosis Made by the Doctors in Hakkâri Public Hospital."

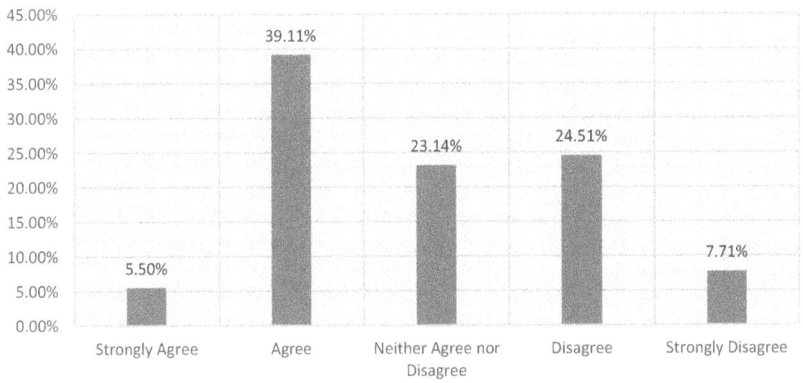

Figure 14. Responses to the Statement "I Always Trust the Results of Tests and X-Ray, Ultrasound and MR Imaging."

questionnaires still continued to say that they would recommend the hospital to others and choose it again themselves. The answer is not complex: they had no feasible alternative.[20] Hakkâri Public Hospital is the only hospital in the city, and the closest better alternatives, in Van, are 200 km away. Here one might recall Pierre Bourdieu's words on the conditions that incline people to "make a virtue of necessity":

> Because the dispositions durably inculcated by objective conditions ... engender aspirations and practices objectively compatible with those objective requirements, the most improbable practices are excluded, either totally without examination, as *unthinkable*, or at the cost of the *double negation* which inclines agents to make a virtue of necessity, that is, to refuse what is anyway refused and to love the inevitable.[21] (Emphasis original.)

In other words, the sense of inevitability does not strictly require but nevertheless tends to push people to learn to be satisfied with and rationalize what is inevitable. This is demonstrated in Figure 15, which reveals that respondents with higher monthly household incomes were more dissatisfied with the hospital. The more able they were to go to other hospitals in other provinces, the less inclined they were to be satisfied with the healthcare provided in Hakkâri.

In other words, when people in Hakkâri city go to Hakkâri Public Hospital, they do not do so because they specifically prefer that hospital over other private or public hospitals or because it has been suggested to them by their friends or neighbors. Rather, they go there because they have no choice.

To conclude, we can speak of a serious trust problem as an important determinant of Hakkârians' experience with healthcare provision at the central hospital and thus—reasonably by extension—in the province generally. No less than half of the respondents have serious doubts about the fundamentals of healthcare provision in Hakkâri, as shown here in regard to the medical capabilities of the doctors and accuracy of medical tests and analyses. These doubts considerably determined the level of patient satisfaction, as illustrated below with a focus on the daily exhibition and operation or the practice of the distrust.

5.2.1.2 Distrust at Work

Nicola Berry describes a seemingly strange case of patient dissatisfaction in Guatemala. Poor and ethnically excluded Mayan people there are inclined to see even routine biomedical procedures of hospitals as disregarding them, which they frame as "not being attended [to]."[22] Refusing explanations that just cite ignorance, Berry's ethnographic research shows that the not-being-attended-to discourse "recapitulates a significant trope in the historical relationship between poor Mayans and the predominantly Ladino Guatemalan state," a relationship that "has been marked by the exclusion of the Maya ... from land, legal, political, educational, and economic resources." That is why, Berry concludes, "patients and their families arrive [at] the hospital primed to be suspicious rather than trusting, worried that doctors are gatekeepers rather than aides."[23]

There is a clear parallel between the patient dissatisfaction in Guatemala with that unearthed here in Hakkâri. Hakkârians' belief that their lives are

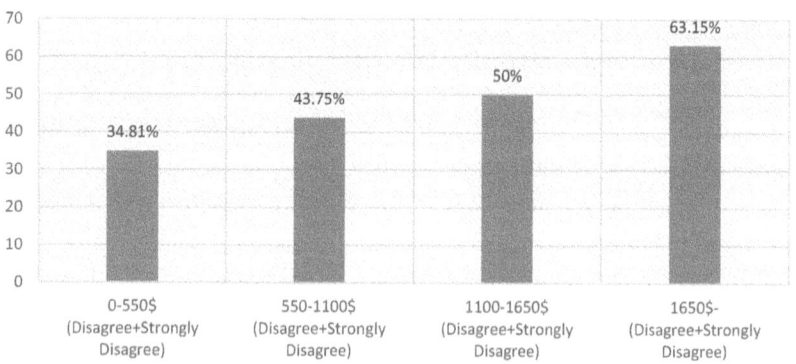

Figure 15. Responses to the Statement "I am Fairly Satisfied with the Healthcare Provision of Hakkâri Public Hospital."
Note: 1 USD = c. 1.8 TL (May 2013).

The Persistence of Patient Dissatisfaction as a Mass Phenomenon | 191

insufficiently valued by the Turkish state guides their experiences with the medical establishment as a prejudgment. It is not a groundless prejudice but rather a sort of inclination to see and respond to—thus prejudge—things as conditioned by a ready understanding based on past experiences. And indeed, this does appear to have been one of the main reasons for the persistence of Hakkârians' dissatisfaction with their healthcare provision at the end of the AKP's first decade in power.

Two local witnesses may be called on to testify to this. The first was a specialist who had been working for a few months at the Hakkari Public Hospital when we met; the second was a member of staff who had previously worked in the patient rights unit of the hospital and hence was familiar with the patients' psychology and issues involved. They both confirmed the fragility of patients and the underlying trust problem. The specialist spoke thus:

> Hakkârians have a problem. They have a prejudice—"The state does not send doctors to us, it doesn't like us," etc.—so one should avoid approaching them in a rough manner. I can even say that if you're not relaxed, they're likely to suspect that an ethnic problem lies behind your manner and actions. They're very fragile. The first thing the patients need is to feel they're appreciated. These people have experienced many things. If you don't give food to a child for a long time and finally give him food, he'll still be angry at you. The people are like this child. Even in a simple case, they easily burst with anger.

One may note here that despite her sympathetic stance toward the patients, the specialist still could not avoid a patronizing perspective and saw the patients' responses as a *childish* anger. The former employee of the patient rights unit spoke thus:

> The people used to get health services under very difficult conditions. They used to be transferred [to other provinces]. Sometimes five or six patients would be transferred by a single ambulance. Following the construction of the new building and the appointment of doctors, we now have an unprecedented number of doctors. Starting with the arrival of these doctors, the infrastructure [of the hospital] has begun to change. In this transition period, some citizens still hold onto unconscious feelings ... The disappearance of this prejudice may take some time, for the people have just begun to get these services. Some technological devices have only been bought recently. Attempts are being made to deal with the shortcomings. During this process, there may still be patients who cannot overcome their prejudices resulting from their past [experiences] and who say, "What can one expect from the services provided here?"

Due to their entrenched prejudgments built on past experiences with the medical establishment and the state, patients often did not regard the hospitals of Hakkâri as adequately endowed with the necessary medical facilities or consider the doctors there to be sufficiently experienced to deliver a proper health service. Leaving minor diseases aside, the Hakkâri medical facilities, in the eyes of many patients, were not places where they expected to receive good treatment for their diseases. The low status of the hospitals and doctors in Hakkâri in the eyes of Hakkârians, and specifically of middle and upper-class Hakkârians, was manifest in their lack of philanthropic contribution to the hospitals.

There is a panel on the wall of the ground floor of Hakkâri Public Hospital, the top of which bears the heading, "The Philanthropists Making Donations to Our Hospital." Making donations to hospitals is important in the philanthropic tradition of Turkey, and it is not surprising to see such a panel on the wall. This panel has been there since 2008, and one might expect to see the names of at least a dozen or half a dozen local philanthropists on the panel. But there were none. The panel had remained empty. Presumably, the panel was hung on the wall not so much to honor those who had made contributions as to encourage possible future donors. There had been some donations made to the hospital, like wheelchairs donated by a rotary club from Istanbul, but Hakkârians had refrained from doing so.

Eventually, in 2013, the names of two donors were added to the panel. According to a provincial Director of Health, the main reason for these donations was not a noticeable change in the local stance toward the medical establishment but rather a personal friendship between the General Secretary of the Hakkâri Public Hospitals Union and the two businessmen. A similar situation applied to Yüksekova Public Hospital. Still, nobody had made a donation there by 2013.

If "it is through philanthropy that people affirm what they believe is in the public good and what they think contributes to it,"[24] the lack of philanthropic contribution to the public hospitals of Hakkâri may be taken as a signifier of the low status of public hospitals in the eyes of the people there. For who *would* donate to an institution that is not well regarded? The words of a middle-aged Hakkârian trade-unionist, who was born and bred in Hakkâri city, spoke volumes:

> No patient's companion here has any hope that his patient will recover when he takes them to hospital ... So many go to the hospital for a headache or flu, yet I have never seen a patient expecting to get real treatment for a more serious disease in Hakkâri Public Hospital. In the case of a surgical operation, we instantly begin to think of alternatives like Ankara or Van ... Let's assume

that I am a rich man and my child is sick. If he undergoes an operation here and recovers, furnishing a [hospital] room may come to my mind. Yet because I do not have any such expectation from the hospital, [that] doesn't come to my mind.

This low expectation of obtaining good quality treatment in the hospitals of Hakkâri caused many responses during medical encounters; the most frequently, these took the form of patient transfer demands. Many patients would want their treatment in Van, Ankara, Istanbul, or Antalya instead of in Hakkâri. For them, going to the hospital and being examined by specialists in Hakkâri was no more than the first step of a bureaucratic procedure in order to be treated elsewhere. Almost all the specialists at Hakkâri, Yüksekova, and Şemdinli Public Hospitals complained about the insistent transfer demands of patients and the difficulty of convincing them that the treatment would be given just as well with the available facilities and staff in the local hospital. The words of the following two specialists in Hakkâri should be regarded as a general reflection of the experiences of doctors there.

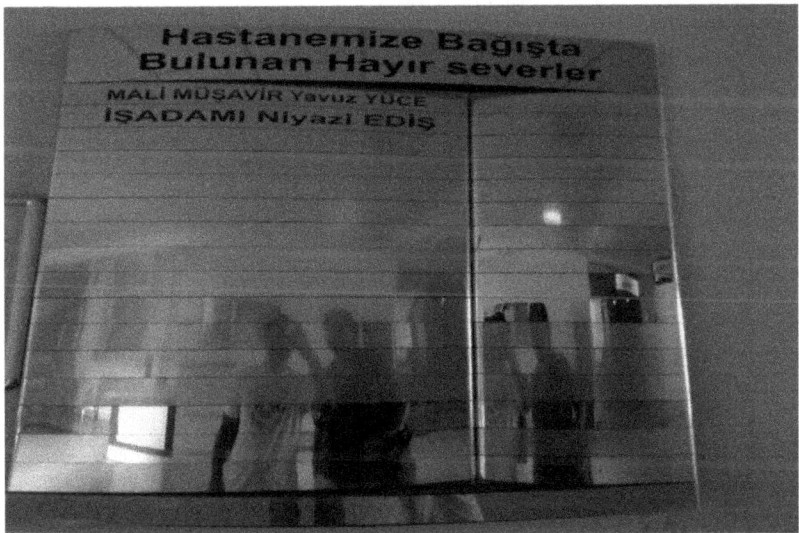

Figure 16. Hakkâri Public Hospital Wall Panel: "The Philanthropists Making Donations to Our Hospital."

Specialist, Yüksekova Public Hospital:

> My problem is that they demand to be transferred to Ankara and Van. Usually, I try not to transfer them and solve their problems here. I transfer the patients only in clear cases of need. They act as if I can't do anything myself and exist here just to transfer the patients to Van where, they think, everything's going to be better, and they'll recover. In this respect, I have a problem convincing the patients.

Specialist, Hakkâri Public Hospital:

> A: It's the city that's decisive. Being in Hakkâri and being examined in a hospital in Hakkâri decreases patient satisfaction to a large extent. They think the state either doesn't provide qualified healthcare to Hakkâri or does it reluctantly, yet the service provided in Ankara and Istanbul is very well qualified ... There's such prejudice. It's impossible to overcome it. [People think that] a patient dying here dies because of many mistakes, but a patient dying in Izmir for the same reason dies despite all necessary treatment being given. You try to improve the conditions of the intensive care unit, bring mechanical ventilators, try to ensure sanitation, improve the conditions of the operating room, etc. Yet, it's very difficult to change the prejudice of the people.
> Q: Do you get many transfer demands from the patients?
> A: Of course! Of course! They always want to go to Ankara or Istanbul, but I only transfer patients when there's a shortage of technical facilities.

The intensity of the transfer demands can be further appreciated through the testimony of the Vice Director of the Provincial Directorate of Social Security Institute, who testified to the extent of the prejudgment of the patients and pressure on the doctors:

> When patients are transferred, we fund the expenses for the transportation, the needs of the patient's companion, and the patient's outpatient treatment. One of the specialists [in Hakkâri Public Hospital] would never mention the reasons for the transfers in the transfer reports of the patients he transferred to other provinces. We informed him that unless he gave reasons for transfers, we wouldn't be able to fund the patients' transfer expenses. Then he said that indeed all of these operations can be performed here, but the patients force him to transfer them, so we suggested that in those cases, he should enter the reason for the transfer as "data analysis and treatment."

In spite of the tangible improvement in the medical infrastructure and health workforce, patients in Hakkâri still insisted on being transferred to other provinces for treatment that could be perfectly well performed in hospitals in Hakkâri. This preference did not constitute an objective evaluation of the positive and negative aspects of the current state of medical services available at the local hospitals but was rather based on the local memory and people's residual impressions drawn from past experiences. Patients assumed that they would not receive the level of treatment in Hakkâri that they would in the western provinces.

In fact, the nature of the biomedical encounter is not one that easily allows patients to make an objective assessment of the available medical facilities and health workforce, as it is characterized by an asymmetry of information depriving them of the expertise necessary to make such judgments.[25] Under normal conditions, when a biomedical encounter in a clinical environment is not determined by dynamics stemming from outside this encounter, the gap between clinical experts and patients is expected to be bridged by the sense of trust called for by the wider trust in the power of biomedicine and expertise.[26] Trust is essential to the workings of the biomedical encounter[27]—as it is, indeed, to the workings of all expert systems of modernity characterized by similar asymmetries of information.[28] Therefore, the weakness of patient trust in a biomedical encounter in a clinical environment is a fundamental deficiency that disrupts its proper functioning, not a secondary lack and peripheral issue.

Insistent transfer demands were perhaps the most striking manifestation of patients' distrust of the medical establishment in Hakkâri, but they were not alone. The convictions of patients concerning the inadequacy of the facilities, specialists, and other health staff determined their approach to these hospitals in other ways, too. The following examples show how the preset convictions of Hakkârians that their lives were not regarded as worthy of care and respect by the state filled the void left by a lack of sufficient knowledge about actual medical procedures and thus (re)produced dissatisfaction. An example is the lack of knowledge of the patients concerning the speed of the medical procedures.

Although many medical procedures, from tests to appointments for MR, tomography, and time spent to be examined by medical specialists, were quicker in the hospitals of Hakkâri than in the crowded hospitals of Turkish metropolises, patients still routinely complained about the speed of the process and adopted a demanding rather than a satisfied response. The case below is recounted by a medical specialist from Hakkâri Public Hospital who had also worked in its management for some months.

Specialist, Hakkâri Public Hospital:

> You can't compare the West [of Turkey] with here. You finish all procedures in a day in Hakkâri. For instance, you can't get a CT scan done in the West for months. Once I sent a girl for a scan, and she came back to my examination room saying, "I'm a student. I was told to come for a CT scan in the afternoon. Is it possible to have the appointment earlier?" Can you believe it? I mean, they're not aware of the favors [we do for them].

Complaints concerning the speed of procedures in the cardiology unit are another instance of this demanding stance. The frustration, bewilderment even, of this next doctor is apparent.

Specialist, Administrator, Hakkâri Public Hospital:

> We have the facilities of big hospitals in cardiology. We have an ECG, an exercise machine. We also have a cardiologist examining patients. A patient in Hakkâri can undergo all these cardiology procedures on the same day. His blood is drawn; its analysis and other cardiology procedures finish on the same day. You can't complete the same process in Istanbul for several months. In Istanbul, you get an appointment for tomography and ultrasound several weeks later. All this proceeds quite fast here, but we still get responses like people asking why an ultrasound requested in the morning was performed in the afternoon. There's constant dissatisfaction. We're not appreciated in spite of all our efforts.

It may be argued that the complaints might not be based on preset convictions and rather resulted from a lack of knowledge on the part of the patients concerning the speed of the same procedures in Istanbul and other cities. Yet this does not explain why the lack of knowledge automatically led the patients to make a negative assumption about the already assumed difference between Hakkâri and the West and led the patients to feel that they were being neglected.

Another, very interesting case exhibits the theoretical proposition that unless the principle structuring the symbolic mediation by which people make sense of facts changes, facts alone cannot alter the principle and may be rather regarded as further evidence confirming the principle which they actually confute.[29] That is, unless the conviction of the patients that their lives are not regarded as worthy changes, contrary facts can still be taken as evidence confirming the conviction.

The following dialogue took place in the waiting lounge of a family health center in Bağlar, a neighborhood of Hakkâri city mostly populated by village evacuees. A resident in the neighborhood—a village evacuee—was asked if he thought that x-ray, ultrasound, MR, and tests take a shorter time in hospitals in western provinces than in Hakkâri. In fact—and unlike many respondents biased by their prejudgments—this man did know that medical tests and procedures were actually carried out in a shorter time in Hakkâri Public Hospital. Yet, after indicating this, he felt compelled to add that it was "most probably because they do not do them properly." That the medical procedures and tests took a shorter time in Hakkâri was, for him, not counter-evidence confuting his conviction but rather proof that reinforced it. It was beyond his imagination that a medical procedure could be performed competently as well as more quickly in Hakkâri than in the West.

Combined with such entrenched prejudgments, patients' lack of knowledge about medical procedures produced constant dissatisfaction that extended to entirely ordinary aspects of medical procedures. Patients might easily find some things offensive and degrading, even in the routine functioning of standard treatments. The complaint by the owner of a small grocery in Hakkâri city about the "inexperienced" doctors of Hakkâri Public Hospital provides a good example of this. After complaining about the doctors at the hospital, who "just prescribe medicine and then brush patients off," he turned his attention to the "inexperienced" doctors, thus:

> And the doctors in the ER don't know anything. They call their friends and ask what they should do for a patient. Can you then trust the knowledge of such a doctor?

What this man regarded as evidence of the inexperience of ER doctors was probably a standard peer consultation procedure to gain the input of other views, knowledge, and experience, which is an essential part of ER work. When a doctor in ER needs or judges such support to be appropriate, they call the specialist on standby duty and inform them about the patient to get advice or, in more serious cases, immediately ask them to come to ER to make the necessary medical intervention. An inexperienced doctor may tend to call on more support than one with many years of service, of course, but no ER doctor can be expected to give top-quality treatment to all emergency patients themselves due to the range of medical issues presented. A request for support—professionally, a "second opinion"—indicates a competent decision-making process. In the eyes of the grocer, however, the ER doctor calling his colleague only reinforced the notion that the doctors appointed to Hakkâri Public Hospital lacked knowledge and experience—with the implication that they were incompetent.

The following case also exemplifies how patients lacking knowledge about medical procedures can be easily led to mistaken conclusions by long-held convictions and negative assumptions.

Specialist, Hakkâri Public Hospital:

> A consultation was demanded from ER for a patient with a leg injury. A relative of the patient came straight into my room and told me that I had to go and examine this person. I was already about to go to ER for the patient. Because I was the only orthopedist examining patients, I said to him, "Give me your name. I'll come to ER in a few minutes." He repeated: "Look at me. You have to take care of this patient. We have rights and things."

In this instance, the doctor's promise to examine the patient in the ER within a few minutes did not convince the patient's companion and was instead perceived as an excuse employed to avoid examining the patient. The patient's companion acted as if the doctor was not willing to examine his patient, as if the examination was an issue for negotiation in which threats and claims might be a valid and successful means of forcing the issue.

A sense of unworthiness grounded in historical relations with the state reproduced dissatisfaction not only by filling the void left by patients' lack of knowledge about medical procedures but also by paving the way for misunderstandings. This could develop from communication difficulties arising through language differences, especially between local Kurdish patients who did not know Turkish well, and Turkish health staff. The experience of a Turkish nurse from Yüksekova Public Hospital provides an example of this.

Nurse, Yüksekova Public Hospital:

> Once when I told the companion of a patient to get their file and then see me [*Dosya çıkart gel*], he interpreted it as me expelling him from the hospital [*Seni hastaneden çıkarıyorum*], which caused some trouble for me.

This misunderstanding was due to the patient's poor command of Turkish, which resulted in his inability to distinguish different meanings of the same verb (*çıkartmak* for issuance [of a form, document, etc.] was taken as *çıkartmak* for expel [evacuate, etc.]). Yet this explanation does not completely account for the misunderstanding since a patient for whom being expelled by a nurse from a hospital during a routine procedure for no obvious reason would be found incredible would not have thought that they actually were being expelled—a misunderstanding would be assumed and the communication checked. Thus, this supposed, completely unreasonable expulsion was not assumed to be incredible at all. On the contrary, it was very much believed, hence responded to.

Developing the general argument of this section, one has to conclude that this individual felt more like a Kurdish person being mistreated by a Turkish state employee than a patient. The situation was similar in other examples when patients did not fully appreciate the service provided or felt impelled to claim their rights. Beneath the discontent and assertion and misunderstanding was the conviction among Hakkârians of their unworthiness in the eyes of the state.

5.2.1.3 The Intricate Relationship between Patient Dissatisfaction, Kurdishness, and Lack of Trust

The conviction of the local people that their lives were relatively unimportant to the state structured patients' relationships with and (re)produced dissatisfaction with the medical establishment. The ever-present "Kurdish issue" would tend to mediate this relationship in various, complicated ways but promote dissatisfaction in all cases. For many Hakkârians, the acts supposed as a disrespect directed at their bodies (their physical, in this case, medical needs) were not unconnected from the disrespect shown to their Kurdishness. In fact, the former was often taken simply an expression of the latter.

When people were asked about healthcare provision in the province, it was quite common for them to start discussing the human cost of the state violence in the province to make their point about how poorly Hakkârians were treated in general—like the patient in the family health center in Merzan who, when asked a question about patient satisfaction with the health services of Hakkâri Public Hospital, took out his wallet and showed me a headshot photo of his deceased father. As a shepherd in Yüksekova, he had been executed by soldiers in 1995. The inseparability for many Hakkârians of the lack of respect—or violation and plain abuse—shown to their identities and to their bodies was nowhere more clearly manifested than in the functioning of the brand new Hakkâri Public Hospital as a metaphor for the reformist Kurdish policies of the AKP.

The terms and words used to criticize Hakkâri Public Hospital—"The hospital is a good building, but it's empty inside," and suchlike—were precisely those used to question the sincerity and intentions of the government's reformist Kurdish policy. The general opinion encountered in Hakkâri was that the Kurdish Opening sounded fine, but really it was a hollow gesture. Through the distinction between the building of the hospital, which seemed to be good, and its usefulness, which was not, Hakkârians expressed their well-established belief that little had substantially changed, that AKP policies were just words and appearances, ultimately empty and devoid of real meaning. They remained unworthy in the eyes of the state—primarily, as Kurds.

The first Rector of the University of Hakkâri was much concerned with the problems of the city and province and paid attention to my research examining one of its weightiest problems. Once, during a social activity organized by the university, he called me to his side to hear my findings and talk them over. I shared with him the experiences of a medical specialist from Şemdinli Public Hospital.

Specialist, Şemdinli Public Hospital:

> They [patients] don't realize who they're talking to. I mean, they think a specialist in Hakkâri is nothing, and a GP in Hakkâri is worse than nothing. This is the logic established in their minds. One even said that if I were a good doctor, I wouldn't have been exiled here from Istanbul! Not all, but most of the patients think like this. They think, "She's come here; she isn't a good [doctor] then. If she were, she'd have stayed in Van or Istanbul." They have this logic and so are against us. And they're ready to make anything into a problem . . .

Emphasizing the patient's accusation that she would not have been exiled from Istanbul if she were a good doctor, this specialist underlined how deeply the conviction that the state does not value them is rooted in the minds of so many Hakkârians and how difficult it was to overcome this conviction. The Rector's response was somewhat mechanical, perhaps reflecting his approach as a physicist: "This conviction can be corrected if—and only if—well-qualified healthcare is provided for years, equivalent to the duration of the poor services in the past that has ended in this conviction."

The reality on the ground was, however, somewhat more complex than that depicted by this developmentalist-linear point of view, which somewhat naively assumed that a steady provision of decent healthcare would nullify deeply held beliefs in the long run. What was not taken into consideration in this assumption was the ethnopolitical attachment to Kurdishness as a variable restructuring the lens through which Hakkârians made sense of the healthcare provisioning and other public services in Hakkâri. The view most widely subscribed to by Hakkârians, that their lives were relatively little valued by the state, led them to read the shortcomings of healthcare provision in the province as more or less related to the political disrespect for their Kurdish identity.

This was evident in the following conversation I shared with an agency worker in a public institution. Let me add that the following interviewee was not one who adhered to her Kurdish identity; she even avoided speaking Kurdish with her daughters in order to prevent them from failing at school, where the lessons were taught in Turkish.

Agency worker in a public institution (Hakkârian female, mid-30s):

> A: There's no treatment ... Our doctors are very bad. We're not happy with them. Again and again, we get the same medicine. They prescribe medicine and painkillers and then brush us off. This isn't treatment ... We complain that our doctors are very bad. They're very, very bad. They don't even examine the patients.
> Q: But also, you have many doctors now compared to the past?
> A: Yes, but they don't seem to know anything. They just prescribe medicine and brush us off.
> Q: Why do they do that?
> A: Probably they think that Hakkârians don't know anything and say, "Who cares? Just prescribe and get rid of them!" Hakkâri has a bad reputation as an unimportant and bad place. It's not. Yes, sometimes our children throw stones, but what can we do? Hakkâri isn't a bad place; it's a good place. They [doctors] think that Hakkâri is a bad place and Hakkârians are bad people.

As indicated in her reference to the children throwing stones—often at the police in demonstrations—this woman saw the root of the doctors' negligence in the reputation of the city as a "bad place," which demonstrated the lack of value afforded the lives of ordinary people and resulted in a political criminalization. And this relatively (by local standards) unpoliticized Kurdish woman was not an exception with an extreme, marginal stance. An employee of the patient rights unit at a hospital in Hakkâri, someone who was familiar with patient complaints and the local psychology, confirmed the prevalence of this conception. In fact, this person also partly shared it, as can be seen in the following exchange.

Employee at a patient rights unit (Hakkârian):

> Because patients lacked many rights for years, this impression among the patients has come into being: "We can't get a quality service because we're Kurdish." When there's a queue, they immediately begin to think in this way. Aren't they right to some extent? Maybe it's a bit better now, but it was really so in the past. So the patients are really anxious ... Almost all the complaints coming to me are similar: "I went in the room, but because I couldn't speak Turkish fluently, the doctor didn't want to listen to me. He prescribed a medicine and then brushed me off," or "Just I was about to enter the room, the doctor

warned me to wait outside." The doctor is right to do so because there is another patient in the room. Yet patients think that something bad is being done.

What would otherwise probably be treated as a doctor's distance, aloofness, and general lack of concern would easily be regarded as evidence of a deeper depreciating attitude. There were two different ways in which Hakkârians linked neglect to attitudes about their Kurdishness. One of these ways was captured in the charge, "You do this, because we are Kurdish," as reported by a specialist in a tone of some anger and astonishment:

> Even in a small case, if you do not meet the expectations and demands of the patients, you can easily hear the accusation that "You do this because we are Kurdish."

The perception is very clear in this response: as arms of the Turkish state, which does not have respect for the Kurdish identity, doctors deliberately do not extend their attention to Hakkârians and are not concerned with their well-being. Patients identify doctors with the state and their bodies with their identity. This is the colonial moment of the doctor-patient encounter in Hakkâri; in the words of Frantz Fanon, "The doctor always appears as a link in the colonialist network, as a spokesman for the occupying power."[30] In other words, in the accusation of "You do this because we are Kurdish," the doctor-patient encounter is more or less a replica of the colonizer and colonized. The following case is typical.

ER Doctor, Hakkâri Public Hospital:

> It was 10 or 11 in the evening, and I had examined more than 300 patients. I felt fuddled ... Anyway, an old couple arrived. From what I remember, the woman said there was a pain in her arm. I asked her how long it had been there, and she said ten or fifteen days. I asked whether the pain was intolerable at that moment. "No," she said. There was a big queue at that time. I lost control and began to shout at her: "Is this the time to come here for an arm which has ached with pain for fifteen days?" Then her husband told me I was oppressing them because they were Kurdish. I tried to explain that it had nothing to do with their Kurdishness; it was about my tiredness and work stress.

The woman's husband did not perceive the rough response of the ER doctor as an impolite and rude response of this particular doctor at that particular time. Rather, he generalized the encounter as an instance exposing the broader ethnopolitical violence employed toward Kurds. He identified the shouting ER doctor with the Turkish state and himself and his wife with Kurdishness.

The following case, in which the father of the patient accused doctors of collaborating with policemen, is another example of patients' sense of having been openly discriminated against due to their Kurdish identity.

ER Doctor, Yüksekova Public Hospital:

Q: Does the social tension in the city have any impact on doctor-patient encounters?
A: Usually, patients are polite, but there are some patients ... There was hematoma in the haunch of a child, so the child had some pain. I called the orthopedist. He came, examined the child, and gave his treatment. The father of the child was saying at that time that he wasn't relieving the pain. "My child is getting worse. Doctors and policemen are in it together. You don't do anything if you can help it." The child had been injured in a demonstration.

It should be added, however, that this was a more extreme case and not the usual way in which Hakkârians referred to doctors' attitudes toward their Kurdishness. A minority, and even then only sometimes, in the crowded atmosphere of ER or during treatment and examination of injured or arrested activists, might be led by the idea that Turkish doctors rendered their anti-Kurdish resentments into an active negative attitude toward patients, "collaborated with policemen," or shouted at patients because they were Kurdish. Figure 17 illustrates the extent to which the questionnaire respondents agreed with the statement that this type of thing would sometimes occur. It was a minority, clearly, but nevertheless a sizable one.

Fully one third of questionnaire respondents expressed the view that they were discriminated against because they were Kurdish. Alternatively, viewing the glass as half-full, three in five expressed the opposite. How should this be interpreted? I would suggest that the dual policy of the AKP, to value and recognize Kurds as service- beneficiaries and devalue and criminalize them as members of an ethnopolitical community, required Hakkârians to rearticulate the terms of the relationship between their Kurdishness and dissatisfaction with the medical establishment. There was a rising awareness on the part of the local people at that time that they *somewhat* mattered to the state and were at least *visible* to the biopolitical eyes of the servant state, albeit not equally valued or visible. The dominant form by which Hakkârians related their dissatisfaction to Kurdishness at this time was guided by the assumption that they did count in the eyes of the state, but not greatly so.

More concretely, one can legitimately argue that a Hakkârian referring to his Kurdishness while complaining of health system around 2010 was most probably talking about their doubts, protests, and demands concerning what they regarded as a *second-class* citizen treatment and responding to *implicit* forms of exclusion, not to the total and deliberate deprivation of health services, direct insults, and offenses. While, for instance, only a third of my questionnaire respondents agreed with the restricted but still sharp expression that "some manners and acts of doctors and nurses . . . sometimes" led them to think that they were not paid satisfactory attention because they were Kurdish, the majority agreed with a similar but more nuanced expression—albeit only just over half—that the doctors adopted a "markedly better" approach to patients with good Turkish language skills (Figure 18).

A few further cases can help to illustrate this understanding that patients complaining about health services with reference to their Kurdishness were articulating their dissatisfaction in relative terms (by comparing their service with that provided to Turks) rather than in absolute terms. The first case discussed below concerns the personal experiences and observations of an ancillary worker employed on minimum wage at the University of Hakkâri. Born and raised in Hakkâri city, she was a high school graduate from a lower-middle-class family, secular, and a moderate supporter of the Kurdish movement.

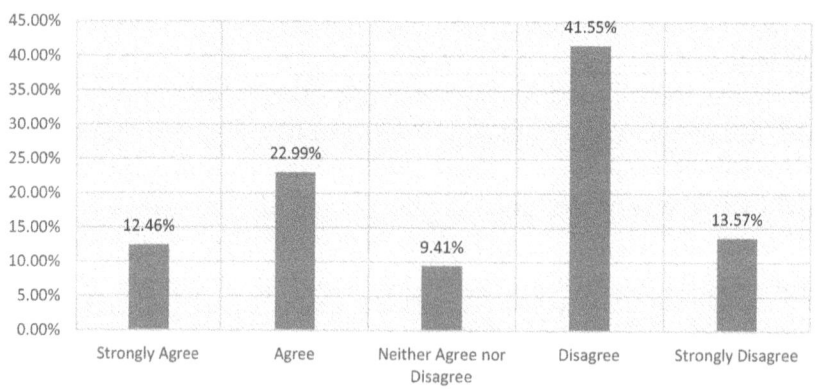

Figure 17. Responses to the Statement "Some of the Behavior and Actions of the Doctors and Nurses at Hakkâri Public Hospital Sometimes Lead Me to Think that I am not Paid Satisfactory Attention because I am Kurdish."

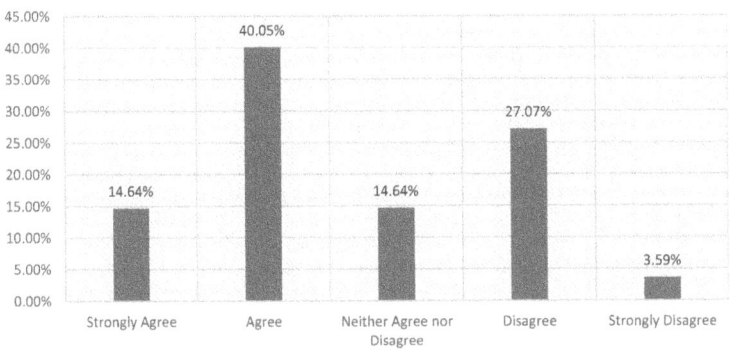

Figure 18. Responses to the Statement "Doctors in Hakkâri Public Hospital Approach Patients Whose Turkish is Better in a Markedly Better Way."

According to her, Kurds were no longer deprived of health services or the victims of hostile acts of health staff due to their Kurdishness. Yet, on the other hand, she was strongly convinced that it was their Kurdish identity and language that caused Kurds to be still deprived of the full attention that Turks and Turkish-speaking patients enjoyed.

Ancillary worker, University of Hakkâri (Hakkârian, female, late 20s):

Q: Is the language issue a problem?
A: Not now, but in the past, it was ... In the past, a midwife might hit a pregnant woman. But even today, if you speak Turkish without any accent, you will get more attention. This is guaranteed. Or if you start a quarrel, you will get more attention, so if you wait quietly and without picking a fight with the doctors or speak Kurdish, their attention decreases.

The complaint by another Hakkârian worker of the university about what he perceived as discriminatory treatment was another manifestation of the protest against having the status of a second-class citizen due to his Kurdish identity. This person was from a village in the central (Hakkâri city) district inhabited by the Jirki tribe, which for many years had cooperated with the state as paramilitaries against the PKK; he was a moderate supporter of the Kurdish movement, used to work for several years as waiter in restaurants in tourist centers, like Antalya, and was employed at the university on the minimum wage.

Worker, University of Hakkâri (Hakkârian, male, late 20s):

> All the doctors coming from outside are prejudiced toward Hakkârians. I personally experienced it. Once, I took my child to the pediatrician in the hospital. The woman behind me in the queue was the wife of a specialist [sergeant] with her child. Because her child was crying so much, I let her go before me. [The doctor] didn't pay even a millionth of the attention to my child that she paid to this woman's child. She just didn't pay the same attention to my child. The doctors behave quite differently with those they see are Turkish.

Again, this man was not a partisan of the Kurdish movement, although also again, he did not conceal his sympathies toward it. In such cases, while referring to Kurdishness when making sense of what they regarded as second-class citizen treatment, people did not do so in the reductionist manner of someone seeking to relate all issues to the cause. They were not fixed on a single perspective, ethnicists who would assume an anti-state stance in all cases; rather, growing up with the daily experience of sovereign violence and indirect state racism was just a fact of life that colored their view of the world.

Another example is similar to those cited above but with a nuance that sheds light on a different aspect of the dominant mode of the articulation of Kurdishness through dissatisfaction with the medical establishment. This involves a handcraft instructor in an interview conducted in the small training center in a Hakkâri city neighborhood largely populated by village evacuees, like her.

Handcraft instructor (village evacuee, female, mid-40s):

> Why do they send inexperienced doctors to Hakkâri? They send inexperienced doctors here; they become professors here and then leave. Why do we have to go to Ankara and Van? [. . .] There are too many cesarean deliveries in Hakkâri. Why do they do cesareans after the second delivery? My mother is eighty years old. Maybe she's gone to seventy deliveries so far [as a traditional midwife], and none of these babies had a health problem. Maybe you heard that the head of a baby was detached [during delivery in the hospital] some time ago. Arms of babies are dislocated. Why do such things take place?
>
> Q: Do you mean that you suspect that these kinds of things occur because of your Kurdishness?
>
> We certainly do. There was a specialist [sergeant]. He used to be in [military] operations. His wife was pregnant. We went to the hospital with his wife. The doctor said to her, "Because you haven't given birth for a long time, I'll take the baby with a cesarean operation." But the woman didn't want a cesarean. Later, her husband came and talked with the doctor, and in the end, the woman had a normal birth. That's when I suspected that

they [doctors] simply just practice on our women. What would have been the case if the specialist's wife was one of us?

The instructor complained about what she regarded as discriminatory treatment that valued Turkish bodies over Kurdish bodies and used the latter as grounds for practice and experiment. Up to that point, her testament had followed that of the more usual unsatisfied patients who argue that, as Kurds, they are given less attention by doctors and generally receive poorer treatment than Turkish patients. But then further comments exhibited an uneasy psychology, a nagging concern culminating in the general question, "Why do such things take place?"

The questions and comparisons raised included a suspicion that Kurds' lives were deliberately risked, treated as doctors' experimental subjects, as medical learning experiences, and so damaged by the state and its health staff. The question about cesarean operations after second deliveries, for instance, was a reference to the circulating doubts that the state aimed to decrease the Kurdish fertility rate (itself based on the growing proportion of Kurds in the population due to their higher birthrate, which had ethnopolitical implications that did prompt some alarmism among Turkish nationalists).[31] Similarly, the instructor did not seem to be convinced that Kurdish babies injured in deliveries in hospitals were harmed by mistake.

This response may be likened to the "You do this because we are Kurdish" response, yet it was different in that the idea that Kurds' lives were deliberately harmed was less an absolute conviction than a (perceived) possibility. The possibility was not strong, but it was an idea she was entertaining with reasons, a conjecture not to be totally dismissed. More generally, also, the people complaining about having been treated as second-class citizens in comparison to Turks due to their Kurdishness had a similar, more or less uneasy psychology. Ultimately, passive indifference to Kurdish bodies (the assumption upon which patients' criticism of second-class citizen treatment was based) and an active disrespect for Kurdish bodies (the assumption upon which the "You do this, because we are Kurdish" response was based) were not two irreconcilably distant stances.

The specific issue of sterilization in relation to vaccination was raised by a midwife who was local to Yüksekova.

Midwife, Yüksekova Health Post:

Q: Have you encountered resistance to the tetanus vaccine?
A: Being Kurdish has helped us. We are telling them in Kurdish that "I myself was vaccinated. You should be, too. It doesn't sterilize." Yet, as far

> as I remember, a woman in a village under the responsibility of Health Post 3 had a miscarriage. [The people] attributed it to the tetanus vaccine and decided to stop being vaccinated.

Just a single case of miscarriage by a woman who had been vaccinated could suffice to reverse the work of local Kurdish professionals and return them to their mindset of "You do this, because we are Kurdish." That is, the women were somewhat ready to be convinced that their lives were beginning to count in the eyes of the state and that the state might do something good for their health, but this development was still vulnerable, reversed by the kind of misfortune that could occur anyway during pregnancy.

5.2.1.4 Conclusions: Dissatisfaction as an Issue of Distrust and Distrust as a Haunting Specter

The words of the head of a pro-Kurdish ecological association and a radical leftist philosopher sum up the argument made in this section.

Head of Cilo Nature Association, Employee at Hakkâri Provincial Directorate of Food, Agriculture and Livestock (Yüksekova, early 50s):

> When it comes to the state, it is a panzer attacking you with a flag on it, a specialist [sergeant], and an armed special police team. I mean, we saw the state as a violent phenomenon. I remember that when the gendarmes came to our village ... Only two gendarmes were enough to gather all villagers and humiliate them ... Violence, violence, violence. However you make sense of it, this last thirty or forty years have accumulated many things in the minds of the people.

> The hospital is a real hospital. Its facilities are good, as well. When I went to [hospitals] in Ankara, I couldn't find the facilities there I find here ... What is missing right now is trust. That's our biggest problem right now; we cannot trust. We suspect they still want to Turkify us by using different methods. That's the biggest problem in our minds right now. It must be overcome. For this to happen, it [the state] needs to assure us.

> Our fragility is that. Is it honest or not? That's the biggest problem right now.

> The state in the minds of the citizens did not die out. There is a [feeling] that that state did not completely disappear, it may revive and come back.

Slavoj Žižek:

> There is no reality without the specter, the circle of reality can be closed only by means of an uncanny spectral supplement .... (what we experience as) reality

is not the "thing itself," it is always-already symbolized, constituted, structured by symbolic mechanisms—and the problem resides in the fact that symbolization ultimately always fails, that it never succeeds in fully "covering" the real, that it always involves some unsettled, unredeemed symbolic debt. This real (the part of reality that remains non-symbolized) returns in the guise of spectral apparitions ... What the specter conceals is not reality but its "primordially repressed," the irrepresentable X on whose "repression" reality itself is founded.[32]

It is unlikely that the head of the Cilo Nature Association would have been familiar with Žižek, of course, but his words on trust and Turkification provide an excellent exemplification of Žižek's argument on reality and specter with reference to the case of Hakkâri. For what better characterizes a specter than someone or something that did not really die and may be revived, to come back and haunt the living once again? Thus, the role of patients' convictions concerning the unworthiness of Kurdish lives in the eyes of the state in their dissatisfaction with health services provided in Hakkâri can be understood as such a haunting specter.[33]

Following this line of thought, the "X" that the AKP reformism of 2003–14 could not or at least did not succeed in burying was Turkish nationalism, the state in the minds of the citizens as the "panzer attacking," the "flag," the "specialist sergeant," and "armed special police team"; in short, the "violence, violence, violence." This reflects the distinction made between the pragmatist and normative aspects of nationalism as enacted by the AKP during this period.

The AKP pragmatically built on the heritage of Kemalist Turkish nationalism, yet it did not give it any place in its ideo-political perspective, the normative aspect of nationalism. Thus, the non-pronounced Turkish nationalism of the AKP—which still persisted in the avoidance of any effective interrogation of the ethnopolitical crimes committed by and in the name of the state, in the ongoing assimilationist policy carried out in public schools, and in the criminalization of Kurdish ethnopolitical claims and its actors—did indeed enable a "return in the guise of spectral apparitions."

Because the violent image of the state established in the minds of Hakkârians as a result of decades-long sovereign violence and indirect state racism did not dissipate completely during the reformist period. Thus, it was constantly lurking, liable at any moment to return in the spectral guise of distrust and continue to haunt the way Hakkârians related to and evaluated the medical establishment. Distrust of the intentions of the medical establishment, of the adequacy of the facilities of the medical establishment, and of the capabilities of the health staff was thus the "uncanny spectral supplement" of the reformed health services, provided in a context in which the new biopolitical emphasis placed on the worthiness of the lives of Hakkârians was not manifest in an explicit denial of Kemalist Turkish nationalism. As the head of Cilo Nature Association perceived, "What is missing ... right now is trust. That's our biggest problem right now; we cannot trust [the state]."

5.2.2 Dissatisfaction as Equal Citizenship

This examination of the persistence of patient dissatisfaction in Hakkâri during the period 2003–14 as a mass phenomenon has demonstrated that if one factor behind this was the widely subscribed conviction that Hakkârians' lives count for little in the eyes of the state, a conviction that had developed over years of sovereign violence and indirect state racism and was further reproduced by the sovereign violence of AKP-style Turkish nationalism, another factor was the refusal of Hakkârians to be degraded by this sovereign violence or indirect state racism.

By indicating the refusal to be degraded by the sovereign violence and indirect state racism, reference is made to the fact that a strong ethnopolitical consciousness had emerged in the previous 30 years, making the dehumanization of Kurdishness increasingly intolerable in the eyes of many Hakkârians. This means that, by 2003-2014, the identification of Kurdishness with backwardness or degeneration was no longer acceptable to them. The resistance had succeeded insofar as a mass self-consciousness or identity has been created.

In present-day Hakkâri by 2013, citizens were proud of their national identity. Babies were given Kurdish names by their parents; shopkeepers used Kurdish names for their shops; Kurdish colors, the yellow, red, and green (*kesk û sor û zer*), once forbidden, were now everywhere, from women's bridal gowns to the football jerseys of the Kurdistan national team worn by teenagers; Newroz, a politicized national festival among Kurds, was celebrated by tens of thousands of people wearing traditional Kurdish costumes; even songs played in weddings were full of praise for the PKK guerillas, Öcalan and Kurdistan; indeed, guerillas were regarded as heroes, and thousands of people would attend their funerals, etc.

Based on the arguments on the rehabilitating effects of anti-colonial struggles,[34] we can conclude that under the leadership of the PKK, Kurdishness has undergone its process of "self-valorization." The "self-valorization of labor" is a phrase coined by Antoni Negri to mean that the working-class struggle against capital is not only built on opposition as refusal and negation but also involves a positive moment in which laborers confirm their capacity to develop new ways of being autonomous from capital. Thus, the self-valorization of Kurdishness is used to capture the idea that the Kurdish struggle against the Turkish state has not only been about resisting Turkish nationalist oppression but also involved a self-constitution, a restoration and confirmation of the agency of Kurdishness.[35]

This is well demonstrated by the fact that the images people would recall from the pre-PKK period to compare and contrast it with the period following were characterized by a total lack of self-confidence, overwhelming fear, and impotence. The narrative of "only two gendarmes" gathering all the inhabitants of a village to line them up, torture, and beat them would be recounted endless times in different forms; "only the boot prints of gendarmes" would be enough to make people change their routes, and gendarmes used to use people as horses to cross a river or a brook.

This self-valorization of Kurdishness as a mood and way of seeing formed the background of a particular type of patient dissatisfaction in Hakkâri; it was what one might call a "citizenly dissatisfaction." It was citizen*ly* in the sense of citizen-like since it was the second-class nature of this status as a relative shortfall that spurred the discontent. This qualifies the assumed attitude as a dissatisfaction with healthcare provision in Hakkâri that referred to the citizenship status and right to healthcare, where the dissatisfaction with services in the province was built on a way of seeing inherent to the claim to "full and equal membership in a political community."[36]

The self-valorization of Kurdishness bestowed upon Hakkârians the self-confidence and sense of respectability to feel and act with and not despite their ethnic differences as full and equal members of society. It thus led them to a sense of full and equal entitlement to healthcare provision. The level and quality of healthcare to Hakkârians perceived themselves entitled was that of the healthcare provided in the relatively developed Turkish provinces in the west of the country, which was much closer to the level and quality of healthcare constitutionally promised to all citizens.

Because of the inherited and lived history, the process of self-valorization that Hakkârians had undergone left them hypersensitive to any shortfall, to the extent of perceiving what was not there, or not necessarily or obviously so. Thus, the patient dissatisfaction that developed in Hakkâri through the early 2000s as a citizenly one involved the sheer incapacity of health services there to sufficiently convince Hakkârians to think that they really were given the quality of treatment that they believed they deserved as full and equal members of society.

It is possible to identify two forms of citizenly patient dissatisfaction in Hakkâri at this time. One was less rhetorical, less abstract, and more subaltern, while the other was more middle-class and informed by the formal language of obligations, entitlements, and the rights of citizenship. These two forms were not always clearly separated from each other, but an elaboration on the distinction affords further insight.

5.2.2.1 Comparison in Space, Not in Time

That a person has to go from Hakkâri to Ankara to have angiography is something shameful. Is not Hakkâri a province like Ankara and Diyarbakır? Why don't they send the device here? Why do I have to look for it somewhere else?

Headman of Keklikpınar neighborhood, Hakkâri city

As stated, it was not unusual in Hakkâri for people dissatisfied with health services to express this with reference to the quality of healthcare provision in Ankara, Istanbul, and sometimes Van. Comparisons made between the experienced "professor doctors" of the western metropolises and the inexperienced, "internship doctors" of Hakkâri "who can't understand disease and [would] put off" patients; contrasts between the other, fully equipped hospitals and those of Hakkâri "whose inside is empty" were frequent; the reality of failed surgical operations in Hakkâri was routinely set against the imaginary of successful treatments in the West where the hospital staff were good-humored and polite as opposed to the "flighty, big-headed, shouting" staff in Hakkâri.

That is to say, the plane in which dissatisfied Hakkârians compared the level and quality of healthcare provision in Hakkâri was spatial rather than temporal. This means they did not compare the actual current situation of healthcare provision in Hakkâri with the poor services provided in the province in the pre-AKP period but with the much better health services provided in other, especially western, provinces of the country—be this higher standard grounded in experience, gossip, or fantasy.

Does this insight merit further interrogation and analysis? One would think that the answer should be a resounding "Yes" if we are to subscribe to critical remarks on how central the denial of coevalness is to the colonizing instincts of modern forms of power, and if we are to situate the comparative intolerance of Hakkârians to any persisting (albeit gradually diminishing) shortcomings of healthcare provision in the tension between the anti-colonial insistence on the "now," on the one hand, and the "not yet" of historicism and narratives of "becoming," on the other.[37]

As Doreen Massey argues, the fundamental maneuver of modernity is to render "coexisting spatial heterogeneity as a single temporal series."[38] By this stratagem, "coexisting heterogeneity is rendered as place in the historical queue"[39] or reduced to the "waiting room of history."[40] In other words, institutions of modernity, including the nation-state, are built on the "denial of coevalness,"[41] that is, the denial of "contemporaneity yet the possibility of difference"[42] and the "affirmation of difference as distance"[43] in time.

Adopting comparisons in space instead of comparisons in time, the respondents and informants contributing to the research presented here can reasonably be said to have occupied a position in which they posited their coevalness with those living in Turkish metropolises served with more developed health institutions and more experienced health staff. By adopting comparisons in space instead of across time, these Hakkârians refused to be given a place in the historical queue of a development narrative. They refused to be addressed as citizens-in-the-making who should compare the old and new periods, realize the progress, and thus appreciate the actual quality of healthcare provision by tolerating some persisting shortcomings. They rather appeared as already-citizens claiming the right to qualified healthcare provision equally and now.

That this comparative perspective was facilitated by an engagement with the idea of equal citizenship is evident in the following dialogue between two University of Hakkâri security guards, both Hakkârians. There was only one security guard at the room at the entry of the faculty building reserved for the building's security guards when I arrived, so I started my interviews with Deniz [pseudonym] alone. Deniz certainly had a critical perspective built on the idea of equal citizenship, one that included judgments and demands borne from the comparative perspective of an equal citizen expecting to have what citizens in Van and Ankara had:

> The doctors here are not usually very good. They're new graduates. They improve their skills here and then leave ... The hospital is a good building. It's big and large. But ... the number of patients per doctor is too high, and the doctors here are not good enough ... Sometimes good doctors arrive as well, but generally we can't trust the doctors. Personally, I don't trust the hospital ... If the number of doctors and medical equipment increased, that would also be good. Why do I have to go to Van? Why do I have to go to Ankara? I want to be able to deal with my health problems in good conditions in my own hometown.

Toward the end of the interview, another security guard, Ismail,[44] entered the room. When I finished the interview, I asked him about the current state of healthcare provision in Hakkâri. Ismail's comments led to the following exchange between him and Deniz:

> *Ismail:* Thank God, it's much better now than before. In the past, doctors used to ignore the patients. There used to be long queues. There were private clinics.
> *Deniz:* If you go to the hospital now, you'll see the same queues in front of the rooms of the gynecologist and pediatrician.
> *I:* Are you crazy? It's good for here. It's good for Hakkâri.
> *D:* Isn't Hakkâri a part of the country? Look at Ankara!
> *I:* Ankara is the capital. Do you compare here with Ankara? [He looked at me with a smiling face as a way of asking for confirmation, as if the other security guard has just said something contrary to the common-sense fact].
> *D:* That's a different point of view. [Deniz withdrew from the conversation.]

Ismail's comparative point of view differed from the comparative point of view of Deniz.[45] While Ismail naturalized the gap between Ankara and Hakkâri via a comparison in time, Deniz blamed the gap via a comparison in space. For Ismail, it was the progress made now compared to the bad old days that mattered, not the relative position of Hakkâri toward Ankara or other western provinces. Ismail spoke from within a developmentalist narrative as a citizen in the making, while Deniz presented as an already fully-fledged and equal citizen.

By making a comparison in space instead of time, discontented patients like Deniz embodied equal citizens claiming the right to equal healthcare provision irrespective of their location. The three Hakkârians quoted below—a student, taxi driver, and local official, none of whom made any explicit references to citizenship—all adopted the comparative perspective of equal citizenship ("this is a province as well") with the depiction of this inadequacy as a degrading attitude, as disrespect toward them ("we are not animals"). The student was interviewed at the University of Hakkâri in an empty classroom of the faculty building. Born and living in a village (in the Hakkâri city district), he was from a poor family whose health insurance premiums were paid by the state and was very angry with the persisting shortcomings of healthcare provision in the area.

Student, University of Hakkâri (from a local village, male, 19 years old):

Why doesn't the Ministry of Health send surgeons to Hakkâri? Why does it appoint bad doctors to Hakkâri? Aren't we humans? They don't pay attention to our health. Doctors here can't do anything. They just transfer the patients to Ankara and Istanbul. Facilities must be provided as well. After all, this is a public hospital, and all equipment should be available here. A device in Ankara should be available in Hakkâri, as well. There should be good doctors in all hospitals. For instance, there aren't many surgeons in Hakkâri. For instance, there aren't many internists in Hakkâri? Why not? Why not?

The taxi driver spoke in the small shanty hut used as a cab stand. Like his colleagues, he was not covered by the GSS because they could not afford to pay the premiums. In his opinion, Hakkâri was a province forgotten by all.

Taxi Driver (Hakkârian, male, mid-20s):

> There's no healthcare provision to be satisfied with. We have to go to Van and Ankara for everything. We can't get an angiography here. This is a province as well. There are people living here as well. The people here aren't animals. Healthcare provision is zero ... My mother is diabetic and has high blood pressure. I took her to the hospital here many times, but there's no explanation, no care, no interest. The people here aren't animals. They'd like a service in their hometown. Why do the facilities [here] lack what's in Van? We'd like to have the same facilities ... This is a province, but it does not have an adequate hospital.

The local official was a municipality clerk. He complained about the appointment of inexperienced doctors to Hakkâri. The comparative perspective entailed by an equal and full citizen stance is less explicit than in the words of the taxi driver and student, but it is evident nonetheless in regard to inequality as an issue of respect.[46]

Municipality clerk, Hakkâri city (from Durankaya town in Hakkâri city district, male, mid-50s):

> Hakkâri has been made into a boot camp with respect to healthcare provision and education. It's a boot camp for doctors and newly graduated teachers. We've never seen a teacher with six years' experience in Hakkâri. Always new graduates come here to get experience. It's seen as a boot camp.
>
> The exile place for all negligent doctors and teachers is Hakkâri. This is a standard punishment method employed by all governments ever. We argue that Hakkâri shouldn't be an exile place.
>
> The surgeons of all bourgeoisies, affluent men, deputies, and ministers in Turkey originated from the East. They did their boot camp here. We served

them as guinea pigs. Look, even saying this is enough to make my hair stand on end, but this is the reality. Many of our relatives died on operating tables while serving them as guinea pigs.

As discussed, complaints about the appointment of "inexperienced" doctors to Hakkâri were closely connected to the historically established and widely shared conviction that the lives of Hakkârians were less worthy of care in the eyes of the Turkish state, but this most popular complaint also involved an equal and full citizen's comparative perspective, assessing the quality of healthcare provision in terms of the "internship doctors" in Hakkâri in comparison to the "professor doctors" concentrated in the western provinces. In the absence of an engagement with the idea of equal citizenship and a spatially comparative perspective, the appointment of newly qualified doctors to Hakkâri via compulsory service law would likely have led to a comparison in time and thus an attitude of gratefulness (as Ismail above).

Those taking a full and equal citizen stance did not limit their criticisms and demands concerning healthcare provision to a comparative list. They went beyond this perspective and formulated their demands based on the gap between what they regarded as the actual needs of Hakkâri and the medical establishment's capacity to meet them. For instance, many people said that a maternity hospital was needed in Hakkâri as soon as possible. They would refer to the high birthrate in Hakkâri and the incapacity of the public hospital to meet demand. The need for a separate children's hospital was similarly much pronounced.

Halil [pseudonym] was a history graduate from Muğla University whose family was politically influential in the local Kurdish movement. He was one of those demanding an additional public hospital for Hakkâri city.

Hakkârian (unemployed history graduate, late 20s, male):

> This [Hakkâri] is a province. Yet we still prefer to go to Van for a good heart treatment. In fact, we have to go to Van. Here we never had enough specialists, nor did they stay long enough. The hospital has never been at a level that meets the needs of this population for treatment, operations, etc. We have a single hospital. It doesn't meet our needs. Why isn't a second hospital made? Why does a poor patient having a heart attack have to go and make payments to the private Lokman Hekim Hospital in Van?

A Hakkârian businessman was asking for both a maternity hospital and a children's hospital:

Businessman (Hakkârian, male, mid-50s):

The Persistence of Patient Dissatisfaction as a Mass Phenomenon | 217

> I am completely dissatisfied with [healthcare provision]. A maternity hospital needs to be opened as soon as possible. There's a restroom next to the gynecology clinic, and everybody sees pregnant women naked while they give birth. It's unacceptable! Also, a children's hospital needs to be opened urgently. I had to take my child to Van because I couldn't get an appointment here. I could take my child to Van, but not everyone can afford it. When I took my child to the ophthalmologist [here], it was the cleaner who checked his eyes … An opening[47] about healthcare provision should be done as soon as possible.

The "opening" here was a reference to the "Kurdish opening." The businessman's usage here when demanding additional hospitals indicates the sharp awareness of Hakkârians of the political dimensions of healthcare provision in the Kurdish region. The following words of a shopkeeper from Hakkâri city who had his shop on the main road of the city also exemplify this demanding stance.

Shopkeeper (Hakkârian, male, mid-50s):

> The people are used to going to Van or Ankara for surgery. My father had heart disease. We took him to Ankara to a professor doctor. He had an angiography there. If those facilities existed here, we wouldn't have gone to Van, Ankara, and Istanbul and had to pay so much money. If we had a fully equipped hospital, we wouldn't need to go elsewhere. Both a maternity and a children's hospital are essential for Hakkâri. A cardiology hospital would also be great.

A sense of appreciation for the improvement of healthcare provision seemed to be completely lacking in these demanding patients. They did not hesitate to make further demands, even unfeasible ones like a separate cardiology hospital in a province with a population of not much more than a quarter of a million people. The immediate explanation for this insistence had partly to do with the continuing deficiencies in the healthcare provision in Hakkâri and the conviction that the lives of Hakkârians were not properly valued by the state, but mostly it was due to the fact that the people making these demands were "already citizens" who felt that they did not need to be grateful for services that they had by right. Thus, they would focus instead on the shortcomings of the service provisioning in terms of their needs and rights.

5.2.2.2 Hakkârians as Rights-Bearing Citizens

> Yüksekova Public Hospital serves around 200,000 people … Given this patient potential, the frequent explosions and firearms injuries due to the

ongoing clashes, traffic accidents resulting from the landscape and inadequate roads and controls, the necessary medical facilities must be available in the hospital and maintained in a functioning state. Expert personnel capable of intervening in urgent patient cases must be employed in the hospital, and the necessary inspections must also be performed carefully. This is the primary and minimum duty of the social state. Because this duty has not been undertaken properly, all officials, from the lowest rank to the top, are under suspicion.

As a citizen and a brother, I believe that the death of my injured brother, whose life could have been saved, cannot be justified on any grounds. I wonder whether my brother would have lost his life in a hospital in Ankara, Istanbul or Van. The answer to this question would reveal that the basic human right, the right to live, was violated by the state institutions and that the constitutional principle of equality was violated in a way that directly threatened human life.

This excerpt is from a petition written by Irfan Sarı, then head of the Yüksekova Union of the Chambers of Artists and Artisans (Yüksekova Esnaf ve Sanatkârlar Odası). As may be gleaned, he was appealing to the patient rights unit following the death of his brother in 2009. His brother had been injured in a traffic accident and died in Yüksekova Public Hospital, where he lost his life due to internal bleeding, which, Sarı argued, went unobserved by the doctors because the tomography machine did not work.

In this petition, we see the usual comparative point of view of Hakkârians who criticize shortcomings of healthcare provision in Hakkâri with reference to the superiority of health services provided in Turkish metropolises, but there is another emphasis here that was generally only implicit. Sarı's letter puts an explicit emphasis on citizenship, the duties and responsibilities of the "social" state, and the state's responsibility to uphold the most basic human right, the right to live. Sarı explicitly assumes and states his citizen status—"as a citizen and a brother"—which is only implicitly present in the comparative gesture. It is as a citizen endowed with rights that he condemns the shortages that led to his brother's death and holds the state's nonfulfillment of its duties responsible, which he regards as ultimately manifesting in a violation of the constitutional principle of equality.

The criteria Sarı relies on, then, to criticize the shortcomings of healthcare provision in Hakkâri are principles concerning rights and duties that are realized in citizenship, the recognition of his place—that of his brother, the local people generally—as full and equal members of society. His criticisms and demands are based on the gap between what is constitutionally promised and is more available elsewhere (in the West) and the actual limits of healthcare provision in

Hakkâri (specifically, Yüksekova). Sarı refuses to tolerate this gap by taking into account the difficult terrain and ongoing conflict between the PKK and the army as excuses; in fact, he does the reverse, demanding positive-discrimination to close this gap and achieve equal citizenship.

The position assumed in the petition was not a standard requirement of the rhetorical strategy used by petitioners to be taken into consideration in official addressees. Nor was the petition addressed to the public or published in a newspaper or website. It was written by a local resident to the hospital's patient rights unit on the death of his brother, for whom no rhetorical strategy could have offered anything further. In fact, it was rather a position assumed by many middle-class Hakkârians more or less actively affiliated with the Kurdish movement as party administrators, NGO activists, and trade unionists. They have been necessarily educated into the vocabulary of politics and the state at the end of years of struggle against the state. As a politically active, leading figure in Yüksekova who had been arrested many times during the 1990s,[48] Sarı was only one among many others for whom the health investment of the government, as with other public investments, did not at all represent a government favor for which citizens should be thankful. Cengiz Şen was another who felt and saw things this way.

The then head of the local branch of the Islamic-leaning Association of Human Rights and Solidarity for Oppressed People (İnsan Hakları ve Mazlumlar için Dayanışma Derneği, Mazlumder), Cengiz Şen was an Islamist, but he was also strongly attached to his Kurdish identity. For example, he did not hold back from telling leading cadres of Haksöz, a pro-government Islamic organization defending the Kurdish policy of the AKP, that "We are not members of the same ummah." His words are important particularly because they demonstrate a way of thinking that does not regard social policies as a counterpart of something that must be somehow returned or as an issue of negotiation whose quality and quantity depend on an agreement between provider and beneficiary. The following words are from the interview I conducted with him in his office:

Q: How would you evaluate the construction of the new hospital and provision of other social assistance?
A: This kind of thing must be provided. If you are a social state, then you have to provide both a hospital and a school for your citizens. You can't flash these things around [i.e., as though they are special]. You tax these people. While providing [these services], it isn't right to flash them around. Positive discrimination must be made for Kurds and the Kurdistan region. Can you compare the streets of Izmit or Bursa with those of Hakkâri? You see the gap between them.

Q: The Prime Minister said in his meeting in Hakkâri that the BDP makes a politics of identity, while the AKP makes a politics of service.
A: What did the AKP do in Hakkâri in the name of service? Nothing!
Q: He was referring to the hospital.
A: It was done by the state, not by the AKP. If the state won't even build a hospital in Hakkâri, then take Hakkâri out of Turkey. As was said by a BDP [deputy], "Take the pasta they give, but don't give your vote to them." Here, the problem of the people is the problem of identity and belonging. I'd like to have a life as Kurd . . . The name of the country can be changed, even. A federal system can be adopted . . .

According to Şen, therefore, health investment and social policy are not political issues, in the sense that they are provided by the social state as a duty, not by the AKP, and to taxpayers, to citizens. Basic social policies like healthcare provisioning are not things that beneficiaries need to be grateful for. The lack of the sense of gratefulness was expressed best, perhaps more than in his call for positive discrimination, in the demanding stance he adopted in the Kurdish issue, with radical suggestions including a change of the name for the country and transition to a federal system.

Another man active in a politically oriented organization was İlkay Şimşek, a Hakkârian teacher in a primary school and head of the local branch of the left-wing and pro-Kurdish Education and Science Workers' Union (Eğitim ve Bilim Emekçileri Sendikası, Eğitim-Sen). His words exemplified a way of thinking shared by other active members of the provincial branch of Eğitim-Sen:

> The physical structure of the hospital may be good. Although doctors don't meet the actual need, they can be regarded as satisfactory when compared to the past. The problem is that all these [services] should have been available in the past. Look at the Declaration of Human Rights. Look at the proclamations of the European Court of Human Rights. The first article of all these documents refers to the right to live, and the second and third articles refer to the citizens' right to healthcare provision. In the Hakkâri case, there was not much healthcare provision here until five or ten years ago. It should have been here, but it was missing. Now, a new physical setting has been built, and a new strategy was developed, but it's been presented to us like it's a favor. That which belongs to us, which we have the right to, has been presented to us like it's a favor.

Şimşek's perspective again illustrates the rights-oriented reasoning that leads citizens to their critical assessment of healthcare provision in Hakkâri. Simply, healthcare provision was missing in the pre-AKP period, which was a violation of their rights. That health services started to be introduced in the AKP period, even if insufficiently, is thus only the return of a right that was effectively suspended in the past, not a good initiative for the AKP to claim credit for. Therefore, it is the actual capacity of healthcare provisioning to meet the right to healthcare provision—not that qualified healthcare provision was largely missing in the past but had since been improved—that Şimşek and his colleagues and many other Hakkârians used as a criterion when evaluating actual healthcare provision in their city and province and region.

5.3 Conclusion: Dissatisfaction as Citizenship Versus Turkishness

This ethnographic examination of the persisting patient dissatisfaction as a mass phenomenon in Hakkâri during the 2003–14 period has plainly revealed a deep issue of trust as a problematic legacy of state-citizen relations in the province and Southeast more widely. Yet the legacy of distrust formed only one aspect of the phenomenon. In fact, the patient dissatisfaction involved another dimension characterized here as *citizenly* patient dissatisfaction.

This nomenclature refers to the incapacity of actual health services in the province to sufficiently meet the expectations of Hakkârians whose expectations were informed by their claim to full and equal citizenship and their experiences by the partial realization of these. For some, this limited result was enough to be content, in the context of the past, for example, while for others it was not, because of or irrelevant of the past. These relatively demanding Hakkârians were discontent with health services that were in any way lacking compared to those provided in more developed Turkish provinces in the west of the country.

Two forms of citizenly dissatisfaction have been distinguished: an implicit and explicit form. The former was enacted by Hakkârians who were unfamiliar with the vocabulary of an official, claim-making form of citizenly dissatisfaction. They would compare the quality and volume of health services provided in Hakkâri with that in the western cities, rather than comparing the present to the past in Hakkâri and appreciating the relative progress in healthcare provision achieved during the AKP period. Adopting space instead of time as a basis of comparison was a complex preference from which we can draw a number of insights. For instance, it undermined the AKP's approach to the Kurdish question insofar as government policy failures rather than successes were observed, predominantly by complaints. The investments were not well returned as political capital.

The spatial, as opposed to temporal, perspective was involved also in the explicit form of citizenly dissatisfaction. This was mostly enacted by educated, middle-class people, usually those affiliated with the Kurdish movement and familiar with the language of official claim-making. Adopting a discourse of references to the duties and obligations of the state, it built on the gap between the state's constitutional promise of delivering qualified healthcare to all its citizens and its actual capacity to meet its promise in Hakkâri. These Hakkârians refused to appear as citizens-in-the-making and thus similarly refused to be merely concerned and satisfied with progress over time. Instead, they felt entitled to the same quantity and quality of health services provided by better facilitated and staffed health institutions in the west of the country as a full-fledged citizenship issue now, as an expression of the right to life, health, and equality.

Dissatisfaction in both the implicit and more sophisticated, formally worked out, and well expressed explicit cases was first and foremost a call for recognition as equals deserving of equal respect and care. It was this emphasis on being recognized and treated as equals without any discrimination or distinction that leads me to class this form of dissatisfaction with healthcare provision as "citizenly"—notwithstanding the fact, that is, that the "implicit" adherents were the majority and there was rather rarely any actual mention of "citizenship" or "rights" by name.

The spatial rather than temporal reference as an inchoate (implicit) expression of the politicized (explicit) rights-based form of citizenliness numbered among the more profound insights it afforded that of a perspective on the structural logic of citizenship. In an unequivocal manner, citizenly patient dissatisfaction in Hakkâri during this period revealed a truth, also asserted by critical social policy scholars, that citizenship is not necessarily a derivative of the nation-state; it does not inherently and always call for a nation-state when it appears. Indeed, as Linda Bosniak argued,

> [T]he automatic correspondence commonly presumed between citizenship and nation-state is unfounded. Citizenship's intimate relationship to the nation-state is not intrinsic but contingent and historical, and the forms and locations of citizenship, as we conventionally understand the term, are more varied than ordinarily acknowledged.[49]

As shown above, the Hakkârian claim to equality with others (their health service with that in the West) implicitly (the spatial comparisons) or explicitly (full and equal citizenship) did not only lead to their dissatisfaction with health services (making the relative progress in time a worthless criterion for assessment). It also prevented them from subscribing to a transition narrative that would incorporate them into the Turkish nation-state as citizens-in-the-making. That those who had been almost totally neglected in Kemalist Turkey began to be embraced in the AKP period and would hopefully be satisfied in the future was insufficient. They were would-be citizens now.

At a higher level of abstraction, what developed through citizenly patient dissatisfaction in Hakkâri was first, the unsettlement of "Turkish citizenship" and, second, the deployment of "citizenship" against "Turkishness," where the former refers to the legally endowed status of equality and being of nation and the latter to the political and national pedagogy of becoming of nation. Thence, we should accept the invitation in the following lines not to be overwhelmed by the "persistent articulation of citizenship as a national question".[50]

> Citizenship has conventionally been viewed as embedded in, or articulated through, three key sets of institutional formations: the state (citizenship as a political status), the nation (citizenship as membership of a community), and the law (citizenship as a juridical status). It seems necessary to loosen these connections, treating them not as the foundational elements or "natural state" of citizenship, but as contingent historical, political and cultural connections, inscribed in and following from different political projects.[51]

In other words, I suggest we take Hakkârians' claim to full and equal citizenship not as a deformed and weak opposing stance calling for or reproducing Turkish nation-state. On the contrary, their claim manifested a refusal to be absorbed into the narrative of "citizens-in-the-making," the narrative with which the Turkish nation-state sought to institute its hegemony over Hakkârians.

Notes

1 See Gritt B. Nielsen, "Peopling Policy: On Conflicting Subjectivities of Fee-Paying Students," in *Policy Worlds: Anthropology and the Analysis of Contemporary Power*, ed. Cris Shore, Susan Wright and Davide Però (New York: Berghahn Books, 2011) and Fiona Wilson, "In the Name of the State? Schools and Teachers in an Andean Province," in *States of Imagination: Ethnographic Explorations of the Post-Colonial*

State, ed. Thomas Blom Hansen and Finn Stepputat (Durham, NC: Duke University Press, 2001).
2 See John Clarke, *Subjects of Doubt: In Search of the Unsettled and Unfinished*. Paper presented at the CASCA Conference, Ontario, May 5–9, 2004; Wendy Larner, "Neo-liberalism: Policy, Ideology, Governmentality," *Studies in Political Economy* 63, no. 1 (2016): 5–25 and Pat O'Malley, Lorna Weir, and Clifford Shearing, "Governmentality, Criticism, Politics," *Economy and Society* 26, no. 4 (1997): 501–17.
3 Nielsen, "Peopling Policy," 69.
4 Joseph R. Betancourt et al., "Defining Cultural Competence: A Practical Framework for Addressing Racial/Ethnic Disparities in Health and Health Care," *Public Health Reports* 118, no. 4 (2003): 294.
5 John D. O'Neil, "The Cultural and Political Context of Patient Dissatisfaction in Cross-Cultural Clinical Encounters: A Canadian Inuit Study," *Medical Anthropology Quarterly* 3, no. 4 (1989): 327.
6 See Nicole S. Berry, "Who's Judging the Quality of Care? Indigenous Maya and the Problem of 'not being attended,'" *Medical Anthropology Quarterly* 27, no. 2 (2008): 164–89; Annette J. Browne and Jo-Anne Fiske, "First Nations Women's Encounters with Mainstream Healthcare Services," *Western Journal of Nursing Research* 23, no. 2 (2001): 126–47; Frantz Fanon, *A Dying Colonialism* (New York: Monthly Review Press, 1965) and Sannie Y. Tang and Annette J. Browne, "'Race' Matters: Racialization and Egalitarian Discourses Involving Aboriginal People in the Canadian Health Care Context," *Ethnicity and Health* 13, no. 2 (2008): 109–27.
7 See Joseph R. Betancourt et al., "Defining Cultural Competence"; Anabell Castro and Ester Ruiz, "The Effects of Nurse Practitioner Cultural Competence on Latina Patient Satisfaction," *Journal of the American Academy of Nurse Practitioners* 21, no. 5 (2009): 278–86; Pedro J. Lecca et al., *Cultural Competency in Health, Social & Human Services: Directions for the 21st Century* (Florence, KY: Routledge, 2014).
8 Terry L. Cross et al., *Towards a Culturally Competent System of Care: A Monograph on Effective Services for Minority Children Who Are Severely Emotionally Disturbed* (Washington, DC: CASSP Technical Assistance Center, Georgetown Univ. Child Development Center, 1989), 7.
9 Donald L. Horowitz, *Ethnic Groups in Conflict* (Berkeley: University of California Press, 1985), 7–8.
10 Fanon, *A Dying Colonialism*, 121–46.
11 See David Arnold, "Smallpox and Colonial Medicine in Nineteenth-Century Medicine," in *Imperial Medicine and Indigenous Societies*, ed. David Arnold (Manchester: Manchester University Press, 1988); David Gordon, "A Sword of

Empire? Medicine and Colonialism in King William's Town, Xhosaland, 1856–1891," *African Studies* 60, no. 2 (2010): 165–83; Richard C. Keller, "Geographies of Power, Legacies of Mistrust: Colonial Medicine in the Global Present," *Historical Geography* 34 (2006): 26–48.

12 This category includes young unmarried women living with their families who are not employed or students; these women can be categorized as hidden unemployed.

13 1 USD = c. 1.8 TL (May 2013).

14 This can be followed in the statistical yearbooks of the Social Security Institution.

15 "Aylık İstatistik Bültenleri," *Sosyal Güvenlik Kurumu* (Social Security Institution), accessed January 11, 2022, https://veri.sgk.gov.tr/.

16 Ibid.

17 Türkiye İstatistik Kurumu (Turkish Statistical Institute), *Yaşam Memnuniyeti Araştırması 2013* (Ankara: TÜİK, 2014), 212–13. The Turkish Statistical Institute has been conducting life satisfaction surveys since 2003. As none of these surveys, but that of 2013, classifies data on a provincial basis, it is not possible to detect the yearly fluctuations in 2003–13 at the level of patient satisfaction in *Hakkâri*.

18 Annette Jo Browne, "First Nations Women and Health Care Services: The Sociopolitical Context of Encounters with Nurses" (Ph.D.thesis, University of British Columbia, 2003), 207–8.

19 İsmail Karaman, *Hakkari Raporu* (Ankara: DPT, 1978), 1.

20 As the coordinator of the quality management unit who was responsible for implementing the questionnaires confessed, because the questions concerning hospital preferences of patients "do not fit the medical reality of *Hakkâri* where there are no alternatives" she could not implement them in a proper way.

21 Pierre Bourdieu, *Outline of a Theory of Practice* (Cambridge and New York: Cambridge University Press, 1977), 77.

22 Berry, "Who's Judging the Quality of Care?"

23 Ibid., 181.

24 Robert L. Payton and Michael P. Moody, *Understanding Philanthropy: Its Meaning and Mission*, Philanthropy and Nonprofit Studies (Bloomington: Indiana University Press, 2008), 60.

25 See Michael Calnan and Rosemary Rowe, *Trust Matters in Health Care* (Maidenhead: Open University Press, 2008); David Silverman, *Communication and Medical Practice: Social Relations in the Clinic* (London: Sage, 1987); Antonella Surbone, "Telling the Truth to Patients with Cancer: What is the Truth?" *The Lancet Oncology* 7, no. 11 (2006): 944–50.

26 See Michael W. Calnan and Emma Sanford, "Public Trust in Health Care: The System or the Doctor?" *BMJ Quality & Safety* 13, no. 2 (2004): 92–97; Bruce Guthrie, "Trust and Asymmetry in General Practitioner-Patient Relationship in the United Kingdom," in *Researching Trust and Health*, ed. Julie Brownlie, Alexandra Greene, and Alexandra Howson (London: Routledge, 2008).

27 See Julie Brownlie, Alexandra Greene, and Alexandra Howson, ed. *Researching Trust and Health*; Mark Hall et al., "Trust in Physicians and Medical Institutions: What Is It, Can It Be Measured, and Does It Matter?" *Milbank Quarterly* 79, no. 4 (2001): 613–39; David Mechanic and Sharon Meyer, "Concepts of Trust among Patients with Serious Illness," *Social Science & Medicine* 51, no. 5 (2000): 657–68.

28 Anthony Giddens, *The Consequences of Modernity* (Cambridge: Polity, 1990).

29 A striking formulation of this argument can be found in Slavoj Žižek's discussion on the case of anti-Semitism in Nazi Germany: "An ideology is really "holding us" only when we do not feel any opposition between it and reality—that is, when the ideology succeeds in determining the mode of our everyday experience of reality itself. How then would our poor German, if he were a good anti-Semite, react to this gap between the ideological figure of the Jew (schemer, wire-puller, exploiting our brave men and so on) and the common everyday experience of his good neighbor, Mr. Stern? His answer would be to turn this gap, this discrepancy itself, into an argument for anti-Semitism: "You see how dangerous they really are? It is difficult to recognize their real nature. They hide it behind the mask of everyday appearance—and it is exactly this hiding of one's real nature, this duplicity, that is a basic feature of the Jewish nature." An ideology really succeeds when even the facts which at first sight contradict it start to function as arguments in its favor." Slavoj Žižek, *The Sublime Object of Ideology* (London and New York: Verso, 1989), 49–50.

30 Fanon, *A Dying Colonialism*, 131.

31 In the website of the Center of Kurdistan Strategic Studies, which was affiliated with the Kurdish national movement, it was reported in 2013 that a civil servant employed at the Hakkâri Governorship had stated that the MoH had asked them to start implementing "sterilization vaccines" to women over 18 years old as soon as possible; this was taken as evidence of the worries of the Turkish state about the rise of Kurdish population. "Kürt Nüfus Soykırımı Güncelleniyor," Nergîz Botan, last modified March 15, 2020, https://www.lekolin.org/kurt-nufus-soykirimi-guncelleniyor/.

32 Slavoj Žižek, "The Spectre of Ideology," in *Mapping Ideology*, ed. Slavoj Žižek (London and New York: Verso, 1994), 21.

33 For a perspective referring to the term "specter" while conceptualizing the fact that the horror of 1990s has not yet become a part of past in the political memory of Kurds, see "1990'larda Kürtler ve Kürdistan Konferansı," Nazan Üstündağ, accessed January 5, 2022, https://www.youtube.com/watch?v=C3uIDIqHv20.

34 Frantz Fanon, *The Wretched of the Earth* (New York: Grove Press, 1963).

35 See Antonio Negri, *Time for Revolution* (New York and London: Continuum, 2003).

36 Thomas Humphrey Marshall and Tom Bottomore, *Citizenship and Social Class* (London: Pluto Press, 1992), 50–51.

37 Dipesh Chakrabarty, *Provincializing Europe: Postcolonial Thought and Historical Difference* (Princeton, NJ and Oxford: Princeton University Press, 2008), 6–11.

38 Doreen B. Massey, *For Space* (London and Thousand Oaks, CA: SAGE, 2005), 68.
39 Ibid., 69.
40 Chakrabarty, *Provincializing Europe*, 6–11.
41 Johannes Fabian, *Time and the Other: How Anthropology Makes Its Object* (New York: Columbia University Press, 1983), 37–70.
42 Harry D. Harootunian, *Overcome by Modernity: History, Culture, and Community in Interwar Japan* (Princeton, NJ: Princeton University Press, 2000), xvii.
43 Fabian, *Time and the Other*, 16.
44 Pseudonym.
45 Later, I learned that Ismail was one of numerous victims in Hakkâri of the absolute poverty of the old, pre-AKP period healthcare provisioning. Because his wife had had a serious problem during a delivery 25 years previously that could not be handled by the health facilities and staff available locally, she was taken to Van where her uterus had to be removed to save her life. Ismail's case supports the general argument here that dissatisfaction was an issue of perspective; in the absence of a strong engagement with the idea of equal citizenship, the sufferings of the past may become reasons for a comparative satisfaction in the present with the actual quality of healthcare provision received (which, though still far from ideal, is at least much improved).
46 For the arguments asserting that citizenship as a status cannot be dissociated from the notions of dignity and equality, see Nancy Fraser and Linda Gordon, "Contract Versus Charity: Why There Is No Social Citizenship in the United States," *Socialist Review* 22, no. 3 (1992): 45–67; Charles Taylor, "The Politics of Recognition," in *Multiculturalism: Examining the Politics of Recognition*, ed. Amy Gutmann (Princeton: Princeton University Press, 1994), 25–73; Liah Greenfeld, *Nationalism: A Short History* (Washington, DC: Brookings Institution Press, 2019), 13–32.
47 By "opening" he refers to the reform process and negotiations for peaceful settlement of Kurdish issue, popularly known as "Kurdish opening." His using the word "opening" when demanding the further improvement of healthcare provision in *Hakkâri* was not accidental. It indicates the inseparability in the minds of many Hakkârians of value ascribed to their bodies and to their identities.
48 He later became mayor of Yüksekova—but was taken under custody in 2019 on terrorism-related charges, dismissed by the Interior Ministry, and imprisoned for 5 months (the Ministry replaced him with a centrally appointed "trustee").
49 Linda Bosniak, *The Citizen and the Alien: Dilemmas of Contemporary Membership* (Princeton, NJ: Princeton University Press, 2006), 5. Quoted in John Clarke et al., *Disputing Citizenship* (Bristol: Policy Press, 2014), 111.
50 Clarke et al., *Disputing Citizenship*, 107.
51 Ibid., 57.
52 TÜİK, *Seçilmiş Göstergelerle Hakkari 2013*, 98.

6

The Compulsory Public Service of Doctors (CPSD) in Hakkâri

This chapter focuses on the compulsory public service of doctors (CPSD), one of the most important aspects of the improvement of healthcare provision in Hakkâri province. As a policy that sent thousands of Turkish GPs and specialists to Kurdish provinces they had never desired to visit, the CPSD forcibly inserted them into a Kurdish reality that was alien to most. The local terrain, the language and culture of the people, and their politics were all different. The CPSD created an encounter with the unfamiliar in which newly trained professionals found themselves rather like foreigners in their own country.

The focus on the CPSD in Hakkâri in this chapter is the nature and limits of this encounter. Did the experience of this posting turn into a sort of "contact zone," in the phrase of Marie Louise Pratt, where "subjects previously separated by geography and history are co-present, the point at which their trajectories now intersect?"[1] Did the experience of this encounter pave the way for a ground where "relations among colonizers and colonized, or travelers and 'travelees,'" were characterized by "co-presence, interaction, interlocking understandings and practices," not "separateness?"[2] More explicitly, did it lead to a mutual recognition through which the doctors fulfilling compulsory service could make sense of the complex issue of persistent patient dissatisfaction and respond to it in an adequate way? Addressing these questions facilitates a consideration of the limits of the assimilation strategy of the AKP.

For a variety of factors, including the design of the CPSD, the ideological background of the doctors, and the difficult living conditions in Hakkâri, the experience of those appointed to serve in Hakkâri was marked by a sense of endurance. Experiencing Hakkâri as endurance alienated them from the dynamics of place, and this alienation from the locality and its people and culture prevented them from developing an adequate understanding of the dynamics of patient dissatisfaction. This, in turn, could easily lead them to adopt essentialist explanations and reproduce discriminatory practices. In other words, Turkish doctors appointed to Hakkâri by the CPSD law formed an expatriate community in terms of their isolation from and disengagement with the host environment and sense of superiority over the locals.[3]

6.1 CPSD, the Production of National Space, and the Kurdish Question

It must be emphasized that neither the geographical maldistribution nor compulsory service of doctors is unique to Turkey. The former is a worldwide phenomenon, especially in underdeveloped contexts, known and discussed as a rural-urban imbalance in the distribution of doctors. This is well demonstrated in the following three cases from three continents—Nicaragua, Bangladesh, and Ghana in the Americas, Asia, and Africa, respectively—reflecting this major health workforce challenge in the Global South at the end of the twentieth century.

In 2000, half of the available health personnel of Nicaragua were concentrated in Managua, the capital, while only one-fifth of the whole population lived in the city. Similarly, in 1998, while four metropolitan districts of Bangladesh had 35 percent of all doctors, they hosted only 15 percent of the country's population.[4] Most strikingly, in Ghana, two-thirds of the population lived in the rural regions in 1997, while almost nine in every ten (87.2 percent) of the doctors were concentrated in the urban regions.[5]

Compulsory public service, meanwhile, has been a common policy adopted by states across the world since the first half of the twentieth century as a cost-effective way of handling the problem of geographical imbalance in the distribution of doctors. Mexico initiated a compulsory medical service program as early as 1936, with medical students obliged to perform a six-month rural service in order to obtain their degree.[6] In 1970, Ecuador installed the *medicatura rural*, making a year of rural service obligatory for all graduates of medical schools.[7] Elsewhere, Thailand adopted compulsory medical service in 1968,[8] and South Africa in 1998,[9] while graduates of government-run medical colleagues in India have been obliged to perform a one-year compulsory rural service since 2007.[10] These are but a few of the many examples of this practice introduced by states across the world.

As for Turkey, the compulsory service requirement of doctors is performed as a state employment policy applied within the context of a long-standing, proactive social strategy, mostly in administration and education, as well as medicine. In medicine, the Turkish Republic has always had a shortage of doctors since the early years of the foundation period, both GPs and specialists, in rural areas generally and across eastern and southeastern Anatolia in particular. The doctors have been (and remain) concentrated in the major urban areas of the western region, especially Istanbul, Ankara, and Izmir, and have generally avoided working in the eastern provinces. A comparison between the provinces of Ankara, housing the capital, and Ağrı, in the northeast and predominantly Kurdish, is indicative of this historical, socio-geographical (urban-rural and western-eastern) divide.

In 1960, there were 2,560 patients per doctor in Ankara and 23,800 in Ağrı, at a comparative (Ankara:Ağrı) ratio, therefore, of around 1:9.[11] By 1975, these patient figures had decreased but disproportionately, favoring Ankara over Ağrı; the former now had 543 patients per doctor but the latter 13,758, for a ratio of about 1:25.[12] By 2002, the imbalance had reduced, but not to the extent even of returning to the old figure; in the case of specialists, for example, the approximate ratio was 1:14, with 1,746 people per specialist in Ankara and 24,228 in Ağrı.[13] This last figure alone, of over twenty-four thousand people for each specialist—of *any type*—indicates the scale of the problem in the East.

Just as with civil servants and teachers, however, the unequal distribution of doctors has never been merely a social justice issue, and the CPSD, similarly, was not just a simple instrument of social policy. Because Kurds make up the majority of the population in the eastern provinces, the issue of the distribution of doctors in Turkey has always been regarded by the state as a problem of belonging and identity as much as one of social justice. That is why İsmet İnönü, one of the co-founders of the Turkish nation-state and the then prime minister, wrote in his famous *Eastern Report* of 1935 that "as a government, we must regard health services as the most effective political and economic measure."[14] It was thus driven by political considerations that the socialization of health services was initiated in a Kurdish province (Muş) in 1963—to the cost of the success of the policy, in fact, since medical infrastructure and other conditions were unsuitable;[15] and thus it was also that the leader of the 1980 junta subsequently issued a CPSD law in 1981 to make "the presence of the state visible in all parts of the country"[16] and invariably referred to the law in his propaganda speeches delivered in the Kurdish provinces; and so it was, then, that Prime Minister Erdoğan asked the electorate in Hakkâri during the national election campaign in 2011 to choose between the AKP's politics of service and the BDP's politics of identity, having listed, item by item, the improvements made by the government to healthcare provision in the province.[17]

Healthcare provision in the Kurdish region has always been a key component in the production of the national geography of Turkey as a homogeneous unit. Along with and as a part of other state employer techniques of compulsory service, including universal (male) military service (*askerlik*), CPSD laws have been a prevalent method in this production process. Albeit in varying forms and with some interruptions, they have nevertheless always been part of the government's agenda. Five CPSD laws have been issued throughout the Republic's history, four imposing compulsory service on all new graduates and one on free boarding students, the first in 1923 and the last, which is still in force, in 2005:

1. The Law on Compulsory Service of Doctors (Law 369, 1923–32);[18]
2. The Law on the Abolishment of Compulsory Service of Those Doctors Who Graduate from the Faculty of Medicine as of 1932 and the Obligations of Free Boarding Medical Students (Law 2000, 1932–88);[19]
3. The Law on the Requirements of the Recruitment of Medical Personnel in State Organization (Law 5979, 1952–54);[20]
4. The Law on the Obligation of State Service of Some Health Personnel (Law 2514, 1981–2003); and[21]
5. The Law on the Amendments of the Basic Law on Health Services (Law 5371, applicable since 2005).[22]

All CPSD laws, including the recent AKP version, have functioned as a form of social policy instrument through which national space has been (intended to be) produced. The idea of a homogeneous "being of nation" has been aimed at by CPSD laws in spatial terms, chiefly by sending doctors to the remotest parts of the country in order to prevent the unjust geographical distribution of doctors from undermining the idea of the unity of the nation. The CPSD introduced in 2005 was no exception.

The assumption guiding all CPSD laws and related regulations has been that doctors overwhelmingly prefer to avoid working in eastern Anatolia due to the hard living conditions that prevail there (which includes doctors from the region, who are looking to improve themselves and for better lives for their families). Reaching for a national space, these laws and regulations defined eastern Anatolia as an area of multiple deprivations. They set doctors' salaries and the duration of their service in the region so as to make it easier for doctors to endure the hardships of life there. In other words—and somewhat paradoxically—in attempting the production of eastern Anatolia as just another part of the homogeneous national space ("being of nation"), the CPSD laws and related regulations constructed eastern Anatolia as a different area of multiple deprivations (the region thus given a place in the hierarchical scale of "becoming of nation"—i.e., at the bottom), and thus pushed doctors in eastern Anatolia to produce the region as one understood and experienced through the prism of endurance.

In order to proceed to the analysis of the CPSD instituted by the AKP as a means of production of national space, it is necessary, therefore, to clarify the concepts "production of space" and "production of space as endurance."

6.2 Unitary Theory of Space as a Key to Understanding Doctors in Hakkâri

This chapter employs as a guiding theoretical perspective the "unitary theory of physical, mental and social space" as developed by Henry Lefebvre.[23] This is a "unitary theory of space" arrived at through a dialectical criticism of Cartesian dualism of the external realm of the material and the internal realm of the human consciousness. With his dialectical insistence on conceiving things in their totality, Lefebvre rejects this dualistic epistemology, which necessarily implies a refusal to take space as a "passive surface, a tabula rasa that enables things to 'take place' and action to ground itself somewhere."[24]

According to Lefebvre, it is not the "things in space" but the actual "production of space" that should be brought into focus. This epistemological shift entails not a bridging of the terms of duality in a more relational conception but rather a complete replacement of duality with a "spatial triad" referring to the "triple determination" of the production of space.[25] These three determinations comprise the following:

1. The conceived space of technocrats, policymakers, planners, bureaucrats, professionals, scientists, and capitalists, which is abstract, hence quantitative, measurable, and homogenizing, and which is dominant, as "tied to the relations of production and to the 'order' which those relations impose . . .";
2. Perceived space, referring to the actual reality surrounding us, the external world of Cartesian dualism, that is, the space that we take as given in our everyday lives; and
3. Lived space, referring to "space as directly lived through its associated images and symbols, and hence the space of 'inhabitants' and 'users,'" which is qualitative and affective, and under constant threat of assimilation into the first two determinations.[26]

These three moments, in relation to one another and in varying proportions, all contribute to the production of space, and it is through their interaction that the production of Hakkâri as endurance is here conceived.

6.3 Production of Space as Endurance: Nothing to Be Discovered, but a Bundle of Problems to Be Passively Managed

Defined in the dictionary as "the ability to withstand hardship or adversity," and especially "the ability to sustain a prolonged stressful effort or activity,"[27] endurance evokes the idea of remaining unchanged and standing firm against an external and ultimately temporary hardship. What is at stake in endurance is not recognizing challenge as internal to an assumed subject-position and following it to the end—which necessarily forces the subject to move toward new identifications, as occurs, for instance, while coming to terms with trauma—but rather the fortification of the challenged subject-position via the defensive externalization of that challenge.

Given that all subject-positions ultimately "depend on the differential system"[28] of the symbolic order, it is possible to make a further argument that what is fortified during the course of endurance by the externalization of challenge is not only the challenged subject-position itself but also and further the very symbolic order enabling this subject-position. Endurance, one can say, is an excellent instance of fantasy in the sense of the term developed by Žižek: a structure that transposes the "inherent impossibility" of symbolic order "into an external obstacle"[29] and thus works to ensure the very consistency of symbolic order and prevent its disintegration.[30]

In the idea of endurance as fantasy, I suggest, is a sense of there being nothing unknown to the enduring subject. Everything already has a place in the differential system secured by endurance fantasy. Crucially, this means that in the production of space as endurance, "the sense of discovering the other"[31] is *missing*. Endurance refers to a relationship with that which is endured in which interaction plays no part. Fundamentally, there is no openness to possible new identifications, no opportunity of expansion and enrichment or even incorporation. Only distance is possible, in the form of dominance, perhaps, or just misunderstanding and misapprehension—or none at all. As for the *content* of endurance fantasy, endurance is an instrumentalist fantasy, meaning that what the enduring subject deals with are not ideological, political, or cultural problems. The enduring subject is not concerned with the complexity, contextuality, and embeddedness of difficult challenges but merely with the temporary hardship itself. Through the lens of endurance, hardship is a hardship, a problem, a threat—nothing else— made bearable at all only by its temporary nature, the knowledge or *precondition* that it will pass.

Endurance fantasy is also an instrumentalist fantasy because the enduring subject does not fight against difficulties to overcome them. The sole or at least primary object of concern is the "fulfillment of days" or "the passing of time." The enduring subject essentially constructs the alien space as a bundle of problems to be passively managed for a fixed period of time as a process of escape, the ultimate and overriding objective, not as problems to be tackled, implying some kind of commitment. On the contrary, the commitment is to the end-date, to the chalking off of days, to the return, to "home."

The lack of place attachment stands at the center of the production of space as endurance. Although the prison and punishment metaphor of the chalking of days gets at the temporal aspect of endurance, the expatriate community parallel may be better for the spatial aspect, especially in colonial contexts and the ways of relating to host societies. As one of the clearest examples of lack of place attachment, this reveals some of the decisive considerations preventing temporary inhabitants from developing an attachment to their environment.

Two key features of expatriate communities are "their transiency in the host society and their relatively privileged status in it."[32] The expatriate is first and foremost "a 'transient' who comes for a specific job or mission and will leave upon its completion."[33] This means that the expatriate's "presence in a foreign land is normally characterized by permanent impermanence."[34] Unsurprisingly, "this transiency reduces the readiness and even the opportunity for adaptation to, and integration into, the host environment."[35] Then, in a further step, the sense of superiority on the part of ex-pats in the colonial sense of the term is further emphasized by the cultural and economic gap between them and locals. The inequality between the colonial and host society reinforces the ex-pat's indifference to the host environment. Hence, the expatriate lives in a bubble. As Cohen notes, "expatriate communities carve out for themselves ... an ecological sub-system of their own which, though it is not necessarily a geographically separate area, still serves to segregate the expatriate community from the host society."[36]

These ideas concerning endurance as the production of space—with a focus on the temporariness and passage of time, assuming distance, implying nonengagement, and fixating on the future departure—and the characteristics of expatriate communities—including transience and the sense of superiority—tell us much about the nature of relationships that Turkish doctors established or rather failed to establish with Hakkârians, their patients.

6.4 The Production of Hakkâri as Endurance as the Outcome of a Trialectical Relationship

In 2003, the AKP removed the CPSD law issued by the military regime in 1981, which had been suspended in 1995 and reintroduced in 2002. The reason for the annulment was that the last 22 years had revealed the impossibility of establishing a geographically balanced distribution of doctors by the policy of compulsory duty employed. Instead, the government adopted the employment of *contract* doctors to overcome the shortage in deprived areas—but they experienced a serious failure in the attainment of this goal also. Therefore, with reference to the uneven distribution of doctors among the provinces and specifically the shortage of doctors in eastern Anatolia, in June 2005, the AKP government pushed through the Assembly a modification of the Basic Law on Health Services that made compulsory public service obligatory for all newly qualified specialists and GPs.

The current CPSD law borrows the classification of the DPT plan published in 2004 that categorized every district in the country into six groups, based on a socioeconomic development index.[37] The groups were assigned varying service obligation durations, thus:

In towns-villages in sixth region districts: 300 days;

In towns-villages in fifth region districts, and in sixth region district centers: 350 days;

In towns-villages in fourth region districts, and in fifth region district centers: 400 days;

In towns-villages in third region districts, and in fourth region district centers: 450 days;

In towns-villages in second region districts, and in third region district centers: 500 days;

In towns-villages in first region districts, and in second region district centers: 550 days;

In first region district centers: 600 days.[38]

Essentially, doctors were now required to work in a state-appointed position for between 1 and 2 years, dependent on the socioeconomic development of the location of the job; the worse the place, the shorter the posting. The level of self-sacrifice (LS) expected from doctors was equalized to prevent injustice according to the following logic:

600 * LS in R1 = 550 * LS in R2 = 500 * LS in R3 = 450 * LS in R4 = 400 * LS in R5 = 350 * LS in R6.

In constructing this equation, the state produced a national geography mapping out the amount of time spent in a place as a measurement of self-sacrifice. Thus, there was a replacement of space by time. In Lefebvrian terminology, this constituted an abstraction of concrete space by the conceived space of policy designers.[39]

Of course, one cannot assume that the model described applies to all doctors doing compulsory service. A certain clarification has to be made concerning the law's reduction of the whole of Turkey to the temporal length of endurance through different levels of self-sacrifice, for it is not only conceived space itself but also and rather a *trialectical relationship* of conceived, perceived, and lived spaces that produced this space.

What could have made sense were the whole country to have had a certain minimum standard of living was flawed in the sense that Turkish doctors looked forward to working in the much more prosperous, developed areas (designated by the law as first and second regions). There were rarely many empty posts in these areas. When doctors were appointed to the first, second, and third regions for their compulsory service, they generally did not count the days. Indeed, specialists in these places tended to continue to work in the same post even after fulfilling their obligations, while GPs in the same places would typically stay and only leave their postings because they had passed the Medical Specialty Exam (Tıpta Uzmanlık Sınavı, TUS), not because they had finished their compulsory service. Indeed, that remains the case since the AKP's CPSD is still in place, and the socio-geographical fundamentals are not greatly changed.

The trialectical relationship between conceived, perceived, and lived spaces produces space as endurance in the "undeveloped" and "distant" Kurdish districts, and certainly in the districts of Hakkâri. Four factors are addressed in the following sections of this chapter, two of them pertaining to perceived space and two others to lived space, which, in relation to the conceived space of the CPSD law, have contributed to doctors not recognizing Hakkâri city, the provincial capital, as an entity in its own right to be discovered and instead led them to assume an instrumentalist stance toward the city.

6.4.1 Space as Perceived by Doctors

Doctors' perceptions and experience of space is characterized here in terms of a minimalist sense of problems and degradation, on the one hand, and as dangerous and strange, on the other.

6.4.1.1 Hakkâri City as a Bundle of Problems and the Degradation of Doctors to a Bare Life

Doctors appointed to Hakkâri city do not encounter a city that has organically developed, however poorly, according to its own dynamics and in relation to the needs and demands of its inhabitants. Rather, they find themselves in a sort of Panopticon structured by concerns of security and control. That is certainly the case now, just as it was also at the time of the research carried out for this study.

Hakkâri city is the result of a project executed in a very short time span during the mid-1990s that had ejected thousands of people out of their rural homes and into a small town wholly surrounded by high mountains that were studded with watch towers. The result had been huge problems resulting from the large gaps, still unclosed, between the infrastructure designed and the topography appropriate for a small-town population, on the one hand, and the new urban reality squeezed and crowded by the addition of new neighborhoods, on the other.

The everyday lives of Hakkârians by 2014 were characterized by several problems. In addition to the infrequent, intermittent tap-water supply, winter air pollution quality due to coal smoke, poor quality sewage system that only covered two-fifths of the city (see Section 1.3.1.3), there were constant and sometimes lengthy power cuts, almost no public spaces or parks where people could spend their leisure time, and there was a shortage of apartments due to both the mountainous topography of the city and the lack of sufficient public housing. The latter was a reflection of the absence of benevolent instruments until recent times, except for that reserved for the army and police.

For doctors posted in Hakkâri city, the difficulty of finding comfortable accommodation, and then the generally poor living conditions regarding air quality, water and power cuts, only compounded the remoteness of the location, the uneasy atmosphere of everyday life, their deprivation of Turkish middle-class consumption patterns, and a different social and cultural environment and lifestyle that made them "outsiders." The following examples gathered between 2008 and 2014 reveal how these hardships were experienced by the doctors in their daily lives.

GP (employed at the Provincial Directorate of Health):

> There are no places to go. We only have Governorship Park. The municipality doesn't work. Everywhere is full of garbage ... I mean, it isn't a good place in terms of environmental conditions. For instance, the tap water is extremely dirty, and there are constant water cuts. It was available every other day and only for two hours in the evenings when I was in Tekser. We had to choose between washing clothes and washings dishes in these two hours. We used to fill bottles with water. Half of the kitchen was full of bottles with water. I don't think that anybody has witnessed such a torture.

GP (employed in a health post in Hakkâri City):

> I still remember it quite well. One of the most powerful figures of the country, you can guess who, was saying on TV that there is public housing reserved for doctors in Hakkâri. No, no. We didn't have any. I stayed in very bad places with mice.

This was a life, the quality of which did not extend much beyond than satisfaction of basic needs. Manifestly, the experience was awful, a "torture" indeed—even if this hardly endurable reality that one might not think "anybody has witnessed" was rather like just the everyday lives of local people. Regardless, in the words of the Provincial Director of Health, it could not be regarded a real, decent-quality life:

> Q: What are you going to do after you finish compulsory service?
> A: I've undertaken a responsibility. I can't go as I wish, leaving things uncompleted. [But] I already have a life outside Hakkâri and will certainly go back to it one day.
> Q: You said you'll go back to your life one day. Do you regard the time you pass here as not a part of your life?
> A: Unfortunately, no, I don't. If you're appointed to do your compulsory service in Zonguldak,[40] for instance, you can continue working there even after compulsory service. But not in Hakkâri.[41]

The daily reality of Hakkâri city reinforced the sense of endurance among doctors posted in Hakkâri. Doctors had few reasons to problematize the "temporary hardship" category of the endurance fantasy constructed by the law. It is unsurprising, therefore, that it was the management of time in a passive mood rather than an attempt to discover and engage with the city that characterized the way that doctors (re)produced the city. Their civic engagement was so weak that I found only two among dozens of doctors who were active in an NGO. Membership of other organizations and participation in the activities of unions was also very low. The experience of a Hakkârian GP and member of the left-leaning health workers' union SES is striking:

> I'm a member of SES ... The people [Turkish doctors] are afraid of the labor union, especially in Hakkâri. We doctors who are members of the SES in Hakkâri once started a campaign to ensure the reach of doctors to all corners of Hakkâri. We also tried to get the participation of a pediatrist or a gynecologist. We thought that the participation of specialists would increase the trust of the patients, but not one of them joined us, none of them.

A Kurdish GP who had been the provincial head of the Van-Hakkâri Medical Chamber for a period confirmed the low level of Turkish doctors' civic engagement:

> They're not willing to unionize. Professor Çetin Kotan and I went to the hospital to inform and unionize them. There were 20 or 25 specialists sitting and chatting in the garden of the hospital in the lunch break. They didn't even stand up out of courtesy when they saw Çetin Kotan, who's a professor, after all. They didn't listen to what he told them. They were just gawking. None of them listened to him.

Turkish doctors' indifference to Kurdish was another example of their lack of engagement with civic life and the city more widely as well as in a professional context. Although almost all the doctors recognized the significance of Kurdish in the doctor-patient encounter, as the head of the Hakkâri Branch of Kurdi-Der (an association that teaches Kurdish) explained, the total number of Turkish doctors attending the Kurdish lessons given by Kurdi-Der between 2010 and 2013 did not exceed ten in total.

Almost all doctors were content with the palliative, non-professional solutions to the problem of language in their relations with patients. Thus, the secretaries of each specialist in the public hospitals, who would be locals, from Hakkâri, were expected to act as translators as necessary, even though they had received no education on the ethics and requirements of this task. It was not uncommon for patients with a poor command of Turkish, mostly women and the elderly, to go to the hospital with one of their relatives who knew Turkish, mostly their sons or daughters. Bilingual Hakkârian patients in the queue would also be asked for their help in translating.[42]

The socialization pattern of assigned doctors also exemplified their nonengagement with the city. They would be unwilling to meet new people outside their immediate environment, which was typically made up just of their medical colleagues. They would form a close community whose interaction with the wider city was negligible—in the words of one specialist doctor, they lived "like a commune." The result resembled an enclave of ex-pats. It is thus unsurprising that a specialist, who had just completed his mandatory military duty when we met, talked as if he were still a soldier living in barracks isolated from normal life when depicting the everyday gap between him and ordinary Hakkârians, or "civilians."

Specialist, Hakkâri Public Hospital:

> I usually spend time with my colleagues, for example, with the plastic surgeon, the gynecologist, general surgeons. I don't spend time together with civilians. They don't have any need to meet with us either. For instance, I don't know the interior design of the apartments of my landlord or my neighbors.

The specialists were concentrated in a few buildings in the city center, went back and forth between the hospital and their apartments, and spent their leisure time almost exclusively with colleagues at one another's homes.[43] On some weekends, they would go to Van, wander, sit in cafes, and do their shopping. When they left their posts, they would hand over their apartments, just as they had been initially handed over to them, complete with the same furniture, to the newly arriving specialists There was no significant investment made in the home. Then, they would leave the city with a single piece of luggage, just as they had arrived.

As for the GPs, they would devote all their free time to studying for the TUS exam to be rid of compulsory service and away from Hakkâri as soon as possible. Since doctors doing their compulsory service did not have to complete the rest of it if they passed, the TUS was effectively their escape and license to proceed with their lives as well as a passport to the higher ranks of their professional career.

In short, relations with the city and the people were largely determined by the instrumentalist logic of day-counting and not by any means characterized by a sense of adventure, let alone of discovering the other. These were the words of a specialist interviewed alongside his Hakkârian friend Salim [pseudonym]:

- As long as you don't talk about politics, there's nobody you cannot communicate with. You should avoid declaring your political views, for the people are very angry at many things. You can see your secretary throwing stones or shouting slogans in the demonstrations. There is nationalism. If you say you're Turkish, they say "I'm Kurdish." You can't find a common point if you talk with them about Turkishness, Kurdishness, the state, and the PKK. Have we ever discussed these things Salim?
Salim: No we haven't.
- Exactly. If we avoid talking about these things, then there's no problem. But if we discuss them, then we fight, for our experiences are different.
Salim: [Nods his head in agreement.]

Here, the specialist pragmatically takes the opinions of the people, including that of his friend, Salim, regarding the Kurdish issue as a given. Ultimately, he wishes to avoid trouble during his temporary stay in Hakkâri. However, it is also clear that his lack of engagement signifies that he does not regard a change in his own ideas about the Kurdish issue as possible. He does not welcome any possible critique from his friend that might challenge his sense of self, other, the situation; he would rather just not know, ignore the whole thing as if it will go away—since he will, of course. The whole failure to engage is predicated on the impermanence of his situation.

Therefore, the friendship between the specialist and Salim was not really an interactional relationship, in the type of way that may be expected of a "normal" friendship, including the sharing and distancing and criticism of one another's values, ideas, and behaviors. Instead, it had developed under the shadow of the instrumentalist logic in which Salim appeared mainly as a way of helping the passage of time in Hakkâri to go more quickly and less painfully: "If we avoid talking about these issues, then there is no problem."

Put differently, the production of space as endurance structurally reduced the interactional capacity of such relationships as doctors did establish with Hakkârians. Or, the lack of quantity was compounded by a lack of quality. The relationships of assigned doctors with the local people tended to be few and shallow.

Specialist, Şemdinli Public Hospital:

> Sometimes shutters are closed, demonstrations take place, and military stations are raided. The soldiers killed and injured in these raids are brought to the hospital. In these times, everything becomes completely different than normal. When there are demonstrations and incidents, even the people we know we have good relations with pass to one side and us on the other, like the fans of Fenerbahçe and Galatasaray [rival football clubs in Istanbul]. Because they're in one team and we're in the other, we can't go out to the shops and wander around on those days.

Rising political tensions would uncover the truth repressed for the sake of good relations between Hakkârians and the doctors: peaceful and positive contact depended on the silence of both sides on the Kurdish issue. For these contacts to persist, the Kurdish issue had to remain unspoken, even though it was the main determinant of life in Hakkâri, so many essential concerns went unaddressed. It was not accidental that the specialist chose the opposition between the fans of Fenerbahçe and Galatasaray to describe the nature of the opposite stances taken by the doctors and Hakkârians when the political tension rose. What could have described the weakness of the interactional moment in the relations doctors established with Hakkârians better than the opposition between rival fans in which stances are fixed and unopen to any change and negotiation?

In addition to the form of relationships doctors established with Hakkârians, the instrumentalist way of being in the city found its expression best in the "not-so-bad" discourses of the doctors. The words of these two doctors were typical of dozens of others.

GP, Hakkâri City (assigned to a health post):

> In general, I don't have a problem with Hakkârians, the people, the general atmosphere. Contrary to the general opinion and ideas, Hakkâri is not in the Stone Age. Except for eight or ten big cities, in each city, there's one main street

[that is good], while the rest of it is bad. Isn't it? Mostly, it is. There are shortages in Hakkâri, of course, but is it so bad? No, it isn't. It's not a place where you can't live and work.

Specialist, Hakkâri Public Hospital:

I'm not staying at the Doctor's Lodge anymore because I married one-and-a-half months after my arrival. My wife had some reservations about Hakkâri. I told her that Hakkâri isn't too bad a place to live, that living conditions aren't as bad as they're portrayed in the media. I told her the reality and managed to convince her. I rented an apartment, and [we] moved there.

The expression "not so bad" takes on an adjectival usage here that reduces the being of that described to its capacity to meet the expectations of the describing subject. It does not tell us about the particular features of the described object; it is not descriptive. As the negative expressions reveal—like "It's not a place where you can't live and work" and "not too bad a place to live"—the life in question is one that can only be expressed in comparison to minimal living conditions without any remarkable content. It is a bare life, not one that can be expressed in positive terms. "Not so bad" may be taken, therefore, as the motto of the instrumentalist indifference of the doctors to the city. They get by to get out; it can be done. The endurance is possible.

6.4.1.2 Hakkâri as a Dangerous and Uncanny Place

The failure of the doctors to move from the experience of Hakkâri as endurance, to move from the idea of "not so bad" to a perspective on the city as a place to be discovered, is not only related to having to deal with many practical problems around the minimum standards of a comfortable life. Imposed by the spatial design of the law, the endurance fantasy is reinforced also by a sort of "real abstraction." Developed by Alfred Sohn-Rethel, the concept of real abstraction refers to a form of abstraction that is not "thought induced":

[I]t does not originate in men's minds but in their actions. And yet this does not give abstraction a merely metaphorical meaning . . . It exists nowhere other than in the human mind, but it does not spring from it. Rather it is purely social in character, arising in the spatio-temporal sphere of human interrelations. It is not people who originate their abstractions but their actions.[44]

The real abstraction in the current context is one that emerged through the violent history of the state-Hakkârian relations, which constructed Hakkâri as a dangerous, fundamentally foreign place, where the natives are unreliable and generally to be avoided when possible. It is this attitude that was evoked when a GP working in a health post in Çukurca described the anxiety of his family living in a Turkish metropolis. "There were 35 missed calls from my wife, mother, and friends on the day the cell phones didn't work due to the dispatching of troops," he explains. "My mother said she nearly went nuts that day."

In using the term "real abstraction" here, the idea is to go beyond depicting or referring to ideas, representations, or anxieties, and to draw attention to the constitutive power of the criminalizing stigmatizations in the practical relations between Hakkârian and Turk. These were so real in Hakkâri around 2010 that, for instance, it was difficult to see the vehicle license plate of Hakkâri (a number "30" at the end) in the city. Instead, car-owners preferred to acquire a license plate with the code for Istanbul (34), Ankara (06), or at least Van (65), a Kurdish city but less stigmatized, in order to avoid any difficulties. Driving in Hakkâri with a "30" plate should not be a problem, but once outside the province, the car would become a target of suspicion at the army checkpoints, for gendarmes, and others.

Similarly, young Kurdish men would conceal their origins when chatting with Turkish girls on the internet and only confess the truth according to the flow of the chat. The parents of those Turkish doctors appointed to Hakkâri often felt obliged to accompany their sons and daughters to their posting, none of whom were less than 25 years old, to stay and support and keep an eye on them. Hakkârians tended to stereotype Turks arriving in Hakkâri as prejudiced against Kurds. That is why the first things a civilian Turk would most probably hear from Hakkârians would be defensive comments on subjects like the misguided representations of Hakkâri in the Turkish media and what good and hospitable people Hakkârians really were.

During my fieldwork period, for example, the extent of Hakkârians' anger against the Turkish media was such that broadcasting vehicles of the Turkish TV channels were stationed for security on either the governorship or police headquarters grounds. Correspondents were only able to report from within the safety of these places under the protection of the police—a fact that also reveals how the border between the media and the state practically ceased in Hakkâri, even then, during a comparatively "liberal" period. A personal anecdote illustrates how real these abstractions were and how difficult it is to escape from the stigmatizations and stereotypes in Hakkâri.

It was during the early days of my field study, and we were sitting and chatting with a group of Hakkârian acquaintances in the garden of the Teachers' Guesthouse when someone I did not know joined the group. My friends introduced him to me, and told him about my research plans. He was a Hakkârian employed in the municipality governed by the pro-Kurdish party. He asked me where I was from. When I told him that I was from the Black Sea region, notorious in the last few decades for its far-right stance, he directly asked me, "Do you agree that the violence must end at all costs [*ne olursa olsun*]?"

I was, of course, against the violence, yet did not want to give a simple answer to the complexity added by the stipulations "must" and "at all costs." To clarify my position, I attempted to answer him: "The issue is . . ." He interrupted me: "Just say yes or no. Can you say that the violent clashes must end at all costs?"

I insisted on giving my own "yes" answer instead of a simple one. He interrupted me again and again, demanding a straight answer. When he realized that I would not just say "Yes" or "No," he took this as evidence of my avoidance of a positive answer and thus my implicit support of violence: "You Turks can't say that the violent clashes must end at all costs, but we Kurds do say that the violence must end at all costs. We cannot tolerate the death of one more individual, whether he is Turkish or Kurdish."

Although I completely agreed with his condemnation of the violence—even if there still seemed some ambiguity around the "at all costs" (were these to be paid by the state, which just needed to withdraw, and did that allow for a Kurdish violence to enforce it or else require a withdrawal of claims made?)—his opinion of me was already fixed. I was a "Turk" siding with the violent policies of the Turkish state. This case was more than a mere miscommunication and rather a manifestation of the fact that stereotypes and abstractions are often more powerful than reality in Hakkâri—or, they become the reality.

Another example of the reality-building power of abstractions and stigmatizations in Hakkâri, again a case of more than a simple miscommunication, occurred one day while we were sitting in the tea house right across the Rectorate. Baran [pseudonym], one of my friends working as a research assistant at the University of Hakkâri, came from the direction of the Hakkâri Public Hospital, which is 100 m away from the Rectorate, and recounted his story.

The day before, he had studied in his room in the faculty building until midnight and then gone to his apartment, which is in a building far from the city center. The door of the building had been locked, he did not have a key on him, and there was nobody in his apartment to open the door for him. He decided to toss tiny stones at the window of the apartment on the second floor of the building to get the attention of the people in the single apartment whose lights happened to be on at the time. He failed to get them to look out the window and open the door of the building and had to pass the night in a friend's apartment. When he had gone to the building on this morning, the porter had asked whether it had been he who had thrown the stones yesterday night at the window of the apartment on the second floor. When he said "Yes," and explained, the porter narrated the tragicomedy he had caused.

In the apartment at whose windows he had softly thrown small stones was a pregnant woman. Her husband was a specialist sergeant who had happened to be involved in a military operation against the PKK that night. When the pregnant woman heard someone throwing stones at her window, she was horrified. She thought it must be terrorists and ran to the apartment of her neighbor on the third floor, but her condition worsened there, and she had to be taken to the hospital. That is why Baran was coming from the direction of the hospital. He had just been to wish her well and apologize for his thoughtless behavior.

It was only a tragicomedy because it was not a tragedy. Baran's stones triggered a course of events that almost led to a miscarriage. Violence was an everyday reality to be reckoned with, a dark potential threatening the most innocent of gestures, and it is not surprising that doctors inserted into such a situation should have had similar experiences. The following case was recounted by a GP who had been working in Hakkâri city but was temporarily appointed to Çukurca, a border town right at the middle of ongoing clashes between the army and the guerillas. I listened to him in the corridor of the provincial Directorate of Health, where he was waiting for his turn to submit his petition to be taken back to Hakkâri city. This is what he and his colleague experienced in Çukurca:

> Once, we came by a *lahmacun* shop open at four in the afternoon and decided to eat a few *lahmacun*s (a flatbread snack with a minced meat topping)—but the man told us he'd run out. We said, "But you're making some right now, and we don't want more than four or five." The man replied that all the *lahmacun*s he was making were for soldiers, and he didn't have enough ingredients to make *lahmacun*s for us.
>
> In another case, my friend wanted to buy a cigarette, but he was refused, so he asked for another brand, but was refused again. But there were many packets of the cigarettes he'd asked for there, so he asked the man why he was refusing when there were plenty of packets of cigarettes behind him. He said that they'd all been sold to the army. In short, he didn't want to sell. He was taking a stance against him [the friend]. The reason behind this attitude was the political ideas

of someone he'd worked with. Because the people saw him [the friend] spending time with this former colleague, he was supposed to be sharing the same [nationalist] ideas.

Unavoidably, doctors' experiences with the people and Hakkâri were, to a considerable extent, structured by these criminalizing abstractions generated by the accumulative effect of decades of Turkish nationalism. The very real abstractions deprived the doctors of the opportunities necessary for and capability of recognizing Hakkâri as an entity in its own right, as a place that could have much to be discovered, for they isolated the doctors from the social environment. These abstractions thus prevented doctors from meeting new people and hearing stories that could counter and resist the criminalizing representations of Hakkâri. A vicious circle consequently developed, helping to maintain the "temporary hardship" category of the endurance fantasy.

In other words, the abstractions, stigmatizations, and stereotypes prevented doctors from moving from the intrapsychic to the intersubjective, from a fixation on the native as an already-known object of the endurance fantasy to a recognition of them as "a separate and equivalent center of self."[45] Another example of this was demonstrated in a specialist's rejection of his friend's suggestion to pick up what looked like hitchhikers:

> We rented a car in Van and left for Hakkâri. The road was extremely frightening, with deep valleys, high mountains, etc. When we got to Başkale, which is like a gypsy neighborhood, we saw some people hitchhiking. My friend suggested I pick one up. I said, "Are you crazy? We can't trust them." Later, I learned that they wave their hands to mean they have smuggled diesel to sell, not to hitch a ride.

This had occurred during the specialist's first trip to Hakkâri, and reflects the kind of bizarre situation the criminalizing abstractions may give birth to. If the smugglers really had been hitchhikers, the specialist would have missed an opportunity of a warm chat with local people, which might have led to some cracks in the usual representations of the native in his mind. As it was, he merely failed to engage with "smugglers" as, also, just ordinary people.

The following conversation with a GP employed in a TB dispensary also shows how criminalizing abstractions and stigmatizations led doctors to keep Hakkârians at a distance:

Q: What is the psychology of your family like?
A: They're very uneasy. Let me give an example. Recently, when they called the dispensary to talk, they couldn't reach me and heard someone speaking Kurdish—maybe due to a crossed line. Later, I learned that they'd been extremely frightened and even cried and tried to get in contact with me through some other connections. They were worried in case something bad happened to me. They check me every day to find out whether anything has happened to me or not.
Q: What do they suggest?
A: Keep your cell phone with you always, never leave it on silent mode, be careful and cautious, don't pay any attention or get in contact with people other than your friends, choose your friends carefully, this kind of thing.
Q: Do you follow their advice?
A: Sure, sure.
Q: It seems like you don't have any friends from Hakkâri?
A: No, absolutely not.

Again, it would be wrong to suggest that these are *just* abstractions on the part of doctors that prevent them from discovering the city or from relating to it in a way other than endurance. The risks posed by the realities of Hakkâri also reinforce the endurance fantasy, in the sense that they block alternative ways of establishing relations with the city and discourage the doctors from developing any real attachment to the place. Another personal anecdote can provide a further illustration.

One evening, I had finished working and went downstairs to leave the faculty. Outside, right in front of the building, there were panzers, policemen, undercover officers carrying automatic guns, and three or four "scorpion" type armored police vehicles. Some children and young men were shouting PKK slogans behind a simple barricade 300 m away, and there were also 20 or 30 children to the left of the faculty watching. I went back to my room to get my camera before returning outside to take photos of the incident from 2 or 3 m behind the children. The children turned to me when the camera flash alerted them to my presence. I approached them and told them of my intentions: "Hey, don't take it the wrong way. I'm not taking your photos." They hesitated for a moment and looked at each other.

"Why are you taking photos then?" The young man who spoke was standing 2 m behind me.

"I'm a research assistant in the University," I replied. He continued his interrogation.

"Does a research assistant do such things? What's your department?" I explained that I was a research assistant in the department of management.

"Okay," he said, "Then I'll go to the rector and complain that you take photos [of the demonstrators]." I told him that I was taking photos of the policemen, not the children, and asked what the problem with that was. Implicitly referring to the locals' oft-cited complaints concerning criminalizing representations of Hakkâri in the Turkish media—which focused almost exclusively on the clashes and protests at the expense of the other aspects of life and natural beauties of Hakkâri, he responded: "Why are you taking photos of policemen? Isn't there anything else than policemen? Take the photo of the uplands and beautiful places."

His tone was confrontational and his style overbearing. I had to explain further. "I'm a sociologist. I am not only concerned with such things. I am writing a dissertation on healthcare provision in Hakkâri." I also added that "I'm a member of Eğitim-Sen," hoping that my membership of a left-leaning and pro-Kurdish labor union might calm him down. In fact, I was quite unsuccessful, and his anger grew to the point of threatening me.

"How can you be a member of Eğitim-Sen? Someone will stop you. Don't be surprised if someone stops you," he added menacingly. I decided to proceed more aggressively.

"Look, my name is İlker. What is yours?" He avoided saying his name. I continued. "I'm a sociologist. If you knew me, you'd be sorry."

Then he tested me by giving names of some instructors to see whether I knew them. Our loud discussion caught the attention of some policemen. They were looking at us. To end the discussion, I said, "Okay, I won't take any more photographs."

One of the children then intervened. "You already have enough photos," he said. I told the youngsters I would not use these photos, returned to the building quickly, and went back to my faculty room to calm down and wait.

A few months later, I saw the same young man in the office of the students' association of the University of Hakkâri, where I went to conduct interviews with the students. It transpired that he was a student of the university. "If I remember correctly, we had a bit of a confrontation a while ago, didn't we?" I asked, hoping to receive an apology for his rude behavior. Instead, he took a cool stance and did not back down.

"I thought that you were a police captain and tried to see whether you had a gun on your hip," he replied, before adding, "If it had been someone else instead of me, he might have acted differently than I did."

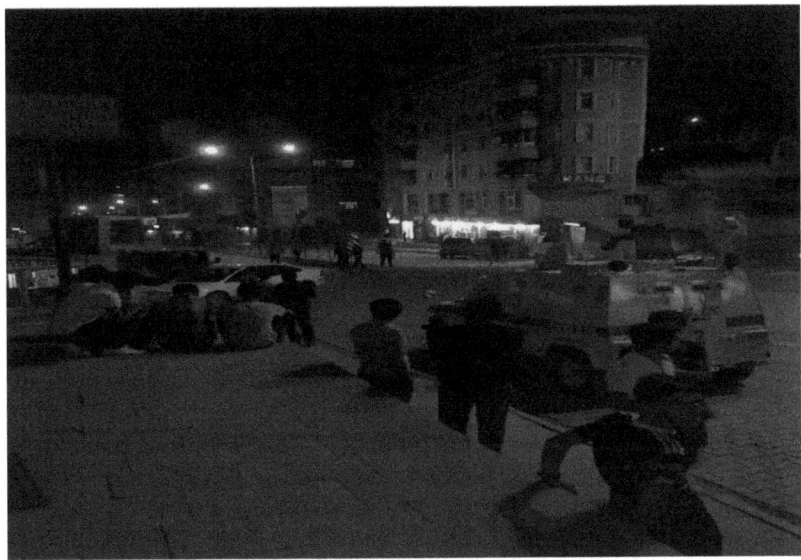

Figure 19. Children Watching Clashes between Demonstrators and the Police.

Again, one should not misperceive the realities on the ground and make assumptions, such as that the student's interrogative style and threats on that night, or his later behavior, reflected the immature extremism of youth radicalism. In fact, as I was later to learn, he had lost relatives in the Yoncalı village massacre in 1989, when three villagers were brutally killed while mowing grass and then burned by a commando troop, and 20 years later, he had been arrested in KCK operations, when his nose was broken in the arrest, and he spent months in different prisons. There were also lawsuits filed accusing him of being affiliated with the PKK and the KCK. In short, up to that point in his life, Turks had not been there to listen to and understand him but rather to collect evidence, to judge and punish. His response to me—on both occasions—was therefore based on his suspicion that I was a police captain documenting the identity of the protesters, which—to him—was a likely scenario.

The burden of history on our encounter—the regional, local, and his personal history—forced me to stop my research on that occasion. This problem also affected the few attempts by doctors to go beyond instrumentalism and recognize Hakkâri as a real entity to be engaged. The real risks posed by the harsh either/or reality of Hakkâri—local or outsider, Turkish or Kurdish, pro- or anti-violence, etc.—may prevent them from relating to the city in a way other than through endurance. This was the case, alas, in the failed attempt of a specialist to run a Scout group there:

> I'm a Scout master, so I thought I could do some scouting here. I went to the Provincial Directorate of Youth and Sports and introduced myself. I told them that I was a Scout master and would like to do scouting. They looked at me like I was crazy. They did actually know what scouting was. They said that it used to be done in the past. Anyway, they promised to help me, but also advised me not to go camping. They thought it might be dangerous. Their suggestion to me was rather to do camping in the military zone. But it just wasn't possible to do scouting like this.

There are numerous such examples. A GP employed in a health post in Hakkâri city told me that he and his wife used to go to restaurants located in Depin, at the entry to the city, on weekends in the early days of their arrival in the city. Then, some policemen were shot dead in Depin, and they stopped going there and to other places outside the center.

The "security" issue can even limit doctors' routine interventions in issues related to their profession. When asked whether they were concerned with, for instance, the fundamental healthcare (and illness prevention) issue of the sanitary conditions of the city, such as the absence of garbage containers, a specialist replied that this was a security issue and none of their business. "Therefore, we do not intervene in the affairs of the municipality," he concluded, and the subject was closed.[46]

6.4.2 Lived Space

Here, the focus on space as lived with its everyday realities is presented in terms of doctors' elitism and their sense of imprisonment.

6.4.2.1 Elitism toward Hakkârians

That the doctors cannot move beyond the endurance fantasy and face Hakkâri as an entity in its own right is also due to the subjective aspect of the production of space, that is, images and symbols that mediate doctors' lived experience of Hakkâri. In this aspect, one should initially refer to the nationalist elitism of doctors. For many doctors in Hakkâri, it is in the early phases of a transition to modernity. Therefore, they associate Hakkâri with backwardness and regard it as a latecomer not worth knowing.[47] These are the words of a specialist from Hakkâri Public Hospital:

Urbanization started in the western part thirty or forty years ago. We were nomads before that. What occurred in the west thirty years ago is only now taking place in Hakkâri. They are learning the urbanization and the Western logic of collective life now. What was established in the West [of Turkey] thirty years ago is just beginning to be established here. While the earlier generation were shepherds in the mountains, the next became technicians, teachers, and so on. This is a matter of generations. We're in the phase of transition. They resemble our situation of thirty years ago. They're a generation behind us.

Similarly, "the people of the city are in a transition," opines a specialist from Şemdinli Public Hospital. "They're in-between the West and the East, the village and the city. They have a life whose orientation is not clear for the moment." Independently of the official representation of Hakkâri as an area of multiple deprivations, it is already very well known to doctors as a place of shortcomings, lacking development. Therefore, in the rare cases where their relationship with the city is not instrumental, it is entirely possible that the denial of Hakkâri as an entity in its own right still may persist in the shape of elitism.

This is what we can see in the experiences of two Turkish specialists working in Hakkâri Public Hospital. They were exceptions in the sense that they were actively engaged in civic and public life in Hakkâri. One of them had founded an NGO organizing fun and educational activities for Hakkârian children. The other was broadcasting a radio program on a local radio station and also giving her support to the NGO founded by her colleague. Their ways of being in Hakkâri were not structured by instrumentalist logic of endurance and day-counting, yet they still failed to establish a real, friendly dialogue with Hakkârians.

When I met them in a room in Hakkâri Public Hospital, they complained of not being properly understood and appreciated. Rather than serving as a bridge, their activities further reinforced the gap between them and Hakkârians. Their attempts backfired in such a way that, as the founder of the association put it, they were even suspected of being affiliated with the state intelligence services:

> They [Hakkârians] really don't understand what we're trying to do. They always look for hidden agendas and hidden interests. We don't expect anything, but we don't expect ungratefulness either. I get upset and my motivation is broken ... People say that we're the MİT agents, that I'm connected to JİTEM ... None of this is true.

Some of these suspicions of a hidden agenda behind the social activities of these specialists reflect the prejudgments of Hakkârians unused to being addressed in a compassionate way through NGOs led by the state employees. More fundamentally, however, the main body of the problem most likely had to do with the one-sided and elitist nature of the relationship these specialists tried to establish with Hakkârians. Theoretically, from the Turkish nationalist point of view of these specialists, they had things to give to and teach Hakkârians but had nothing to learn from them, reflecting also the tradition of Turkish bureaucratic authority based on the "distinction of state officials from *halk* (the common people)."[48] Practically, this is supported by the essentially patronizing perspective evident in the following words.

Specialist, Hakkâri Public Hospital:

> I believe that just as there are flowers on the balcony of my apartment in Istanbul, so too they should be on the balconies of the apartments here. Some habits in I*stanbul* should be transferred to people here . . . For instance, when I first arrived, I used to wear clothes that met the standards here; later, I thought that it is not they but I who should set the standards. Then with some minor changes, I started to wear the clothes that I'd wear in Istanbul. When I spoke on the phone before I came to here with the father of a female specialist who had resigned after fifteen or twenty days working in Yüksekova, he told me to have my hair cut very short, dye it a dark color, and not attract attention. This is the point of view adopted toward this place. Go there, do not attract attention, and come back.[49] This is not my personal choice. They should adapt to me, because it is me, not they, who knows the truth.

As the final sentences reveal, the self-confidence is almost religious, with a sense of missionary zeal. Or perhaps with a heavier tone, we might read the self-sacrificing attempts to contribute to civic and public life in Hakkâri as an activism weighed down by the "white man's burden" problematic. Certainly, there was no evidence of an attempt to go beyond the established Turkish nationalist stigmatizations and stereotypes concerning Hakkârians.

The way in which these specialist doctors situated themselves toward Hakkârians was further revealed by a disagreement we had at a particular moment of our interview when I cited the Turkish serial *One Turkey* (*Tek Türkiye*) broadcast during 2007–11 on Samanyolu, then the TV channel of Gülenists (a powerful, clandestine religious organization that had facilitated the capture of the state from the Kemalists by the AKP during the first decade). *Tek Türkiye* was mainly based on the story of a struggle in a Kurdish village between a doctor working hard and self-sacrificingly to serve the poor and uneducated people and the PKK and its cruel affiliates exploiting and benefiting ignorance of Kurdish people. The story is full of Turkish nationalist clichés, simplistic stereotypes, and absurd dichotomies, presenting the struggle as a good versus evil morality tale. When I cited the serial in our interview, I did not enter my mind that my secular interviewees might identify with the doctor of *Tek Türkiye* and subscribe to its perspective, but that was the case:

İlker:	There is a serial, *Tek Türkiye*, on Samanyolu. The protagonist is a doctor working in a village in the southeastern region . . .
Specialist 1:	Here, the people hate this serial. You can question this hate. Do you know why they hate it? [Spoken as though expecting that I would be surprised by hearing about this.]
İlker:	But the serial is really so bad, I can understand this anger. [I did not imagine that the specialists might not problematize the absurd and racist clichés of *Tek Türkiye*, especially as they were in direct relationship with Hakkârians on a daily basis].
Both:	Why? [This was the moment we realized that our assumed consensus on Hakkâri and Hakkârians did not actually exist.]
İlker:	Because . . . the people in it aren't realistic. It's full of clichés, it's a caricature [I held back from openly giving my opinion that it was a colonialistic, racist serial, which would have ended the interview and risked my field work, but the atmosphere in the rest of the interview became tense.]
Specialist 2:	That [Hakkâri] is a caricature, sure. We call it *"Vizontele"* [a comedy movie set in a small Kurdish town in the 1970s that experiences television for the first time]. That's *Vizontele*, indeed [meaning that there was nothing wrong with the way Hakkâri was depicted in *Tek Türkiye*].
Specialist 1:	But the reason why the people don't like the serial is that it denigrates the PKK. Ask them why they don't like it. They don't watch it on purpose. They don't like it on purpose. That's the reason. It supposedly makes them [Kurds] look bad [meaning that the artistic value of the serial could be problematized, but only a PKK affiliate would claim that the serial misrepresents reality in this political sense].

Such Turkish nationalist elitism in Hakkâri did not always appear so explicitly in doctors' testimonies. A less explicit manifestation of the superior indifference of doctors to the situation of Hakkâri shows how this stance was adopted by a large majority of doctors in Hakkâri: The doctors I interviewed frequently used pejorative terms like "ignorant" (*cahil, bilinçsiz*) and "uneducated" (*eğitimsiz*) when speaking of Hakkârians. In the transcripts of my interviews with the doctors, the word "*cahil*" occurs 28 times and "*bilinçsiz*" 21 times. Some doctors who otherwise adopted a cautious stance (by avoiding making judgments and simply paraphrasing the language and ideas of official brochures, regulations, or laws) still did not hesitate to make statements such as "We need to go down to the level of the people."

6.4.2.2 Hakkâri as an Open Prison

In addition to the role of elitism in the production of Hakkâri as an experience of endurance, one should also refer to the role of images and symbols engendered by the sense of deprivation and loss on the part of the assigned doctors. Given the topographical isolation of Hakkâri and its geographical distance from most of the country, the deprivations and shortcomings faced by the newly arriving GPs and specialists having to stay there for at least a year often resulted in a strong sense of claustrophobia and being cut off from the world.

Specialist, Hakkâri Public Hospital:

> I'd already made contact with some people working here as teachers via one of my acquaintances before I arrived. They welcomed me in Van and took me to Hakkâri. It was evening when we arrived . . . It was dark, and I felt stuck. "I'm stuck here. What should I do now?" That was my first feeling. I wanted to jump and get out of here, but I realized I couldn't and cried without any specific reason.

This sense of deprivation and loss led doctors to experience and live Hakkâri as an open prison and render their presence in Hakkâri into a sort of confinement—especially as they could not leave Hakkâri as they wished and at will.

Specialist-Administrator, Yüksekova Public Hospital:

> Q: What do you do in your leisure time?
> A: Nothing, zero. We come here in the morning, work all day, go back home, lock the door of our apartments, and rest. We try not to go outside or to the market as much as possible. We only go outside for shopping to buy vital needs and then go back to our home.
> Q: Are you afraid?
> A: I am, but also I don't enjoy touring around. There are already no places to see. Anything can happen at any moment, as well. Internet, cell phone, computer, TV . . . That's all . . . It's precisely an open prison. Ours is nothing short of an open prison.

The harsh geographical conditions of Hakkâri played a powerful role in the construction of this sense of confinement. The mountainous landscape surrounding Hakkâri and its districts reinforced the sense of isolation as the high mountains and deep valleys became metaphorical prison walls in the minds of the doctors. For example, a GP who worked in Çukurca and Hakkâri city said the following:

> Frankly, the journey from Van to Hakkâri is very interesting. Between Van and Hakkâri the geography is very mountainous. You feel like you're entering into another world ... When we were going to Hakkâri by bus, we came across a tank. I'm not exaggerating. Psychologically, I had started to motivate myself two weeks ago, saying to myself that I was coming to a problematic place where conditions are harsh. What annoyed me were the high mountains that make you feel that you are in a prison, as if they're coming for you. The mountains are so high. If you get claustrophobia, you then have a serious problem here. You're surrounded by high, rocky mountains. You're in a hole and can't see the horizon clearly. There's nothing but mountains. It upsets your psychology. It's like Alcatraz. You feel like you're in a prison. The real problem started with my passage to Çukurca ... Çukurca is a very small place. There are constant power cuts. Sometimes the mobile phone network collapses throughout the whole district for three days. You get depressed when you have power cuts five or six times a day. I felt like I was in prison there. Everywhere is surrounded by mountains. You can't go anywhere ...

The sense of living in an open prison, particularly the sense of claustrophobia and containment, can clearly play a powerful role in the production of space as an experience of endurance.

6.5 Essentialist and Discriminatory Discourses and Practices of the Doctors

The production of Hakkâri as endurance impacted significantly on doctor-patient encounters. The instrumentalism associated with endurance did not only qualify the way of being of doctors in Hakkâri but also, in the absence of any intersubjectivity, served as the normative model according to which the doctors judged the attitudes of the patients. The projection of instrumentalism onto the patients almost inevitably resulted in essentialist discourses on the patients. The persistence of the widespread dissatisfaction with healthcare provision in Hakkâri on the part of the patients did not make sense to the doctors, for whom the improvement in the capacity to meet the healthcare needs was the central fact and beyond dispute.

This is not to say that doctor-patient encounters in Hakkâri were exclusively informed by the expatriate background or otherness of Turkish doctors manifesting only in essentialist and discriminatory discourses and practices. But essentialist and discriminatory discourses and practices employed by Turkish doctors in Hakkâri were commonplace, and that was closely linked to the ways of seeing inherent to the production of Hakkâri as endurance.

GP, Yüksekova health post:

> I don't want to work here, this isn't Turkey. This is Kurdistan, and I don't want to serve the Kurdish people. All of the people here are PKK supporters. Tayyip nourishes the Kurds. He delivers money to the children [referring to the conditional cash transfers]. Why doesn't he deliver money to the children in the West?

Specialist, Hakkâri city:

> A: In the past, I didn't know the goals of the people here so well, the general characteristics of the Kurdish people. I was really ignorant about them. Now, I think I understand their character better, the causes of Kurdish people and their real goals ... My point of view changed. It's less artificial. It's different from the one that's manufactured by the media ... I don't like it here. I hate this place.
> Q: How do people approach doctors?
> A: In general, they respect us, but this respect is related to their character. It's a fake respect.
> Q: Fake respect?
> A: Sure, sure. Because they need us, they respect us in appearance. On the other hand, they attack the people they don't need [referring to security forces].

The first doctor quoted above was planning to resign, but neither expressed an unusual attitude or experience of life for the doctors assigned to the province. Doctors tended to imply essentialist discourses on patients concerning their ignorance and implicating their Kurdishness. Even those doctors not using explicitly essentialist terms when speaking about patients did not offer counter-evidence. As the vocabulary many of them used surrounding Hakkâri ("terrorism," "terror region," "PKK terrorism," along with "backward," "ignorant," etc.) shows, their first-hand "experiencing" of Hakkâri typically did not elicit a considerable break in their perspectives, which were largely informed by the convictions of mainstream Turkish nationalism. And on the occasions when they did break through the standard Turkish nationalist conditioning, as in the case above, it could be to just more deeply experience their isolation and difference.

The assumption widely shared by critics of the role the Turkish media has played in the Kurdish issue was that if the Turkish people living in the western part of the country understood the reality of the Kurdish region, they would not support the violent Turkish nationalist policies of the state. This was not the case, however. Most of the Turkish doctors experiencing Hakkâri first-hand in an unmediated fashion would maintain the Turkish nationalist convictions they went with. Some would go even further and develop more essentialist stigmatizations or racist stereotypes only deepened by the conviction of "experience."

According to Cohen, the tendency on the part of ex-pats to maintain stigmatizations and stereotypes about their hosts is mainly due to the fact that they have daily contact with only a very limited section of the local people under very specific conditions, which is not at all representative of life in the society at large. These meetings and connections, moreover, are influenced by the superior status of ex-pats:

> [D]espite his prolonged stay in the host country, the expatriate ... is largely cut off from the social reality of the country of his sojourn and often oblivious to it. The opinions and attitudes of expatriates to their hosts are in no small degree formulated from their contacts with a variety of subordinate service personnel, such as servants, chauffeurs, and gardeners ... No wonder, then, that their experiences not only do not change their old prejudices and stereotypes about the natives of the host country but often give birth to new ones ... Unsophisticated natives often reinforce the stereotypes of the expatriates by submissive or servile behavior, or by the uncritical acceptance of the superiority of the expatriates and emulation of their life-style, which sometimes assumes grotesque forms.[50]

Cohen's remarks shed light on important aspects of the issue here. Yet his explanation is partly an apologetic insofar as it shifts the responsibility of ex-pats' stigmatization of hosts to the side of the hosts. Alternatively, we might remember the warnings of John Wallach Scott, that experiencing reality as such is not possible: "experience is a linguistic event (it does not happen outside established meanings)."[51] Scott refuses "a separation between 'experience' and language" and instead emphasizes the "productive quality of discourse."[52]

Following Scott's refusal, the persistence of Turkish nationalist convictions by doctors in Hakkâri and the prevalence of essentialist discourses on patients should be taken as inherent to the production of Hakkâri as endurance. As indicated (above), the sense of discovering the other and openness to possible new identifications is missing in the production of space as endurance, which refers to a relationship with that which is endured in which interaction has no part, while the instrumentalist rationality involved means that the enduring subject constructs space in terms of problems to be passively managed for a temporary period. These two characteristics of the production of space as endurance independently and together pushed doctors to adopt essentialist discourses on patients and even sometimes employ discriminatory treatment to them. The following section identifies and analyzes two forms of these essentialist and discriminatory discourses and practices.

6.5.1 Discriminatory Treatment of Political Suspects

One outcome of the production of Hakkâri as endurance manifest in the doctor-patient encounter was the discriminatory treatment of political suspects. This could be clearly seen in the role played by doctors in the juridical process concerning those accused of affiliation with the PKK. As a legal requirement, everyone taken into custody needed to be taken to hospital immediately following their detainment in order to document whether they had been ill-treated during the detainment process. This issue has always been a problem in Turkey; cases in which doctors were threatened or attacked by policemen merely because they wanted to record evidence of ill-treatment used to be routinely reported (especially before the late-1990s, before the EU-accession process, when the torture of political detainees was the rule rather than exception).

Turkish doctors in Hakkâri, just as in other Kurdish provinces, often failed to document the ill-treatment of political suspects during the detainment process. This was either because these doctors held a strong anti-PKK stance—which cannot be thought independently of the lack of any interest in discovering the other (Hakkârians, "terrorists") and openness to possible new identifications—or because they wanted to avoid trouble with the police during their temporary stay. This latter point surely is again entwined within the construction of Hakkâri as a bundle of problems to be passively managed for a certain period of time.[53]

Clear support for the Turkish security forces was evident in the following two cases of voluntary collusion between doctors and the police. The first pertains to ill-treatment of the imprisoned cousin of one of my Hakkârian colleagues from the University of Hakkâri:

> My cousin was a PKK guerilla. Although he gave himself up to the security forces voluntarily last year, he was still tortured, so much that he should have been given a medical report stating that he wouldn't be able to do anything for five or six months. But when the police took him to the hospital, the doctor examined him in the room reserved for the police in the ER, not even in his room. When my cousin told him that if he reported the torture, he'd submit it to the court, the doctor declined to document the evidence of the torture, saying, "If you didn't deserve it, they wouldn't have done it."

A statement from a Hakkârian ER doctor based at Yüksekova Public Hospital also confirms that doctors assuming an anti-PKK stance actively collaborate with the police in the juridical process concerning PKK suspects.

> Q: Some doctors have told me that patients in Hakkâri are prejudiced against doctors?
> A: Of course, they're prejudiced. When there's an incident, there's unrest in the city; children throw stones and commit crimes, and so on. In the end, it's the judges and attorney generals that are authorized to punish them, not policemen or doctors. Nobody can beat them, rough them up, swear at them. My job is to examine and give treatment to patients. If a doctor from the West mistreats a child when he's brought in by the police for examination in the hospital after he's been taken under custody for throwing stones at them, this is wrong.
> Q: Are there such cases?
> A: Yes, it happens, and it happened in the past as well. If you have a stethoscope round your neck and you tell a child that they speak too much, they're terrorists, and this scenario goes on many times over years, a prejudice comes into being among these people that those coming from the West do not understand them, that they call them terrorists. There have been such doctors. One of them was even my colleague ... He worked together with me in the ER. There were such doctors in health posts as well. They used to mistreat the children and rough them up together with the police. They wouldn't treat everyone equally.

Turkish doctors do not always willingly volunteer to collaborate with the police, such as when they just do not want any trouble during their temporary stay and so are unwilling to resist illegal demands. A Hakkârian nurse working in a health post in Yüksekova reported such a case of passive complicity as a non-commitment to the situation:

> The policemen broke the arm of a child during a demonstration two or three years ago. I was a trainee then in a health post in Hakkâri [city]. The policemen came to the health post to talk with the doctors. They ordered me to leave the room, but even before I left the room, they told the doctors, "You have to sign this document stating that you did not examine this child." What could they do? They were doctors and were frightened. They signed the document. They [the police] had the same document signed [by doctors] in other institutions. In the end, the police managed to arrange a clean bill of health for the child.[54]

Exceptions should also be cited, although they may only serve to prove the rule. For example, a nurse from Yüksekova working in a health post there explained that one of the former directors of the district Health Directorate had once ordered doctors not to examine the children injured in incidents: "This led to a big quarrel in the health post when a doctor argued that she couldn't know where patients come from and would examine everyone entering the health post, whoever they were." The resistance was short-lived, however, as the director then opened disciplinary proceedings against her.

6.5.2 Paradigmatic Forms of the Essentialist Discourse on Patients: "Hungry Piranhas"

The production of Hakkâri as endurance produced essentialist discourses and discriminatory practices not only by guiding the reproduction and intensification of doctors' anti-PKK stance or their avoidance of trouble as the primary concern. In fact, this was a relatively minor aspect of the essentialist discourses and discriminatory practices employed by the Turkish doctors. The main body of these discourses and practices rather had to do with the fact that enduring doctors could not make sense of the dissatisfaction of the patients, predominantly because they were neither familiar with Hakkârians' way of reasoning nor had any strong desire to be so. In this regard, the stigmatization of patients became a useful and easy way of both making sense of the "strange" dissatisfaction of patients and escaping from the burden of feeling impelled to seek ways to confront the dissatisfactions.

Specialist, Hakkâri Public Hospital:

Q: Does the social tension in the city have an effect on the doctor-patient encounter?

A: Yes, for instance, now I need to write my name on the standby list. This is the last day for it. I need to submit my name to the list for my standby duty. But if I leave the room to write my name, some motherfucker immediately will go to complain about me. The people are malevolent toward us.

Q: It is said by your colleagues that it is difficult to ensure patient satisfaction in Hakkâri.

A: Of course. The people here approach the things as if we have a secret agenda and are malevolent toward them. Do they use the medicine prescribed by us or not? For instance, when we say that surgery is required, patients still say, "I'll go to Van." They don't trust us. They're malevolent toward us. I'm not generalizing, but a few exceptions won't be enough to save us if there's a big revolt [lit.: "social explosion"].

This specialist appears to have misinterpreted all the symptoms of the patients' conviction that their lives counted for little in the eyes of the Turkish state as manifestations of the "malevolence" he felt directed at Turkish doctors. He does not seem to have been aware of—or was unprepared to take into account—the fact that the negative prejudgments of the patients might have been engendered by their prior experiences with the medical establishment and state apparatus. He did not realize or allow for this as explaining patients' perceptions of the absence of a doctor from his room during work hours as neglect and a cause for complaint, the belief that the doctors in Hakkâri were too inexperienced to be trusted enough to use the medicine they prescribed, and the conviction that the hospitals in Hakkâri were insufficiently equipped for surgical operations. Instead, the doctor, like many of his colleagues enduring the situation, adhered to existing stereotypes that situated the responses of patients in an established discourse.

Again, accusing patients of acting in bad faith was a striking but not the dominant form of the essentialist responses given by doctors concerning the dissatisfaction of patients. The dominant, even paradigmatic form of essentialism was rather the perception of patients as ungrateful, greedy, and unappreciative of the labor and self-sacrifice of the doctors. Lacking any identification with and thus attachment to Hakkâri, doctors doing compulsory service there were thus largely guided by an instrumentalist rationality of endurance. Their existence in the province was no more than an interruption in their personal career and a suspension of "normal" life. For them, days in Hakkâri were something that merely passed, or did not. This was a life characterized by the logic of day-counting. The instrumentalism of endurance was not only what they performed; in the absence of any intersubjectivity, it commonly served the normative model according to which they judged the attitudes of patients. It was as if the misery of the living conditions in Hakkâri prevented the alternative of living there on any terms other than those of endurance.

Hakkâri Public Hospital, Specialist:

> In the end, you have to compare the present with the past. In the past, there wasn't a single specialist. All patients used to be transferred. Now all kinds of operations are performed. All patients are given treatment.

Crucially, as discussed, this sort of assessment was precisely *not* the usual way that the patients evaluated healthcare provision in Hakkâri. The disconnection between the two approaches was not recognized because the assigned doctors did not have so much more communication with their patients than with other Hakkârians outside the hospital. They simply did not know what the problem was, for the same reason that they did not deeply consider it or rather care to consider it and actively enquire into it—because, ultimately, all they were doing was enduring their CPSD assignment.

As a result, the instrumentalism of endurance was projected onto the patients through essentialist discourses on their ungratefulness and greed. The persistence of widespread dissatisfaction with healthcare provision did not make sense to the doctors given the huge improvement in the capacity to meet local healthcare needs, who believed patients should adopt a grateful and tolerant stance by comparing the deprivations of the past with the facilities of the present—and by enduring, just they did, the inevitable shortcomings of life in Hakkâri.

A step-by-step illustration of the formation of essentialist discourses on the ungratefulness and greed of the patients can be given with the following two examples. The first refers to an event that occurred in the Hakkâri Public Hospital ER and is recounted by a specialist who witnessed it:

> Once a girl came to the ER. She'd been injured by a pin. It wasn't possible to treat her here as the pin had gone in deep. You can find the exact position of the pin in these cases only if you have a scope. It's a very simple operation when you have a scope, but not having one made it impossible to find and take the pin out. Was it an urgent case? No. A pin in your leg doesn't kill you. Yet the patient insisted on being transferred to Van by ambulance. In order for an ambulance to be used for the transfer of patients, it has to be an emergency. If you transfer such a patient by ambulance, the number of ambulances available

for urgent cases decreases by one. This was all explained to the patient, and she was almost convinced that an ambulance was unnecessary. However, a journalist there provoked her and called someone. Even the provincial Director of Health and the Governor were informed about the situation. In the end, she was transferred to Van [by ambulance] on the Governor's decision. What was said there was: "You're not transferring me because I'm Kurdish. Isn't it a state ambulance? Why don't you use it for me?" What could the Governor do against these arguments?

Here, there was a clash of two different stances. The specialist took the prevailing conditions as given; as the equipment was missing, the number of ambulances was limited, and the case was not urgent, then what was to be done was clear—advise the patient to go Van by her own means. This stance, it may be noted, was itself derivative of the instrumentalist rationality of endurance, which corresponded to the passive management of the conditions of the city (i.e., which were also taken as given). The position taken by the girl and the journalist was quite different. They regarded the absence of a scope as a problem they should not have to deal with (endure) by their own means, but rather an issue for the state, which was obliged to provide health services equally to all its citizens and should thus find a solution to its own shortcoming, not the victim of the shortcoming. That is why, I believe, they insisted on demanding an ambulance for the transfer.

That the insistence on the transference by ambulance was made from an equal citizen's perspective is clear from the refusal to be discriminated against for being Kurdish and claim of the ambulance as a civic prerogative (since it belongs to the state). From the point of view of the specialist, however, the insistence of the patient and the journalist was medically unjustified, wasteful, and unreasonable. It seemed childish and immature. It was unsurprising, therefore, to hear her just 2 min after finishing telling this story that she felt Hakkârians complain about everything, lack any sense of gratitude, and exploit the medical establishment.

The second case pertains to the experience of a farmer from a village in Hakkâri city district:

> I took my child to Hakkâri Public Hospital to have him examined by a dermatologist. His appointment number was 50, but we were a bit late, so I went in the doctor's room to find out when they'd accept us to the room. I was led out the room. When I looked at the screen, I saw that those patients whose appointment numbers were 10 and 70 had already been examined. I realized they accepted patients to the room arbitrarily. I went in again and objected to

the way they accepted the patients to the room. Then the doctor shouted at me, "You Hakkârians complain about everything! Even if your child dies, I won't look after him!"

Normally, patients were given an appointment via a telephone call or website, but patients given an appointment would not always arrive at the hospital at the appointed time. This occurred frequently in Hakkâri, where a considerable part of the population still lived in rural areas. Therefore, patients would be called to the room not always according to the appointment number they held. The secretaries might call patients already there instead of waiting for the arrival of a patient who was late for their appointment, and someone looking at the screen showing the list of patients accepted to the room could easily think that the system was arbitrary—which seems to have been how the patient understood the situation in this case.

Patients in Hakkâri were inclined to read the procedures they encountered through the prism of a negative conviction. This patient's repeated attempts to object to the queuing system cannot be understood independently of this grievance. On the other hand, according to the doctor, who appeared not to appreciate how the patient saw the situation, the patient's objection was no more than another instance of the usual baseless dissatisfaction with the medical establishment shown by all Hakkârians. This was then framed in the established discourse on the essential insatiateness of Hakkârians who "complain about everything."

In this discourse, which emerges either as a misunderstanding of another misunderstanding, as in the latter case, or through an inability to make sense of a dissatisfaction arising from concerns about equal treatment as citizens, as in the former case, the patients were accused. The application of energy to gain insights into another type of explanation was not exhibited, or a desire to do so or even a conception of that possibility. Instead, words and phrases like "ungratefulness" (*tatminsizlik/takdir etmemek*), "exploitation" (*sömürü*), "spoiled" (*şımarık*), and "hungry piranhas" (*aç piranalar*) were generously expended, as in the excerpts below.

Specialist, Hakkâri Public Hospital:

> Their point of view is that "these doctors have to take care of us, it's their duty, and we don't need to appreciate their work." Of course, it's true that it's our duty to take care of them. Yet the attitude of people in the West toward doctors in terms of appreciation is different from here. You know doctors are given many gifts everywhere, especially after surgical operations. For instance, there was a urologist in the hospital here who used to do ten operations a day. When

I asked, he said that he was only given a gift once every year and a half. We don't expect to receive gifts, but they even don't say, "May God be pleased with you!" and thank us, let alone give gifts.

Specialist, Hakkâri Public Hospital:

> Let me say that they've forgotten the past, how they were oppressed, how they were ill-treated. Look at the facilities made available to them. These facilities, these physical conditions are missing even in Istanbul. I see that these people have begun to get used to them … They've become used to the services so much that they claim they have the right to things that indeed they do not have the right to … Some of them have started to become spoiled.

The following words are especially important since they were expended by a provincial Director of Health. Therefore, they should not be taken only as the expression of a personal idea but read also as the expression of a view that was widely held at the top levels of the local administration of state healthcare services:

> I myself have started to think, after I became an administrator, that the people we try to provide healthcare for are exploiting our work and showing ingratitude toward us. I still think that everyone has a right to full healthcare, but we are extremely overworked here while trying to provide people with this right. By way of a simple example, I would cite a case when 20 people injured in a traffic accident were brought to the hospital. All the specialists and even the provincial Director of Health were there and worked until midnight. You can't see such mobilization in another city; yet here, a relative of a patient says to the provincial Director of Health that it is he who's responsible if something should happen to the patient. Access to healthcare is, of course, a right. Yet, it's not the right of anybody to threaten doctors. I think that people should be educated about these issues. I've been feeling recently like they are hungry piranhas, and the more you give, the more they want. They're never satisfied.

These discourses accusing patients of being greedy and exploiting the state have real effects on the treatment of patients. One former provincial Director of Health told me that, in the past, although some patients were severely disabled, they were officially and deliberately assigned low disability ratings so as to make them ineligible for social assistance, which was reserved for severely disabled people:

> Q: It's said that there is a big demand for disability reports, that doctors are forced to give high disability ratings to patients.

A: Yes, but the reverse can occur as well. Sometimes the reports that should be given weren't given in the past. The former Vice Head Physician used to always ignore the ratings assigned by one of the members of the committee to ensure the overall disability rating remained below 90 percent. Obviously, he regarded the money assigned to the claimants as detrimental to the state.

Another reflection of this prejudiced response to "greedy" and "exploiting" patients in the doctor-patient encounter can be seen in the results of the complaints officially submitted to the patient rights unit of Hakkâri Public Hospital (serving after 2005 as part of the neoliberal and customer-oriented transformation of the national healthcare system). In 2013, 44 complaints were discussed by the patient rights committee, three-quarters of which pertained to doctors, but none were upheld. The number of patient complaints in 2013 ultimately regarded as a case of patient rights violation, therefore, was zero.

When we look at the overall state of the results of patient complaints submitted to the patient right units of all public hospitals in Turkey for that year, we see that the ratio of patient complaints ultimately regarded as a case of patient rights violation to all complaints was around 10 percent. In 2007, 2008, 2009, 2010, and 2011, the rates were 11, 18, 13, 11, and 12 percent, respectively.[55]

This discrepancy can be partly explained by the professional solidarity of doctors guided by the sense of protecting their accused colleagues. According to the general secretary of the Hakkâri Public Hospitals Union, the patient rights units in Hakkâri had a poor performance because the doctors would cover for each other. Given the weakness of the engagement of doctors with Hakkâri—the endurance factor—the level of doctors' sympathy with patients is relatively low, while doctors' professional solidarity with colleagues is high. Yet, this still does not account for the extremeness of the case, for why not even a single patient complaint among 44 (with 33 involving doctors) was not upheld.

The secret of the extremeness of the case lay in the totalizing gesture, as occurred in the case recounted by the provincial head of the SES employed in Hakkâri Public Hospital. He once told me that "the deputy chief physician used to write 'canceled' on each patient complaint file. When I objected and said 'You should follow the procedure,' he answered with, 'That's my way of doing things.'"

What led the deputy chief physician to cancel all patient complaints in advance without even transferring them to the patient rights committee for further interrogation goes beyond the requirements of professional solidarity. It concerns the prior belief of doctors in the groundlessness of the patient complaints. This then returns us to the essentialist discourses by which the doctors in Hakkâri make sense of patient dissatisfaction, complaints, and demands as instances of a local lack of appreciation, which extended to the broader region-to-country relationship and the valuation of the people themselves, as they well knew.

6.6 An Exception: Nursing and Midwifery Professionals

The essentialist discourses of Turkish doctors on the demanding stance and dissatisfaction of Hakkârians mainly had to do with the lack of sympathy with Hakkârians or ability or desire to consider possible new identifications, and this disengagement with Hakkârians was sustained, beyond the varying forms and levels of Turkish nationalism among the doctors, by the instrumentalist logic of endurance and day-counting. This argument can be cross-checked with the analysis of a tendency among Turkish nursing and midwifery professionals and other health workers (technicians, clerks, ambulance drivers, etc.) as distinct from Turkish GPs and specialists with respect to their stance toward Hakkârians. Unlike the main body of Turkish doctors, some of the Turkish nurses, midwives, technicians, and clerks in the hospitals, health posts, and family health centers in Hakkâri did manage to go beyond the problematic of endurance. They did establish dialogue and cooperation with Hakkârians, acquire new perspectives and leave old ones, and thus develop an understanding and sympathetic stance toward complaints and anger of Hakkârians.

The difference between these two groups of Turkish health professionals can be partly ascribed to the (somewhat) higher class habitus of the GPs and specialists and more working-class habitus of the rest, making the latter more tolerant than the former of the harsh conditions of Hakkâri. The main reason behind this difference seems to have been the difference between the conditions of employment of doctors and other health professionals.

Whereas the doctors fulfilled their compulsory service obligation in Hakkâri over between 300 and 450 days to leave for a better post in another province, the main body of the other Turkish health professionals there were contract-based workers and not given the option of leaving Hakkâri for a post in another province. Many of the nurses, midwives, clerks, and technicians had been already working for years in Hakkâri when I met them in the field. For them, Hakkâri was much more than a temporary hardship that they had to endure for a short period of time to go back to their routine; it was their life, at least for the indefinite future. Therefore, the way in which they were related to the local area, the region, and the people had a different dynamic to the instrumentalist logic of day-counting.

The longer the health workers stayed in Hakkâri, the more Hakkârian they became; and the more Hakkârian they became, the abler they were to see things from the locals' point of view and—crucially—win the *trust* of patients. This is clearly evident in the words of a group of Turkish nurses and midwives in the Yüksekova-2 Health Post (Figure 20), all of whom had come from Turkish cities to work as contract personnel. Referring to my question concerning the resistance of women of reproductive age to the tetanus vaccine, the conversation ran thus:

Nurse-A: When we first came, we had a lot of trouble. But that was a long time ago, nearly five years. Over time, people got to know us, we got to know them, they got used to us, and we got used to them. The sense of trust increased as the bond between us grew stronger.

Me: Other problems?

Nurse-A: Compared to other health posts, this one has less problems because we've all been working here for five years. That's not the case with other health posts. The people know us, even our names.

Nurse-B: They even know where we're from.

Nurse-A: When we first came, they were hiding the children in the barns, but now they themselves bring them. For example, a woman said to me today, "We made a lot of mistakes then by not allowing our children to be vaccinated," and now she says, "All our children should be vaccinated." So the mentality has changed in Yüksekova. They bring their children to us as soon as they are born.

The transformation appeared to be reciprocal. While winning the trust of the people they served, some of these health workers gradually managed to sympathize with Hakkârians and see things from their point of view. Their paradigm shifts sometimes reached such levels, we can say, that even their firmly established anti-Kurdish or anti-PKK stances were destabilized. For example, a Turkish nurse who had been working in Yüksekova for 5 or 6 years avoided calling the PKK-affiliated street demonstrators in the neighborhood "terrorists" and was even proud of being respected by the demonstrators. Referring to the violent street clashes between the PKK supporters and the police in the neighborhood, she said the following:

The clashes make us nervous, and we get upset. Frankly, when I first came here, I wondered what I was doing here. But now, we're not afraid of the clashes. I can go home by walking through the clashes because they [the protesters] do not attack me. They even look out for us. They tell us where the clashes are happening and suggest alternative routes. They offer to go with us. They really like us and our health post.

A technician at the Yüksekova Central Health Post had not only developed his ability to empathize with Hakkârians, which was not exceptional among the nursing and midwifery and other health professionals in Hakkâri, but so strongly identified with Hakkârians that he did not avoid engaging in a polemical exchange with one of his colleagues, a Turkish nurse who was in Hakkâri for a short period of time as the wife of a policeman. He tried to correct her criminalizing claims on Hakkârians, thus indicating, indeed, that experiencing Hakkâri as endurance and as a contact zone corresponded to two irreconcilable forms of relationship with Hakkârians.

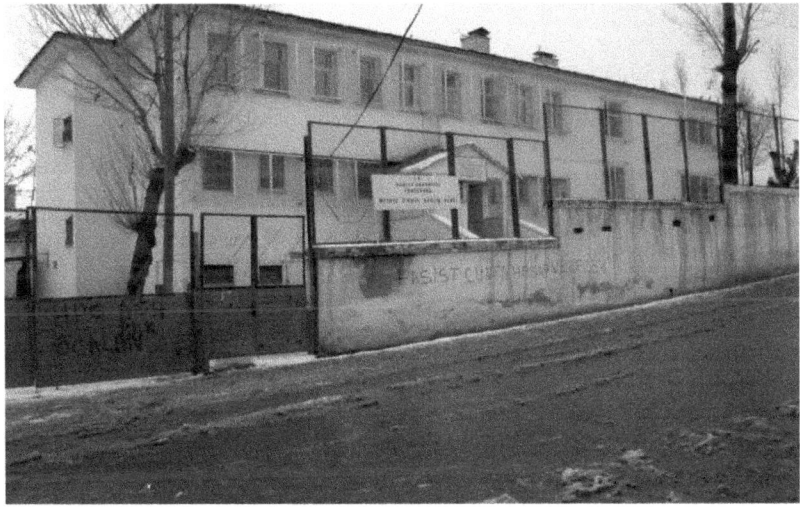

Figure 20. Yüksekova Central Health Post-2.
Note: This health post building previously belonged to the army. The army left it after the village evacuations (enforced by the army), which resulted in the development of new neighborhoods around the building and its targeting during clashes between the security forces and the highly politicized inhabitants of the new neighborhoods. The graffiti on the wall of the building reads: *Faşist cunta hesap verecek* (The fascist junta will pay).

> *Technician:* When we came here in 2005, vaccination rates were around 30 to 40%. It's recently increased to 95%
> *Question:* What was that resistance about?
> *Technician:* Usually, a staff member here used to stay for a year and then leave, so integration and trust could never be developed. However, I've been working here for five years and met many people. I went to their homes, shared their meals, and invited them to my home as well. They know that I wouldn't do anything wrong by them, so trust is created between us ... Also, that [tetanus vaccination] campaign was implemented in 18 provinces, and all of these 18 provinces are Eastern provinces. If the same campaign had been done in the West as well, it wouldn't have been a problem.
> *Question:* It is claimed that some health posts are targeted by demonstrators?

At that moment, a nurse present in the room intervened. She was one of the nurses whom I had seen before the interview in the room of the local Director of Health along with two other nurses. Asserting their status as wives of policemen, they had all asked the Director for exemption from the scheduled fieldwork in the villages, which they had argued might have been risky for them.[56]

> *Nurse:* Yes, I heard about it. [They threw stones] at Health Post 1.
> *Technician:* No, it wasn't Health Post 1. Something like that happened in 2005, but in fact, they weren't pelting it with stones.
> *Nurse:* Come on! That recently happened there.
> *Technician:* A few children might have thrown stones in the big clashes, but ...
> *Nurse:* I heard about it.
> *Technician:* In 2005, a child was shot around Health Post 2 [during the demonstrations]. He was taken to the health post but died there. Then the people there got agitated. But I haven't yet heard of a single case where health staff have been targeted on purpose.
> *Nurse:* I heard that last year, they threw stones at the ambulances.
> *Technician:* Such things may happen in clashes. This also happened in 2005. But they had a reason. They thought we were carrying police in the ambulance.

While the technician sympathized with Hakkârians to see things from their point of view, corrected criminalizing misrepresentations, and even understood why sometimes demonstrators would throw stones at the ambulances, the nurse merely repeated and reproduced the Turkish nationalist stigmatizations of Hakkârians circulating in the media as the backdrop to received wisdom and everyday consciousness. This disagreement between the nurse and the technician had its roots in two different ways of being in Hakkâri. One was rooted in living, the other based rather on enduring.

6.7 Conclusion

This chapter has examined the way of being of doctors in Hakkâri, mostly living in Hakkâri city and mostly posted there on compulsory service, not as a career preference. The doctors in Hakkâri experienced this province primarily as an exercise in endurance. This resulted in an unbridgeable gap between patients, who were often dissatisfied with healthcare provisions as a result of the sense of being discriminated against and engagement with the idea of equal citizenship, and doctors, who could not make sense of the persistence of patient dissatisfaction with the medical establishment in Hakkâri despite the remarkable progress there in recent years.

Doctors, especially the Turkish medical specialists, struggled to make sense of this dissatisfaction because they lived as an expatriate community, socially and culturally isolated from the host environment. They could and would not establish real relations with the patients or go beyond projecting their own way of being, the instrumentalist rationality of endurance, onto their patients. In other words, the experience of Hakkâri as an encounter typically failed to create any kind of a "contact zone" between the doctors and the local people. The gap between the two was filled by the doctors, not occasionally and contingently, but fairly consistently by essentialist discourses accusing patients of being greedy, ungrateful, and exploiting the medical establishment.

Notes

1. Mary Louise Pratt, *Imperial Eyes: Travel Writing and Transculturation* (London and New York: Routledge, 2008), 8.
2. Ibid.
3. For a comprehensive account of the characteristics of expatriate communities, see Erik Cohen, "Expatriate Communities," *Current Sociology* 24, no. 3 (1977).
4. Pascal Zurn et al., "Imbalance in the Health Workforce," *Human Resources for Health* 2, no. 1 (2004): 8.

5 Gilles Dussault and Maria C Franceschini, "Not Enough There, Too Many Here: Understanding Geographical Imbalances in the Distribution of the Health Workforce," *Human Resources for Health* 4, no. 1 (2006): 2.
6 Arthur J. Rubel, "Compulsory Medical Service and Primary Health Care: A Mexican Case Study," in *Anthropology and Primary Health Care*, ed. Jeannine Coreil and J. Dennis Mull (Boulder: Westview Press, 1990), 138.
7 Anthony Cavender and Manuel Albán, "Compulsory Medical Service in Ecuador: The Physician's Perspective," *Social Science & Medicine* 47, no. 12 (1998): 1937.
8 Suwit Wibulpolprasert and Paichit Pengpaibon, "Integrated Strategies to Tackle the Inequitable Distribution of Doctors in Thailand: Four Decades of Experience," *Human Resources for Health* 1, no. 12 (2003): 12.
9 Steve Reid, "Community Service for Health Professionals: Human Resources," *South African Health Review* (2002): 136.
10 *The Hindu*, 18 Nov 2007.
11 Ragıp Üner and Nusret Fişek, *Sağlık Hizmetlerinin Sosyalleştirilmesi Ve Uygulama Planı Üzerinde Çalışmalar* (Ankara: SSYB, 1961), 146.
12 Devlet İstatistik Enstitüsü (State Statistical Institute), *Türkiye İstatistik Yıllığı 1977* (Ankara: DİE, 1977), 86.
13 Marko Vujicic, Susan Sparkes and Salih Mollahaliloğlu, "Health Workforce Policy in Turkey: Recent Reforms and Issues for the Future" (working paper, World Bank, Washington DC, 2009), https://openknowledge.worldbank.org/handle/10986/13784.
14 Serap Yeşiltuna, ed. *Atatürk ve Kürtler: Resmi Kanun, Kararname, Rapor ve Tutanaklarla* (Istanbul: İleri Yayınları, 2007), 481.
15 Asena Günal, "Health and Citizenship in Republican Turkey: An Analysis of the Socialization of Health Services in Republican Historical Context" (Ph.D. diss, Boğaziçi University, 2008), 220-28.
16 *Milliyet*, October 22, 1981.
17 "Recep Tayyip Erdoğan'ın 21 Mayıs 2011 tarihli *Hakkâri* Mitingi Konuşmasının Tam Metni," Recep Tayyip Erdoğan, last modified January 4, 2022, https://tr.wikisource.org/wiki/Recep_Tayyip_Erdo%C4%9Fan%27%C4%B1n_21_May%C4%B1s_2011_tarihli_Hakkari_mitinginde_yapt%C4%B1%C4%9F%C4%B1_konu%C5%9Fma.
18 *Etıbbanın Hizmeti Mecburiyesi Hakkında Kanun*.
19 *1932 Senesinden İtibaren Tıp Fakültesinden Neşet Edecek Tabiplerin Mecburi Hizmetlerinin Lağvı ve Leyli Tıp Talebe Yurduna Alınan Tıp Talebesinin Tâbi Olacakları Mecburiyetler Hakkında Kanun*. The law was officially canceled in 1988 on the grounds that it was no longer applicable (other regulations had made it obsolete). Here one must cite the 1978 regulation (*Mecburi Hizmet Yükümlülüğünün Krediye Dönüştürülmesi Hakkında Yönetmelik*) providing for compensation for compulsory

service obligation and the 1983 regulation (*Yurt İçinde Mecburi Hizmet Karşılığı Öğrenci Okutma ve İhtisas Yaptırma Yönetmeliği*) standardizing the rules and duration of the compulsory service obligations of the various civil service sections.

20 *Tıp Mensuplarının Devlet Teşkilâtında Vazifeye Alınma Şartlan Hakkında Kanun.*
21 *Bazı Sağlık Personelinin Devlet Hizmeti Yükümlülüğüne Dair Kanun.* The law was amended three times; first in 1986 and last in 1995. In 1995, the compulsory service imposed on specialists was suspended until 2000, when the suspension was prolonged for another 2 years and extended to compulsory service for general (non-specialist) doctors.
22 *Sağlık Hizmetleri Temel Kanunu, Sağlık Personelinin Tazminat ve Çalışma Esaslarına Dair Kanun, Devlet Memurları Kanunu ve Tababet ve Şuabatı San'atlarının Tarzı İcrasına Dair Kanun ile Sağlık Bakanlığının Teşkilat ve Görevleri Hakkında Kanun Hükmünde Kararnamede Değişiklik Yapılmasına Dair Kanun.*
23 Henri Lefebvre, *The Production of Space* (Oxford and Cambridge, MA: Blackwell, 1991), 21.
24 Andy Merrifield, *Henri Lefebvre: A Critical Introduction* (New York: Routledge, 2006), 107.
25 Ibid., 108, 111.
26 Lefebvre, *The Production of Space*, 33, 39.
27 "Endurance," http://www.merriam-webster.com/dictionary/endurance.
28 Laclau, *Emancipation(S)*, 52.
29 Judith Butler, Ernesto Laclau, and Slavoj Žižek, *Contingency, Hegemony, Universality: Contemporary Dialogues on the Left* (London: Verso, 2000), 100.
30 "Symbolic order": society is impossible because "antagonism and exclusion are constitutive of all identity. Without limits through which a (non-dialectical) negativity is constructed, we would have an indefinite dispersion of differences whose absence of systematic limits would make any differential identity impossible. But this very function of constituting differential identities through antagonistic limits is what, at the same time, destabilizes and subverts those differences." Laclau, *Emancipation(S)*, 52.
31 Jessica Benjamin, "An Outline of Intersubjectivity: The Development of Recognition," Supplement, *Psychoanalytic Psychology* 7 (1990): 41.
32 Cohen, "Expatriate Communities," 17.
33 Ibid., 18.
34 Ibid.
35 Ibid.
36 Ibid., 77.
37 Bülent Dinçer and Metin Özaslan, *İlçelerin Sosyo-Ekonomik Gelişmişlik Sıralaması Araştırması* (Ankara: Devlet Planlama Teşkilatı, 2004).
38 Republic of Turkey, *T.C Resmi Gazete*, no. 25866, July 5, 2005.

39 It might be suggested that it is paradoxical to still speak of the production of space while, on the other hand, arguing that concrete space is replaced by the passing time of endurance; the replacement of space by time can also be read as an active production of *indifference* to space, but the expression "indifference to space" may be misunderstood as invoking the Cartesian assumption (that space precedes the human subject); therefore, the replacement of space by time via CPSD law is expressed in terms of the production of space as endurance. For an insightful discussion concerning indifference to space, see Alan Latham, "Powers of Engagement: On Being Engaged, Being Indifferent, and Urban Life," *Area* 31, no. 2 (1999).
40 A city and province in the western Black Sea region of Turkey.
41 *Milliyet*, August 28, 2010.
42 There was no translation problem in most of the family health centers as most were staffed with Hakkârian GPs.
43 A guest house for doctors with 30 beds, right across the *Hakkâri* Public Hospital, was opened in 2009. It was intended to host newly appointed doctors in their early arrival days until they find an apartment. However, I was told that some doctors stayed in the guest house during their whole working period in *Hakkâri*.
44 Alfred Sohn-Rethel, *Intellectual and Manual Labour: A Critique of Epistemology* (Atlantic Highlands, NJ: Humanities Press, 1978), 21.
45 Benjamin, "An Outline of Intersubjectivity," 35.
46 It is claimed garbage containers are used for the placement of bombs.
47 For a discussion on Turkish elitism toward the Kurds, see Welat Zeydanlıoğlu, "The White Turkish Man's Burden: Orientalism, Kemalism and the Kurds in Turkey," in *Neo-Colonial Mentalities in Contemporary Europe? Language and the Discourse in the Construction of Identities*, ed. Guido Rings and Anne Ife (Newcastle upon Tyne: Cambridge Scholars Publishing, 2008), 155–74.
48 Elif M. Babül, "Training Bureaucrats, Practicing for Europe: Negotiating Bureaucratic Authority and Governmental Legitimacy in Turkey," *PoLAR: Political and Legal Anthropology Review* 35, no. 1 (2012): 31.
49 Notice that the advice "Go there, do not attract attention, and come back" is the very definition of the instrumentalist approach.
50 Cohen, "Expatriate Communities," 69.
51 Joan W. Scott, "The Evidence of Experience," *Critical Inquiry* 17, no. 4 (1991): 793.
52 Ibid.
53 M. Fayik Taşkın, ed. *Sağlık Kurultayı Belgeleri (3-4-5 Aralık 2010, Diyarbakır)* (Diyarbakır: Aram Yayınları, 2012), 92.
54 See https://www.youtube.com/watch?v=UT9Gk3tkGsk.
55 "Hasta Hakları Uygulamaları İstatistikleri," *Sağlık Bakanlığı* (Ministry of Health), accessed January 13, 2022, https://shgmhastahakdb.saglik.gov.tr/TR-4771/hasta-haklari.html.

56 Due to security concerns, as far as I could see, the nurses and midwives who came to Yüksekova as wives of policemen and military personnel appointed there were mostly employed in the Yüksekova Central Health Post as it was close to the police headquarters and away from the neighborhoods where most people lived.

7
Discussion

What opinion-makers and party administrators do not understand is the change in the state.

Muammer Türker, former Governor of Hakkâri

and Secretary of the National Security Council

In relating the chapters to one another to draw together and extend the arguments, the discussion here is carried out at two levels (as indicated in the introduction). The first level is mainly of interest to scholars of Turkish and Kurdish studies. Reflections on the research findings further analyze their implications for the limits of the AKP's state-nationalism in the 2003–14 period studied. The second level pertains to the global and comparative implications of the research, which primarily concern the dynamics of ethnopolitical challenges in multiethnic societies and the subsequent state strategies deployed to contain these challenges.

7.1 Patient Dissatisfaction and Essentialist Discourses as Limits of Turkish State-Nationalism

Returning to the original question posed on the assimilation and containment strategy employed by the AKP until 2014, it can be argued that the dissatisfaction of patients with the quality of healthcare provision in Hakkâri at the time, and the essentialist and discriminatory discourses of the doctors on the supposed ungratefulness and greediness of the patients, both shed light on its limits. During my fieldwork period, healthcare provision was not peculiar among the benevolent policies employed in Hakkâri with regard to the dissatisfaction of Hakkârians with services and, indeed also, to the disappointment on the part of the state agents with this dissatisfaction.

As indicated by the words quoted below of Muammer Türker, then Governor of Hakkâri, the very form of the dissatisfaction with the state's health provisioning (citizenly disaffection, and dissatisfaction and disaffection as prejudgment) together with the disappointment of the state agents (accusing Hakkârians of being ungrateful) was common to prevailing dissatisfactions, disaffections, and disappointments around public services generally in the city:

> The state tries to compensate for its negligence in the past ... It has introduced extraordinary positive discrimination measures into Hakkâri over the last ten years ... The Ministry of Environment and Forestry has undertaken the responsibility of the construction of a sewage system, potable water network, and treatment unit of Yüksekova. Unfortunately, people see it as an "obligation of the state." No, it is just taking on an additional responsibility. If I avoid undertaking these constructions, nobody can hold me responsible. It is not my duty.
>
> The construction of roads, schools, and hospitals does not automatically solve anything. There's a generation that hates the state. We have to win them over. Although you improve everything, the images of the past do not easily disappear. The police who have stones thrown at them today are the police of a previous decade. The state they [the stone throwers] are angry with is the one that was the perpetrator of "murders by unknown perpetrators." It is the state that bombed Umut Bookstore in Şemdinli, tortured people, and evacuated villages. What opinion-makers and party administrators do not understand is the change in the state.[1]

The first part of this quotation speaks of citizenly dissatisfaction and the second of the strength of the conviction that the state still did not regard the lives of

Kurds as very worthy of care and respect. Notice also the not-so-implicit pedagogical disappointment of the former governor. By 2011, when this opinion was published in a government-friendly national newspaper, neither the dissatisfaction with public services nor the anger and incomprehension on the part of the state agents in the face of the reluctance of the people to compare past and present and thus appreciate the improvement was peculiar to any particular sector of public services delivered in Hakkâri. And indeed, there is nothing very surprising in all the anger and incomprehension, given the homology between the doctors' approach to the patients and the AKP's approach to Kurdish "service-beneficiaries."

The disappointment of the AKP in its failure to weaken the mass support in Hakkâri for the Kurdish movement replicated on a wide (managerial) scale the disappointment of the doctors at the everyday (service provision) level. Both disappointments resulted from an inability to lead Hakkârians to compare the improvement in the present with the deprivations of the past, realize the transition and development, and appreciate the change. And both projected the instrumental rationality of endurance onto Hakkârians. While the enduring doctors performed this as a projection of their own mode of being onto patients, the AKP did it in addressing Hakkârians as citizens-in-the-making as a part of its development and transition fantasy.

In this context, the speech delivered by then Prime Minister Erdoğan in 2011 in Hakkâri city is revealing in its expression of the discursive package with which the AKP employed its assimilation strategy:

> Compare Hakkâri of eight and a half years ago with present-day Hakkâri. My brothers in Yüksekova, Şemdinli, and Çukurca would listen to Kurdish music in secret. Mothers could not speak Kurdish with their children. Nobody would talk about Ahmedi Xani, and Mem-u Zin was forbidden ... Today the Ministry of Culture and Tourism publishes Mem-u Zin. One state TV channel broadcasts in Kurdish 24 hours a day. Who made these reforms? Which party made these reforms? We made these reforms and will continue to make better ones. Today the University of Hakkâri organizes the International Congress of Kurdology, the Congress of Kurdish Women, and the Congress of Kurdish Language and Literature in the 21st Century. Who founded this university?
>
> Do you know how much we invested in healthcare provision in Hakkâri? 120 trillion, 120 trillion. We completed the construction of two family health centers ... and also initiated the construction of five family health centers and completed their construction quickly. There were no tomography or MR machines in the public hospitals of Hakkâri. Now we have two tomography

and one MR machine ... Do you know how many dialysis machines there were in Hakkâri before us? There were six ... Now there are twenty dialysis machines available. How many 112 [emergency ambulance] stations were there in Hakkâri before us? Only one. And now? Fourteen ... Do you know how many ambulances there were in Hakkâri? One. And now? Twenty ... I am asking my Kurdish brothers: will you vote for service provision or the politics of identity? I believe that doing the right thing, as you are expected to do, my Kurdish brothers will vote for the politics of service. There were ten specialists before us, and now that has risen to 96.[2]

Here, Erdoğan projects the objective rationality of a bare life onto Hakkârians. He tries to deprive Hakkârians of the subjective, of their experiences, histories, and ideologies, namely the "politics of identity," which he supposes prevents them from looking through the lens of objective rationality of bare life and noticing the tangible, measurable improvement. The Hakkârians addressed in the electoral speech are not addressed as subjects, with subjectivities and stories of their own, who deserve to be recognized and whose share in the transformation process should be acknowledged. The sole actor in this narrative is the Turkish state that employed violence in the past and now "changes" in the present. The people appear in the scene only as victims of state violence and recipients, at best as passive agents called in a pedagogical way to move on from the images of the past:

> I ask for my brothers in Hakkâri to appreciate the reality from now on. I ask for my brothers in Hakkâri to question the politics of violence from now on. I ask for mothers in Hakkâri to own their children from now on and call them back from mountains ... I ask for you to make a distinction between the followers of the politics of identity and the followers of the politics of service from now on.[3]

In short, the place reserved for Hakkârians in this discourse is no more than a move from objects of sovereign violence, *homo sacer*, a type of bare life, to (if they collaborate) objects of the politics of service, service-beneficiaries, another type of bare life—or, to objects of the Anti-Terror Law, once again *homo sacer*, if they insist on pursuing the politics of identity, as was shown in KCK arrests.

The limit of the assimilation and containment strategy of 2013–14 can be expressed, then, as the extent to which Hakkârians could be (re)produced as objects of a developmentalist pedagogy, achieved by dividing them into their bare and qualified lives and then privileging the former while criminalizing the latter through recourse to the depoliticizing contrast between the politics of service and the politics of identity. As discussed with reference to the doctors' disappointment with the patients' persistent dissatisfaction, and as the electoral failure of the AKP shows, this limit should be taken seriously, at least for the following two reasons.

First, full recognition of their Kurdishness was actually a prerequisite of any possible change in many Hakkârians' perception of and approach to public services. This was because they were convinced by their life experience that their Kurdish lives were viewed as less valuable in the eyes of the Turkish state. Consequently, being asked to make a choice between the politics of identity and the politics of service just did not resonate with many Hakkârians. They claimed access to proper public services as an issue of equal recognition. This was not open to negotiation or a weapon that could be used against their political subjectivity.

Second, this limit should be taken seriously because the citizen in the making, the single subject-position offered to Hakkârians by the developmentalist pedagogy, was in serious contradiction to the lived reality of many Hakkârians who appeared as *already* citizens. The claim to qualified healthcare provisioning and other public services *now* and *equally* from the point of view of these fully-fledged citizens was quite irreconcilable with the developmentalist pedagogy of Erdoğan calling on Hakkârians to adhere to the objective rationality of bare life and appreciate the positive change for now as citizens-in-the-making.

In short, the limit of the strategy followed during 2003–14 was the limit reached in an attempt to carry out a sort of politics of redistribution that was not a moment of full recognition. It was rather a sort of politics of redistribution that tried to convince Hakkârians to be content with a situation that fell short of full respect to their identity and bodies.[4]

To elaborate on this argument, we might proceed with the famous conceptual distinction expressed by Donald Winnicott between "object-relating" and "object-usage." Winnicott argues that "object relating is an experience of the subject that can be described in terms of the subject as an isolate." In relating to an object, the object exists as "subjective object," "projective entity," and "a bundle of projections," to the extent that it means something only from the stance of the subject. It is just "a phenomenon of the subject."[5] It does not have a life of its own independent of the subject.

As for object-usage, "usage cannot be described except in terms of acceptance of the object's independent existence, its property of having been there all the time." What is needed for the object-usage to occur "is the subject's placing of the object outside the area of the subject's omnipotent control; that is, the subject's perception of the object as an external phenomenon, not as a projective entity, and in fact the recognition of it as an entity in its own right."[6]

To proceed through this distinction, we can conclude that Hakkârians (Kurds) as imagined by the pre-2015 strategy of Erdoğan and the AKP were perfect examples of "a bundle of projections" that lack lives of their own independent of the state; they owe their agency—which occupied a space between "being victims of the state violence" and "appreciating the positive change of the state"—completely to the state that had enabled this agency by its violence in the past and positive change in the present. The secret of what made the AKP's approach to Hakkârians and Kurds generally during this period a Turkish nationalist one—independently of, and even despite, its democratic reforms and health investments—resided precisely in this gesture: the implicit degradation of "Kurdishness" by approaching Kurds as if they did not have a separate history independent of their relations with the Turkish state, as if the existence of Kurds counted only to the extent that they were part of the narrative of the democratization of the Turkish state. Patronizing and pedagogical language was therefore inherent in and integral to this unequal encounter of the state and the Kurds.

The problem was that a considerable part of Hakkârians did not want to be projective entities of the Turkish nationalism of the AKP. They did not want to be judged, advised, or patronized, for they thought they were already deserving of full care and respect as entities in their own right. In other words, they demanded to be recognized in the sense that recognition is first and foremost "to accept and respect the other as an end in herself such that controlling, dominating, and manipulating behaviors are inappropriate."[7] The implicit and explicit emphasis placed on equal and full citizenship by Hakkârians as reported here, therefore, should be read in the first place as a desire for a position that prevents anybody from addressing them from a superior one or from advising them to be content with anything short of full respect of their identities and bodies.

We can conclude, then, that the limit of the strategy of the AKP approach during the first decade of their rule was, in the last instance, rooted in the unbridgeable gap between addressing the Kurd as an object, a projective entity of Turkish nationalist fantasy, and recognizing the Kurd as a subject in their own right, as someone who "has a separate and equivalent center of self."[8] More concretely, the improvement of public services in Hakkâri during the 2003–14 period should be regarded as an attempt to render people as pedagogical objects and bare lives by translating their everydayness into a moment in the linearity of the transition and development narrative of the Turkish state-nationalism. This attempt, however, largely failed to construct a hegemony in the face of the subjectivities of the already-citizens; the subjectivities and histories excluded from this narrative continued to haunt the pedagogical narrative in the very performance of citizenship in Hakkâri, played out in this instance as dissatisfaction with public services and thus, ultimately, dissatisfaction with the AKP and its brand of Turkish nationalism.

7.2 The Issue of the Rationality of Ethnopolitical Challenges: Gains and Losses

Beyond the issues of Turkish nationalism and Kurdish identity, what lessons can we generate from the failure of the AKP's benevolent assimilation strategy in Hakkâri and in the whole of the Kurdish region in 2003–14? To which theoretical discussions does the failure of the AKP strategy lead us? One might suggest many theoretical discussions, yet, in all cases, the issue of the (ir)rationality of ethnopolitical challenges comes to the fore. The failure of the AKP's assimilation strategy was a striking violation of the commonsensical assertion that the more benevolent and the less violent an assimilative power, the weaker will be the ethnopolitical discontent. Indeed, the more benevolent, less violent politics did not prevent the Kurdish movement from reaching the peak of its strength, both in Hakkâri and in other Kurdish provinces.

To expect a more benevolent and less violent an assimilative power to result in weaker ethnopolitical discontent is to assume that ethnopolitical challenges are built on an instrumentally rational basis. Tom Nairn in *The Break-up of Britain* made this argument in Marxist terms (when he recognized the irrational and passionate aspects of nationalism but highlighted the rational core of nationalism as a response to uneven development).[9] A more explicit expression of the argument can be found in Anthony Birch's works.

According to Birch, "the extent to which ethnic and cultural minorities are content with their situation of political integration in a larger state depends on the balance of advantages in any particular period."[10] This is why, according to Birch, minority nationalisms were weak in the first half of the twentieth century when, for instance, most of the citizens of "Quebec, Scotland, Wales, and Brittany believed that the benefits they derived from their membership of the Canadian, British, and French states outweighed the cultural and other sacrifices involved," while these sort of minority nationalisms intensified in the postwar period when "the balance of advantage between the sizable multipurpose state and the small community has changed to the disadvantage of the sizable state."[11] This balance shifted due to the emergence of international organizations (the IMF, World Bank, NATO, etc.) liberating ethnic groups of the necessity to tolerate cultural and political sacrifice in order to enjoy the economic and military stability, security, and facilities enabled by membership of a larger state.[12]

The arguments put forward by Michael Hechter also exemplify this approach. Hechter argues that "it stands to reason that the members of peripheral nations may be willing to sacrifice some self-determination to profit from inclusion in a larger, albeit multinational, state. This willingness undercuts the demand for sovereignty. The demand for sovereignty among peripheral nations, therefore, varies with its net benefit."[13] More examples could be added, but in the end, the argument of the rationalist approach is not a complicated one: the emergence and strength of ethnopolitical challenges depend on the calculus of advantages and disadvantages of being incorporated into a sizable state.

7.2.1 The Lessons of Hakkâri

It is clear that the findings of this study of Hakkâri do not confirm the rationalist approach to ethnopolitical challenge. The Kurdish movement reached the peak of its power in Hakkâri and the wider Kurdish region when the usual state violence toward Kurds generally and thus Hakkârians was at its lowest point in a generation and when the state's capacity to meet the basic needs of Kurds/Hakkârians was similarly unequaled (albeit it still insufficient). If this is not to be regarded as another confirmation of the essential irrationality of nationalism as "a passionate assertion of the will,"[14] then the case of Hakkâri may assist in identifying some of the limitations of the rationalist approach.

The first issue that needs to be emphasized about the rationalist approach is that it retrospectively projects the concept of the nation backward in history. This approach problematically suggests that nations are natural entities that exist prior to the emergence of nationalist movements or to the decision to form nationalist movements where the advantages of secession/autonomy outweigh the advantages of political loyalty. The major drawback of this objectivist understanding of the nation is that it leads us to ignore the subjective aspect of nation. This research can thus help elucidate two particular manifestations of this drawback.

First, the above argument does not take into account that the ethnopolitical way of seeing is historically determined.[15] This is revealed in the analysis of patient dissatisfaction in Hakkâri. It thus does not allow an objective "bird's eye" view from which to view the "advantages" or "disadvantages" of the situation as they "really" are. The historically established belief that their Kurdish lives are undervalued by the Turkish state led Hakkârians to a pessimistic way of seeing the state in which the disadvantages were much more visible than the advantages.

This way of seeing made the rational calculation of advantages and disadvantages as if from a bird's eye view impossible, not only by its selective biases but also, albeit to a lesser extent, by a misperception of "advantages" as "disadvantages."

Secondly, an ethnopolitical way of seeing may not permit an objective view of these "advantages" or "disadvantages," not just because of its historically determined nature. As a specific and normative way of seeing the world, the ethnopolitical way of seeing involves a substantive rationality that applies "certain criteria of ultimate ends ... and measure[s] the results of the action ... against these scales of 'value rationality' or 'substantive goal rationality.'"[16] Given that the ultimate end of any ethnopolitical challenge is to institutionalize the ethnopolitical unit as an entity on its own right, albeit not necessarily in a secessionist form, it can be said that things appear advantageously to the substantially rational ethnopolitical gaze only to the extent that they confirm the ethnopolitical unit as an entity on its own right, and things become disadvantageous only to the extent that they deny that confirmation. If Hakkârians had been content with their being as citizens-in-the-making and thus adopted a comparison in time instead of a spatial comparison as their analytical framework and means of assessing the quality of healthcare provision, things that appeared as disadvantages to them would, in all likelihood, have seemed as advantages.

Can we conclude, then, that the (ir)rationality of ethnopolitical challenges cannot be categorically discussed if the ethnopolitical way of seeing is not an "objective" way of seeing? Should we follow Béland and Lecours and agree with their conclusion that, as shown by ethnopolitical movements in Scotland and Quebec that demanded further decentralization of social policy when they were net receivers of territorial transfers, ethnopolitical movements are driven and shaped primarily by autonomous logic of ethnopolitics, not by gains and losses, interests and rationality?[17]

This research implies an acknowledgment of the possibility of speaking of a space for calculus of advantages-disadvantages in the relationship between the state and a minority group. At least, this is implied where and insofar as the relationship is characterized by immense unevenness and dependency, as it was in Hakkâri, and as long as we avoid subscribing to some sort of discursive reductionism claiming that the dominant discursive framework informing a minority's way of seeing can be shaped independently of this unevenness and dependency. We should remember that ethnopolitical movements in Scotland and Quebec have demanded further decentralization of social policy despite being net receivers of territorial transfers, yet without acting in a dramatically "irrational" way by so doing, given that the transfers made were not so massive as to redefine the relationship between the actors as one of dependency.

The findings of this thesis, however, do show that the way that benevolent, less violent politics impinges upon ethnopolitical discontent may be quite different from that predicted by the rationalist theory. One can follow this in the strangeness of the evidence gleaned from Hakkâri when it is viewed from a comparative perspective. I refer to the hybrid nature of ethnopolitical discontent in Hakkâri with the Turkish state: Hakkârians complaining about the insufficiencies of healthcare provision never suggested that healthcare provisioning and other social services would be better had they organized and operated their own healthcare policies independently of the central government.

While the local discontent with the political and cultural policies of the state led them to demand recognition by putting forward their ethnic differences and distinctiveness, their response to the insufficiencies of state healthcare provisions was to demand not autonomy but a more effective state presence. This they did by asserting their citizenship status. Even though the AKP usage of social policy tools as instruments of political control was also subject to criticisms, these censures never progressed into demands for the financial or administrative decentralization of social policy. The total lack of demand for decentralization of social policy in the agenda of my informants applies to both local and central actors of the Kurdish movement. The Kurdish movement, which is especially strong in Hakkâri, has always made insistent demands for political and cultural autonomy—which has been the main thrust of the local, bottom-up activism of the KCK—and yet the decentralization of social policy was not even included at the bottom of the list of demands from the Turkish state gathered in this research.

That the dissatisfaction with healthcare provisioning and other social services does not or at least need not and did not lead directly to demands for the decentralization of social policy distinguishes the Kurdish case from similar ethnopolitical challenges in European and American contexts. Dissatisfaction with social policy in multiethnic Euro-American situations has led to ethnopolitical demands for the decentralization of social policy, as in Scotland/UK, Quebec/Canada, and Flanders/Belgium, among others. The decentralization of social policy is one of the most important agendas of ethnopolitical movements in these contexts.[18]

Is it possible to account for this divergence with a suggestion that the hard, non-discursive reality of economic dependency, which is not experienced by Euro-American ethnopolitical movements, pierces the discursive framework of the Kurdish ethnopolitical vision, forces it to loosen its substantial rationality, and thus makes room for some sort of pragmatism? Is it possible to account for the assertion of citizenship status and the idea of Turkey instead of demands for decentralization of social policy and healthcare organization against the insufficiencies of healthcare provision in the province as a "not-yet" issue or a rhetorical maneuver used to ensure that the demands are heard and responded to by the state?

Perhaps, but the main problem with these explanations is their identification of the ethnopolitical challenge with sub-state nationalism that thus classifies the Kurdish case as a divergence or exception. This is particularly the case given that sub-state nationalist movements are inherently inclined to "bring the mechanisms of solidarity within the boundaries of their national community"[19] as movements in search of instituting the sovereignty (independence) of their nations. In addition to this theoretical reason, my research findings also work against these explanations.

If the lack of demand for the decentralization of social policy, healthcare organization, and the assertion of citizenship status and the idea of Turkey against the insufficiencies of healthcare provision pertained only to the political discourse of Kurdish politicians calling out to the state, these explanations could have made some sense. However, those referring to their citizenship status and the idea of Turkey were generally not only Kurdish politicians calling out to the state. They were mostly just ordinary citizens considering the shortcomings of healthcare provision in the province. Even though they did not need to refer to their citizenship status or make comparisons with (other) Turkish provinces to describe the shortcomings, they nevertheless articulated their dissatisfaction through implicit and explicit citizenship references and provincial comparison. This means that Hakkârians calling for a more effective presence of the state in the field of social policy with reference to their citizenship status while insistently demanding for political and cultural decentralization cannot be identified with ethnopolitical pragmatism. This was a *hybrid* ethnopolitical expression.

Following William Roseberry's loose conception of hegemony, we may do better than to put this hybridity down to inconsistency or a case of pragmatist concession and should rather define it as a case of *hegemony*:

> I propose that we use the concept [hegemony] not to understand consent but to understand struggle, the ways in which the words, images, symbols, forms, organizations, institutions, and movements used by subordinate populations to talk about, understand, confront, accommodate themselves to, or resist their domination are shaped by the process of domination itself. What hegemony

constructs ... is not a shared ideology but a common material and meaningful framework for living through, talking about, and acting upon social orders characterized by domination ... That common material and meaningful framework is, in part, discursive: a common language or way of talking about social relationships that sets out the central terms around which and in terms of which contestation and struggle can occur.[20]

Hegemony as defined by Roseberry refers to neither ideological domination nor ideological consent. It rather refers to the varying capacity of the dominant to inform the range of symbolic and material realities of the dominated. Therefore, if we speak of some sort of hegemony of the dominant over the dominated, it is not so surprising that the challenge of the dominated—here an ethnopolitical challenge—may *spontaneously* call for some or most terms of the dominant—here citizenship and the idea of Turkey.

This cannot be likened to the mechanism at work in the pragmatist concession on the principle of sovereignty of an otherwise nationalist/secessionist ethnopolitical challenge, for the language of the challenge of the dominated under hegemony is hybrid as an expression of the hybridity of the reality of the dominated (being Kurdish and a citizen of Turkey at the same time), not as an issue of concession. According to the results of a survey conducted in June 2010 on "Perceptions and Expectations Concerning the Kurdish Issue," the proportion of Kurds declaring that it was either "important" or "very important" to be defined as "citizens of the Republic of Turkey" (*Türkiye Cumhuriyeti vatandaşı*) was 68.2 percent. Similarly, the idea being mooted at the time that the population be referred to as "Türkiyeli" (lit.: from Turkey or Turkey national) was important to 66.8 percent of Kurds. For only 13–14 percent of Kurds were these identities "unimportant" or "totally unimportant."[21]

We can justifiably argue that even though increasing public investment and social transfers to Hakkâri and other Kurdish provinces during the 2003–14 period did not enable the AKP to establish hegemony in a strong sense of the term, that is, to weaken the mass support for Kurdish ethnopolitical claims, they nevertheless contributed to organizing a tangible world around the ideas of Turkey and citizenship and thus helped establish these ideas in the everyday lives of Kurds. Even though the persistence of patient dissatisfaction in Hakkâri at this time after the considerable improvement of local healthcare provisioning was a failure of the benevolent policies of Turkish state-nationalism, that the dissatisfaction with healthcare provision appeared in the form of "patient dissatisfaction" and the dissatisfied Hakkârian as a "citizen" asking for better healthcare services with implicit and explicit reference to "equal citizenship" may be seen as its success.

Returning, then, to the issue of the (ir)rationality of ethnopolitical challenges, the evidence from Hakkâri cannot be used to defend the indifference of ethnopolitical challenges to gains and losses, that is, to the politics of more benevolence, less violence. Equally, however, this evidence does also lead us to conceive the way that gains and losses impinge upon the ethnopolitical challenge more as a sociological phenomenon occurring at the level of everyday reality than as a political phenomenon emerging through pragmatist calculations of extra-discursive gains and losses.

To sum up, the research findings reported here suggest three reservations with the rationalist argument as an account of ethnopolitical challenge. First, we should pay attention to narratives situating the objective present of the challenge into a subjective past-present-future story. The evidence from Hakkâri shows us that what looks advantageous or disadvantageous to the ethnopolitical gaze cannot be understood independently of this narrative plot.

Second, ethnopolitical challenge refers as much to a specific discourse and structure as to a narrative or temporality. It expresses truths and norms that confirm the ethnopolitical unit as an entity in its own right. As this research clearly shows, an ethnopolitical gaze can classify even those policies whose benefit to the ethnopolitical unit appears self-evident into disadvantages if they do not confirm the ethnopolitical unit as an entity in its own right.

Third, the ground on which the ethnopolitical gaze is shaped is not independent of relations of power. The form of ethnopolitical discontent may be informed by a hegemony of the dominant over the dominated, as the references to citizenship status and comparisons made with Turkish provinces show. The evidence from Hakkâri indicates the possibility that the expression of ethnopolitical discontent with non-secessionist terms does not have to be a "not-yet" issue and pragmatist concession; it may rather signify a case of hegemony.

These reservations may enrich the conceptual toolbox of researchers studying the dynamics of ethnopolitical movements, especially, but not exclusively, in peripheral contexts. They may assist in making sense of unexpected responses and the seemingly irrational preferences of ethnopolitical movements that benefit from yet rebuff benevolent state-nationalist strategies.

Notes

1. *Star*, August 30, 2011.
2. "Recep Tayyip Erdoğan'ın 21 Mayıs 2011 tarihli *Hakkâri* mitinginde yaptığı konuşma," https://tr.wikisource.org/wiki/Recep_Tayyip_Erdo%C4%9Fan%27%C4%B1n_21_May%C4%B1s_2011_tarihli_Hakkari_mitinginde_yapt%C4%B1%C4%9F%C4%B1_konu%C5%9Fma.
3. Ibid.
4. To those who might object to the argument at a theoretical level with the claim that recognition is about difference and identity, not about equality and justice, I would cite arguments on this issue of Axel Honneth in his discussion with Nancy Fraser: "subjects perceive institutional procedures as social injustice when they see aspects of their personality being disrespected which they believe have a right to recognition." See Nancy Fraser and Axel Honneth, *Redistribution or Recognition?*, 132.
5. Donald Woods Winnicott, *Playing and Reality* (New York: Basic Books, 1971), 88.
6. Ibid., 88, 89.
7. Robert R. Williams, *Hegel's Ethics of Recognition* (Berkeley: University of California Press, 1997), 84.
8. Jessica Benjamin, "An Outline of Intersubjectivity: The Development of Recognition," Supplement, *Psychoanalytic Psychology* 7 (1990): 35.
9. Tom Nairn, *The Break-up of Britain: Crisis and Neo-Nationalism* (London: NLB, 1977).
10. Anthony H. Birch, "Minority Nationalist Movements and Theories of Political Integration," *World Politics* 30, no. 3 (1978): 334.
11. Ibid., 334, 335.
12. Ibid. For a similar argument, see Michael Keating, "Nations without States: The Accommodation of Nationalism in the New State Order," In *Minority Nationalism and the Changing International Order*, ed. Michael Keating and John McGarry (Oxford and New York: Oxford University Press, 2001), 19–43.
13. Hechter, *Containing Nationalism*, 117.
14. Elie Kedourie, *Nationalism* (London: Hutchinson, 1961), 89.
15. See André Lecours, "Sub-State Nationalism in the Western World: Explaining Continued Appeal," *Ethnopolitics* 11, no. 3 (2012): 275–77.
16. Max Weber, *Economy and Society: An Outline of Interpretive Sociology*, 2 vols. ed. Guenther Roth and Claus Wittich (Berkeley: University of California Press, 1978), 85–86.
17. Béland and Lecours, *Nationalism and Social Policy*, 139–40.
18. Ibid.
19. Ibid., 193.
20. William Roseberry, "Hegemony and the Language of Contention," in *Everyday Forms of State Formation: Revolution and the Negotiation of Rule in Modern Mexico*,

ed. Gilbert M. Joseph and Daniel Nugent (Durham and London: Duke University Press, 1994), 360–61.
21 Konda, *Kürt Meselesi'nde Algı Ve Beklentiler* (İstanbul: İletişim, 2011), 101.

Appendix

Appendix 1. The Status of the 34 Villages in Hakkâri City (Center) District by the End of 1995

Village (Official Name)	Village (Kurdish Name)	Evacuated	Transferred	Not Evacuated
Ağaçdibi	Kehê		x	
Akbulut	Goranis	x		
Akçalı	Gezne			x
Akkuş	Dêr	x		
Aksu	Billeh	x		
Bayköy	Bayê			x
Bağışlı	Şîvelan (Xezekiyan)			x
Biçenek	Dirêse	x		
Boybeyi	Asingiran			x
Cevizdibi	Bêtkar	x		
Ceylanlı	Welto	x		
Çaltıkoru	Sêvîn	x		
Çaylıca	Berî		x	

(*Continued*)

Appendix 1. Continued

Village (Official Name)	Village (Kurdish Name)	Evacuated	Transferred	Not Evacuated
Yeni Çanaklı	Cemêezu		x	
Çimenli	Cemêbedel		x	
Demirtaş	Ewranis	x		
Doğanyurt	Pîran	x		
Elmacık	Nispas	x		
Geçimli	Rumtik	x		
Geçitli	Peyanis			x
Işık	Nîsê			x
Işıklar	Pirkanis	x		
Konak	Kocanis	x		
Kavaklı	Marînus	x		
Kaval	Qewal	x		
Kaymaklı	Simûrînis	x		
Kırıkdağ	Dêz		x	
Oğul	Tal	x		
Otluca	Xenanis	x		
Ördekli	Kotranis	x		
Pınarca	Balekan	x		
Taşbaşı	Kelêtan		x	
Üzümcü	Dizê			x
Yoncalı	Anîtos	x		
TOTAL (34)		**21**	**6**	**7**

Source: Prepared by an activist of the Hakkâri Provincial Branch of the Human Rights Association (İnsan Hakları Derneği, İHD).

Appendix 2. Health Staff of the Public Health Organization in Hakkâri in 1973

Public Health Institutions	GPs	Dentists	Health Clerks	Nurses	Midwives
Provincial Directorate	1	0	2	0	0
Public Hospital	1	1	1	4	0
Central Health Post	2	0	2	0	2
Üzümcü Health Station	0	0	0	0	1
Durankaya Health Station	0	0	0	0	1
Bağışlı Health Post	0	0	1	0	1
Ördekli Health Station	0	0	0	0	0
Işıklar Health Station	0	0	0	0	1
Geçitli Health Post	0	0	1	0	1
Kaval Health Station	0	0	0	0	0
Beytüşşebap Health Post	1	0	2	0	1
Bölücek Health Station	0	0	0	0	0
Çukurca Health Post	0	0	2	0	1
Güdeşa Health Station	0	0	0	0	1
Uzundere Health Station	0	0	0	0	0
Şemdinli Health Post	1	0	2	0	1
Günyazı Health Station	0	0	0	0	0
Çatalca Health Station	0	0	0	0	0
Uludere Health Post	1	0	2	1	1
Ortabağ Health Station	0	0	0	0	0
Şenoba Health Station	0	0	0	0	1
Yüksekova Health Post	1	0	2	0	1
Uzunsırt Health Station	0	0	0	0	1
Gündere Health Station	0	0	0	0	1
Directorate of Maternal & Infant Health	0	0	0	2	0
Directorate of Tuberculosis Control	0	0	1	0	0
Directorate of Leprosy Control	0	0	0	0	0
Directorate of Trachoma Control	0	0	0	0	0
Directorate of Malaria Control	0	0	0	0	0
TOTAL	8	1	18	7	16

Source: *Cumhuriyetin 50. Yılında Hakkari: 1973 İl Yıllığı.*

Appendix 3. The Number of Out-patients Examined in the Clinics of Hakkâri Public Hospital on One Day (November 11) in Six Consecutive Years (2008–2013)

CLINIC	2008	2009	2010	2011	2012*	2013
ER**	251	620	353	480	336	292
KETEM***	n/a	n/a	2	n/a	1	n/a
Anesthesiology	9	4	n/a	2	5	6
Neurosurgery 1	59	1	n/a	n/a	n/a	n/a
Neurosurgery 2	n/a	n/a	n/a	6	50	64
Endocrinology & Metabolism 1	n/a	n/a	n/a	n/a	16	n/a
Dermatology 1	91	36	57	67	n/a	101
Infectious Diseases 1	n/a	n/a	n/a	n/a	n/a	22
Gastroenterology 1	n/a	n/a	n/a	18	21	33
Physical Therapy 1	32	19	n/a	n/a	n/a	47
General Surgery 1	4	4	2	52	78	n/a
General Surgery 2	30	31	47	n/a	n/a	90
General Surgery 3	34	34	n/a	n/a	n/a	n/a
General Surgery 5	n/a	n/a	n/a	n/a	17	n/a
Ophthalmology 1	79	56	68	61	n/a	n/a
Ophthalmology 2	n/a	43	n/a	n/a	79	n/a
Ophthalmology 3	n/a	n/a	n/a	n/a	n/a	105
Thoracic Surgery 1	0	22	n/a	2	n/a	n/a
Thoracic Medicine 1	28	47	31	32	n/a	51
Thoracic Medicine 2	n/a	n/a	2	n/a	n/a	n/a
Gynecology 1	n/a	80	14	1	n/a	n/a
Gynecology 2	5	39	63	n/a	110	80
Gynecology 3	52	9	n/a	n/a	n/a	83
Cardiovascular Surgery 1	n/a	n/a	n/a	1	n/a	n/a
Cardiovascular Surgery 2	n/a	n/a	n/a	n/a	5	n/a
Cardiology 1	36	5	28	n/a	n/a	56
Cardiology 2	n/a	n/a	n/a	n/a	20	n/a
Cardiology 3	n/a	n/a	n/a	27	23	n/a
Neurology 1	n/a	n/a	27	45	43	86
Otorhinolaryngology 1	62	41	n/a	n/a	n/a	57

Appendix 3. Continued

CLINIC	2008	2009	2010	2011	2012*	2013
Otorhinolaryngology 2	n/a	n/a	n/a	n/a	n/a	55
Otorhinolaryngology 3	n/a	n/a	n/a	n/a	32	n/a
Nephrology 2	n/a	n/a	n/a	n/a	3	5
Orthopedics 1	37	69	11	n/a	103	49
Orthopedics 2	n/a	n/a	n/a	34	2	n/a
Orthopedics 3	n/a	n/a	42	n/a	n/a	59
Psychiatry 1	n/a	n/a	n/a	n/a	n/a	18
Psychiatry 2	n/a	n/a	16	n/a	30	n/a
Pathology 1	n/a	n/a	3	n/a	n/a	n/a
Plastic Surgery 1	16	47	n/a	n/a	n/a	5
Pediatric Surgery 1	22	3	10	n/a	n/a	n/a
Pediatric Surgery 2	n/a	n/a	n/a	n/a	13	n/a
Pediatrics 1	39	18	n/a	n/a	43	n/a
Pediatrics 2	n/a	n/a	28	n/a	n/a	104
Pediatrics 3	n/a	78	62	63	84	1
Pediatrics 4	n/a	78	n/a	68	n/a	n/a
Urology 1	25	n/a	n/a	18	n/a	2
Urology 2	26	50	n/a	n/a	44	62
Urology 3	n/a	n/a	16	n/a	n/a	n/a
Internal Medicine 1	n/a	73	n/a	n/a	2	n/a
Internal Medicine 2	6	n/a	75	n/a	5	n/a
Internal Medicine 3	50	n/a	n/a	59	46	n/a
Internal Medicine 4	n/a	86	n/a	n/a	43	n/a
Internal Medicine 5	n/a	n/a	n/a	n/a	53	97
TOTAL	993	1,616	957	1,036	1,307	1,630

Source: Constructed by the author based on data obtained from Hakkâri Public Hospital.
* November 12.
** Emergency Room.
*** Cancer Early Diagnosis Center.

Bibliography

Newspapers

National

Cumhuriyet
Milliyet
Tercüman

Local

Hakkâri
Hakkâri Ekspress
Hakkâri'nin Sesi
Serxwebûn

Prime Ministry State Archives

BCA BMGMK [Catalogue Number: 030 01/120 765 1].
BCA BMGMK [Catalogue Number: 030 10/180 244 6].
BCA BMGMK [Catalogue Number: 030 10/230 548 10].

302 | Bibliography

BCA CHP [Catalogue Number: 490 01/490 1976 1].
BOA DH MKT [Catalogue Number: 1646/21].
BOA DH.ŞFR [Catalogue Number: 148/24].

Parliamentary Minutes and Official Gazette

Republic of Turkey. *Cumhuriyet Senatosu Tutanak Dergisi*
    Term 1, session 33, volume 63, January 31, 1971.
Republic of Turkey. *Millet Meclisi Tutanak Dergisi*
    Term 8, session 54, vol. 24, February 23, 1950.
    Term 4, session 132, vol. 20, September 14, 1976.
    Term 5, session 115, vol. 4, February 24, 1978.
Republic of Turkey. *T.B.M.M Tutanak Dergisi*
    Term 18, session 6, vol. 14, September 29, 1988.
    Term 18, session 27, vol. 33, November 7, 1989.
Republic of Turkey. *T.C Resmi Gazete*
    No. 9401, September 7, 1956.
    No. 9495, December 28, 1956.
    No. 9529, February 7, 1957.
    No. 9763, November 22, 1957.
    No. 11330, February 9, 1963.
    No. 17303, April 7, 1981.
    No. 18199, October 22, 1983.
    No. 20231, June 24, 1989.
    No. 22240, March 27, 1995.
    No. 22415, September 25, 1995.
    No. 24078, June 13, 2000.
    No. 25866, July 5, 2005.

Websites

Aile ve Sosyal Politikalar Bakanlığı (The Ministry of Family and Social Policies). "Türkiye'de Uygulanan Şartlı Nakit Transferi Programının Fayda Sahipleri Üzerindeki Etkisinin Nitel ve Nicel Olarak Ölçülmesi Projesi Final Raporu." Accessed January 26, 2022. http://www.sck.gov.tr/wp-content/uploads/2020/02/SNT-Program%C4%B1n%C4%B1n-Etkisi nin-%C3%96l%C3%A7%C3%BClmesi-Raporu.pdf

AK Party. "*Soruları ve Cevaplarıyla Demokratik Açılım Süreci: Milli Birlik ve Kardeşlik Broşürü.*" 2010. https://serdargunes.files.wordpress.com/2015/08/acilim220110.pdf

Anadolu Ajansı. "Erdoğan'dan 'bayrak' tepkisi." December 1, 2013. https://www.ntv.com.tr/turk iye/erdogandan-bayrak-tepkisi,4lhAdJc1x0q0vzOrI_3BfA

Bağımsızlık, Demokrasi, Sosyalizm için Yürüyüş. "Tuzluca Olayları Üzerine." Accessed March 13, 2022. https://issuu.com/solyayin/docs/y_75_029/16

Bia Haber Merkezi. "30 Ayda KCK'den 7748 gözaltı, 3895 tutuklama." Accessed March 13, 2022. https://bianet.org/bianet/siyaset/133216-30-ayda-kck-den-7748-gozalti-3895-tutuklama

Botan, Nergîz. "Kürt Nüfus Soykırımı Güncelleniyor." Last modified March 15, 2020. https://www.lekolin.org/kurt-nufus-soykirimi-guncelleniyor

Doğruhaber. "Erdoğan: 'BDP ideoloji siyaseti yapıyor'." Last modified March 10, 2014. https://dogruhaber.com.tr/haber/120489-erdogan-bdp-ideoloji-siyaseti-yapiyor/

Erdoğan, Recep Tayyip. "Recep Tayyip Erdoğan'ın 21 Mayıs 2011 tarihli Hakkâri Mitingi Konuşmasının Tam Metni." Last modified January 4, 2022. https://tr.wikisource.org/wiki/Recep_Tayyip_Erdo%C4%9Fan%27%C4%B1n_21_May%C4%B1s_2011_tarihli_Hakkari_mitinginde_yapt%C4%B1%C4%9F%C4%B1_konu%C5%9Fma

Erdoğan, Recep Tayyip. "Recep Tayyip Erdoğan'ın 1 Haziran 2011 tarihli Diyarbakır mitinginde yaptığı konuşma." Last modified January 4, 2022. https://tr.wikisource.org/wiki/Recep_Tayyip_Erdo%C4%9Fan%27%C4%B1n_1_Haziran_2011_tarihli_Diyarbak%C4%B1r_mitinginde_yapt%C4%B1%C4%9F%C4%B1_konu%C5%9Fma

European Court of Human Rights. "Case of Meryem Çelik and Others." Accessed February 11, 2022. http://hudoc.echr.coe.int/sites/eng/Pages/search.aspx#

Hafıza Merkezi. "Zorla Kaybedilenler Veritabani." Accessed May 5, 2018. http://www.zorlakaybetmeler.org/events.php?city

HPG. "Şehîden Me Rûmeta Me Ne." https://hpgsehit.com/index.php/ehit-kuenyeleri

İHOP. "Human Rights, the Rule of Law, and the Protection of Human Rights Defenders: Report on the Diyarbakır KCK Case." Accessed December 17, 2021. http://www.ihop.org.tr/wp-content/uploads/2011/04/20110414_KCK_ENG.pdf

İnsan Hakları Derneği (Human Rights Association). "Yıllık Raporlar." Accessed March 5, 2022. https://www.ihd.org.tr/td_d_slug_2/

İnsan Hakları Derneği Diyarbakır Şubesi. "1988–2014 Yılları Arası Çatışmalı Süreçte Katledilen Çocuklar Raporu." Accessed November 25, 2014. https://www.ihddiyarbakir.org/

Sağlık Bakanlığı (Ministry of Health). "İstatistik Yıllıkları." Accessed February 12, 2022. https://khgmistatistikdb.saglik.gov.tr/TR-43867/istatistik-yillari.html

Sağlık Bakanlığı (Ministry of Health). "Hasta Hakları Uygulamaları İstatistikleri." Accessed January 13, 2022. https://shgmhastahakdb.saglik.gov.tr/TR-4771/hasta-haklari.html

Sosyal Güvenlik Kurumu (Social Security Institution). "Aylık İstatistik Bültenleri." Accessed January 11, 2022. https://veri.sgk.gov.tr/

Strateji ve Bütçe Başkanlığı: Kütüphane (Library of the Strategy and Budgeting Ministry). https://katalog.sbb.gov.tr/Record/44192

TRT Haber. "Diyarbakır bir Gaziantep Olamadıysa . . ." Last modified January 19, 2013. https://www.trthaber.com/haber/gundem/diyarbakir-bir-gaziantep-olamadiysa-71534.html

Türk Tabipler Birliği (Turkish Medical Chamber). *Doğuda ve Kırda Sağlık*. Accessed August 10, 2013. http://www.ttb.org.tr/halk_sagligi/ges/GES2002.pdf

Türkiye İstatistik Kurumu (TurkStat). "Nüfus ve Konut Araştırması 2011." Accessed January 20, 2022. https://data.tuik.gov.tr/Bulten/Index?p=Nufus-ve-Konut-Arastirmasi-2011-15843

TÜİK Kütüphanesi (TurkStat Library). https://kutuphane.tuik.gov.tr/yordambt/yordam.php

UNDP. "Human Development Report: Turkey 1998." Accessed February 15, 2022. http://www.tr.undp.org/content/turkey/tr/home/library/national-hdrs/nhdr-1998.html
UNDP. "Human Development Report: Turkey 2001." Accessed January 13, 2022. http://www.tr.undp.org/content/dam/turkey/docs/Publications/nhdrs/NHDR2001.pdf
Üstündağ, Nazan. "1990'larda Kürtler ve Kürdistan Konferansı." Accessed January 5, 2022. https://www.youtube.com/watch?v=C3uIDIqHv20
Vujicic, Marko, Susan Sparkes, Salih Mollahaliloğlu. "Health Workforce Policy in Turkey: Recent Reforms and Issues for the Future." Accessed March 5, 2022. https://openknowledge.worldbank.org/handle/10986/13784
Yüksek Seçim Kurulu (Supreme Electoral Council). "Seçimler." Accessed April 3, 2022. http://www.ysk.gov.tr/ysk/GenelSecimler.html
Yüksekova Haber Portalı. "Hakkari'de Heykel Açılımı." Last modified June 20, 2011. https://www.yuksekovahaber.com.tr/haber/hakkaride-heykel-acilimi-53581.htm
Zentürk, Adnan. "Bir Salgını Önlemek." Accessed April 1, 2022. http://www.sdplatform.com/Dergi/224/Bir-salgini-onlemek.aspx

Books and Articles

Agamben, Giorgio. *Homo Sacer. Sovereign Power and Bare Life.* Meridian. Stanford, CA: Stanford University Press, 1998.
———. *State of Exception.* Chicago: University of Chicago Press, 2005.
Ahıska, Meltem. *Occidentalism in Turkey: Questions of Modernity and National Identity in Turkish Radio Broadcasting.* London: I. B. Tauris, 2010.
Ahmad, Feroz. *Turkey: The Quest for Identity.* Oxford: Oneworld, 2003.
Akdoğan, Yalçın. "The Meaning of Conservative Democratic Political Identity." In *The Emergence of a New Turkey: Democracy and the Ak Party*, edited by M. Hakan Yavuz. Salt Lake City: University of Utah Press, 2006.
Akkaya, Ahmet Hamdi, and Joost Jongerden. "Reassembling the Political: The PKK and the Project of Radical Democracy." *European Journal of Turkish Studies* 14 (2012).
Althusser, Louis. *On the Reproduction of Capitalism: Ideology and Ideological State Apparatuses.* London: Verso, 2014.
Altun, Fahamettin. *Hakkari İl Yıllığı, 1967.* Ankara: Gürsoy Matbaacılık Sanayi, 1972.
Anderson, Benedict R. O'G. *Imagined Communities: Reflections on the Origin and Spread of Nationalism.* London and New York: Verso, 2006.
Arnold, David. "Smallpox and Colonial Medicine in Nineteenth-Century Medicine." In *Imperial Medicine and Indigenous Societies*, edited by David Arnold. Manchester: Manchester University Press, 1988.
Arvas, İbrahim. *Tarihi Hakikatler: İbrahim Arvas'ın Hatıratı.* Ankara: Yargıçoğlu Matbaası, 1964.
Aşgın, Sait. *Cumhuriyet Döneminde Doğu Anadolu'ya Yapılan Kamu Harcamaları, 1946–1960.* Ankara: Atatürk Kültür, Dil ve Tarih Yüksek Kurumu, Atatürk Araştırma Merkezi, 2000.

Ateş, Sabri. *Ottoman-Iranian Borderlands: Making a Boundary, 1843–1914*. New York: Cambridge University Press, 2013.

Atmaca, Hüseyin. *Bir Köy Çocuğunun Serüveni: Köy Enstitüsünden Parlamentoya*. Ankara: Abis, 2009.

Avar, Sıdıka. *Dağ Çiçeklerim, Anılar*. Ankara: Öğretmen Yayınları, 1986.

Aydın, Erdem. *Türkiye'de Sağlık Teşkilatlanması Tarihi*. Ankara: Naturel, 2002.

Babül, Elif M. "Training Bureaucrats, Practicing for Europe: Negotiating Bureaucratic Authority and Governmental Legitimacy in Turkey." *PoLAR: Political and Legal Anthropology Review* 35, no. 1 (2012): 30–52.

Bahcheli, Tozun, and Sid Noed. "The Justice and Development Party and the Kurdish Question." In *Nationalisms and Politics in Turkey: Political Islam, Kemalism and the Kurdish Issue*, edited by Marlies Casier and Joost Jongerden. London and New York: Routledge, 2011.

Balibar, Etienne, and Immanuel Maurice Wallerstein. *Race, Nation, Class: Ambiguous Identities*. London and New York: Verso, 1991.

Bauman, Zygmunt. *Modernity and Ambivalence*. Ithaca, NY: Cornell University Press, 1991.

———. *Modernity and the Holocaust*. Ithaca, NY: Cornell University Press, 1989.

Bayrak, Mehmet. *Kürtlere Vurulan Kelepçe: Şark Islahat Planı*. Ankara: Öz-Ge Yayınları, 2009.

Béland, Daniel, and André Lecours. *Nationalism and Social Policy: The Politics of Territorial Solidarity*. Oxford and New York: Oxford University Press, 2008.

Benjamin, Jessica. "An Outline of Intersubjectivity: The Development of Recognition." Supplement, *Psychoanalytic Psychology* 7 (1990): 33–46.

Bennett, Huw. "The Mau Mau Emergency as Part of the British Army's Post-War Counter-Insurgency Experience." *Defense & Security Analysis* 23, no. 2 (2007): 143–63.

Berberoğlu, Enis. *Kod Adı Yüksekova*. İstanbul: Milliyet Yayınları, 1998.

Berry, Nicole S. "Who's judging the quality of care? Indigenous Maya and the problem of 'not being attended'." *Medical Anthropology Quarterly* 27, no. 2 (2008): 164–89.

Beşikçi, İsmail. *Orgeneral Mustafa Muğlalı Olayı*. İstanbul: Belge-Uluslararası Yayıncılık, 1991.

Betancourt, Joseph R., Alexander R. Green, J. Emilio Carrillo, and Owusu Ananeh-Firempong. "Defining Cultural Competence: A Practical Framework for Addressing Racial/Ethnic Disparities in Health and Health Care." *Public Health Reports* 118, no. 4 (2003): 293–302

Bhabha, Homi K. *The Location of Culture*. London and New York: Routledge, 2004.

Bilgiç, Aydın. *Yaslı Gittim Şen Geldim: 1955–1957 Hakkari Anıları*. Ankara: Özsan Matbaacılık, 1999.

Billig, Michael. *Banal Nationalism*. London and Thousand Oaks, CA: Sage, 1995.

Birch, Anthony H. "Minority Nationalist Movements and Theories of Political Integration." *World Politics* 30, no. 3 (1978): 325–44.

Birinci Genel Müfettişlik. *Güney Doğu/Birinci Genel Müfettişlik Bölgesi*. Istanbul: Cumhuriyet Matbaası, 1939.

Bora, Tanıl. "Türk Sağı: Siyasal Düşünce Tarihi Açısından Bir Çerçeve Denemesi." In *Türk Sağı:Mitler, Fetişler, Düşman İmgeleri*, edited by İnci Özkan Kerestecioğlu and Güven Gürkan Öztan. İstanbul: İletişim, 2012.

Bosniak, Linda. *The Citizen and the Alien: Dilemmas of Contemporary Membership*. Princeton, NJ: Princeton University Press, 2006.

Bourdieu, Pierre. *Outline of a Theory of Practice*. Cambridge and New York: Cambridge University Press, 1977.
Breuilly, John. *Nationalism and the State*. Manchester: Manchester University Press, 1993.
Browne, Annette Jo. "First Nations Women and Health Care Services: The Sociopolitical Context of Encounters with Nurses." Ph.D. diss., University of British Columbia, 2003.
Browne, Annette J., and Jo-Anne Fiske. "First Nations Women's Encounters with Mainstream Healthcare Services." *Western Journal of Nursing Research* 23, no. 2 (2001): 126–47.
Bryman, Alan. *Social Research Methods*. Oxford and New York: Oxford University Press, 2012.
Buğra, Ayşe, and Osman Savaşkan. "Politics and Class: The Turkish Business Environment in the Neoliberal Age." *New Perspectives on Turkey* 46 (2012): 27–63.
Butler, Judith, Ernesto Laclau, and Slavoj Žižek. *Contingency, Hegemony, Universality: Contemporary Dialogues on the Left*. London: Verso, 2000.
Calnan, Michael W., and Rosemary Rowe. *Trust Matters in Health Care*. Maidenhead: Open University Press, 2008.
Calnan, Michael W., and Emma Sanford. "Public Trust in Health Care: The System or the Doctor?" *BMJ Quality & Safety* 13, no. 2 (2004): 92–97.
Castro, Anabell, and Ester Ruiz. "The Effects of Nurse Practitioner Cultural Competence on Latina Patient Satisfaction." *Journal of the American Academy of Nurse Practitioners* 21, no. 5 (2009): 278–86.
Cavender, Anthony, and Manuel Albán. "Compulsory Medical Service in Ecuador: The Physician's Perspective." *Social Science & Medicine* 47, no. 12 (1998): 1937–46.
Chakrabarty, Dipesh. *Provincializing Europe: Postcolonial Thought and Historical Difference*. Princeton, NJ and Oxford: Princeton University Press, 2008.
Chatterjee, Partha. *Nationalist Thought and the Colonial World: A Derivative Discourse?* London: Zed for the United Nations University, 1986.
———. *The Politics of the Governed: Reflections on Popular Politics in Most of the World*. New York: Columbia University Press, 2004.
Clarke, John. *Subjects of Doubt: In Search of the Unsettled and Unfinished*. Paper presented at the CASCA Conference, Ontario, May 5–9, 2004.
———. "Welfare States as Nation States: Some Conceptual Reflections." *Social Policy and Society* 4, no. 4 (2005): 407–15.
Clarke, John, Kathleen M. Coll, Evelina Dagnino, and Catherine Neveu. *Disputing Citizenship*. Bristol: Policy Press, 2014.
Clarke, John, and Janet Newman. *The Managerial State: Power, Politics and Ideology in the Remaking of Social Welfare*. London and Thousand Oaks, CA: SAGE Publications, 1997.
Cohen, Erik. "Expatriate Communities." *Current Sociology* 24, no. 3 (1977): 5–90.
Corbridge, Stuart. *Seeing the State: Governance and Governmentality in India*. Cambridge and New York: Cambridge University Press, 2005.
Coşar, Simten, and Aylin Özman. "Centre-Right Politics in Turkey after the November 2002 General Election: Neo-Liberalism with a Muslim Face." *Contemporary Politics* 10, no. 1 (2004): 57–74.
Çörüt, İlker. "An Ethnographic Account of Compulsory Public Service by Doctors in Hakkari: The Limits of the AKP Assimilation Strategy and the Production of Space." In

The Kurdish Issue in Turkey: A Spatial Perspective, edited by Zeynep Gambetti and Joost Jongerden. London: Routledge, 2015.

———. "Ethno-political Subordination and Patient Dissatisfaction: The Kurdish Case in Hakkari during the AKP Period in Turkey, 2003–2013." *Nations and Nationalism* 26, no. 3 (2020): 553–75.

Cross, T. L., B. J. Bazron, K. W. Dennis, and M. R. Isaacs. *Towards a Culturally Competent System of Care: A Monograph on Effective Services for Minority Children Who Are Severely Emotionally Disturbed.* Washington, DC: CASSP Technical Assistance Center, Georgetown Univ. Child Development Center, 1989.

Çağaptay, Soner. *Islam, Secularism, and Nationalism in Modern Turkey: Who Is a Turk?* London and New York: Routledge, 2006.

Çiçek, Cuma. "Elimination or Integration of Pro-Kurdish Politics: Limits of the AKP's Democratic Initiative." *Turkish Studies* 12, no. 1 (2011): 15–26.

Dandoy, Regis, and Pierre Baudewyns. "The Preservation of Social Security as a National Function in the Belgian Federal State." In *The Territorial Politics of Welfare*, edited by Nicola McEwen and Luis Moreno. London and New York: Routledge, 2005.

Darcy, Shane. *Collective Responsibility and Accountability under International Law.* Ardsley, NY: Transnational Publishers, 2007.

Dean, Mitchell. *Governmentality: Power and Rule in Modern Society.* London and Thousand Oaks, CA: Sage, 1999.

Devlet İstatistik Enstitüsü (State Statistical Institute). *1980 Genel Sanayi Ve İşyerleri Sayımı.* Ankara: DİE, 1983.

———. *2000 Genel Nüfus Sayımı:Nüfusun Sosyal Ve Ekonomik Nitelikleri, Hakkari.* Ankara: DİE, 2002.

———. *Ekonomik Ve Sosyal Göstergeler.* Ankara: DİE, 1998.

———. *Gap İl İstatistikleri 1950–1996.* Ankara: DİE, 1997.

———. *Sosyalizasyon Bölgelerinden Derlenen Doğum İstatistikleri 1972.* Ankara: DİE, 1977.

———. *Sosyalizasyon Bölgelerinden Derlenen Ölüm İstatistikleri, 1973–74–75.* Ankara: DİE, 1978.

———. *Tarımsal Yapı Ve Üretim 1990.* Ankara: DİE, 1993.

———. *Tarımsal Yapı: Üretim, Fiyat, Değer, 1995.* Ankara: DİE, 1997.

———. *Türkiye İstatistik Yıllığı 1977.* Ankara: DİE, 1977.

Devlet Planlama Teşkilatı (State Planning Organization). *İl İncelemeleri (Batman, Bingöl, Bitlis, Diyarbakır, Elazığ, Hakkari, Mardin, Muş, Siirt, Şırnak, Tunceli, Van) Ön Raporu.* Ankara: DPT, 2000.

———. *Kalkınmada Öncelikli İller İnceleme Raporu.* Ankara: DPT, 1981.

———. *Kalkınmada Öncelikli Yöreler Raporu 1985.* Ankara: DPT, 1985.

———. *Kalkınmada Öncelikli Yöreler Raporu No: 5.* Ankara: Devlet Planlama Teşkilatı, Kalkınmada Öncelikli Yöreler ve Bölgesel Kalkınma Genel Müdürlüğü, 1987.

———. *Kalkınmada Öncelikli Yöreler Ve Türkiye İçin Seçilmiş Göstergeler 1991.* Ankara: Devlet Planlama Teşkilatı, Kalkınmada Öncelikli Yöreler ve Bölgesel Kalkınma Genel Müdürlüğü, 1991.

Dinçer, Bülent, and Metin Özaslan. *İlçelerin Sosyo-Ekonomik Gelişmişlik Sıralaması Araştırması.* Ankara: Devlet Planlama Teşkilatı, 2004.

Doğan, Erhan. "The Historical and Discoursive Roots of the Justice and Development Party's EU Stance." *Turkish Studies* 6, no. 3 (2005): 421–37.

Dussault, Gilles, and Maria C. Franceschini. "Not Enough There, Too Many Here: Understanding Geographical Imbalances in the Distribution of the Health Workforce." *Human Resources for Health* 4, no. 1 (2006).

Eldem, Edhem, Daniel Goffman, and Bruce Alan Masters. *The Ottoman City between East and West: Aleppo, Izmir, and Istanbul.* Cambridge: Cambridge University Press, 1999.

Eral, Nilgün Arısan, and Atila Eralp. "What went wrong in the Turkey-EU relationship?" In *Another Empire? A Decade of Turkey's Foreign Policy under the Justice and Development Party*, edited by Kerem Öktem, Ayşe Kadıoğlu, and Mehmet Karlı. Istanbul: Istanbul Bilgi Üniversitesi Yayınları, 2009.

Erdost, Muzaffer İlhan. *Şemdinli Röportajı*. Ankara: Onur Yayınları, 1993.

Erinç, Sırrı. *Doğu Anadolu Coğrafyası*. Istanbul: Sucuoğlu Matbaası, 1953.

Fabian, Johannes. *Time and the Other: How Anthropology Makes Its Object*. New York: Columbia University Press, 1983.

Fanon, Frantz. *A Dying Colonialism*. New York: Monthly Review Press, 1965.

Farmer, Paul. *Pathologies of Power: Health, Human Rights, and the New War on the Poor*. Berkeley, CA and London: University of California Press, 2005.

Ferguson, James, and Akhil Gupta. "Spatializing States: Toward an Ethnography of Neoliberal Governmentality." *American Ethnologist* 29, no. 4 (2002): 981–1002.

Fırat, M. Şerif. *Doğu İlleri Ve Varto Tarihi*. Ankara: Türk Kültürünü Araştırma Enstitüsü, 1981.

Foucault, Michel. *The History of Sexuality*. New York: Vintage Books, 1988.

———. "Governmentality." In *The Foucault Effect: Studies in Governmentality*, edited by Graham Burchell, Colin Gordon, and Peter Miller. Chicago: University of Chicago Press, 1991.

———. *Society Must Be Defended: Lectures at the Colláege De France, 1975–76*, edited by Mauro Bertani and Alessandro Fontana. New York: Picador, 2003.

———. *Security, Territory, Population: Lectures at the CollèGe De France, 1977–78*, edited by Michel Senellart. Basingstoke and New York: Palgrave Macmillan, 2007.

Fox, Jon E., and Cynthia Miller-Idriss. "Everyday Nationhood." *Ethnicities* 8, no. 4 (2008): 536–63.

Fraser, Nancy, and Linda Gordon. "Contract Versus Charity: Why There Is No Social Citizenship in the United States." *Socialist Review* 22, no. 3 (1992): 45–67.

Fraser, Nancy, and Axel Honneth. *Redistribution or Recognition?: A Political-Philosophical Exchange*. London and New York: Verso, 2003.

French, David. *The British Way in Counter-Insurgency, 1945–1967*. Oxford and New York: Oxford University Press, 2011.

Gambetti, Zeynep. "Yönetimsellikten Irkçılığa." *Dipnot*, no. 6 (2011).

Gaunt, David. "The Complexity of the Assyrian Genocide." *Genocide Studies International* 9, no. 1 (2015): 92–94.

Giddens, Anthony. *A Contemporary Critique of Historical Materialism*. Vol. 2, *The Nation-State and Violence*. Cambridge: Polity Press, 1985.

———. *The Consequences of Modernity*. Cambridge: Polity, 1990.

Gordon, David. "A Sword of Empire? Medicine and Colonialism in King William's Town, Xhosaland, 1856–1891." *African Studies* 60, no. 2 (2010): 165–83.

Green, Linda Buckley. *Fear as a Way of Life: Mayan Widows in Rural Guatemala*. New York: Columbia University Press, 1999.
Greenfeld, Liah. *Nationalism: A Short History*. Washington, DC: Brookings Institution Press, 2019.
Guha, Ranajit. *Dominance Without Hegemony: History and Power in Colonial India*. Cambridge, MA: Harvard University Press, 1997.
Guthrie, Bruce. "Trust and Asymmetry in General Practitioner-Patient Relationship in the United Kingdom." In *Researching Trust and Health*, edited by Julie Brownlie, Alexandra Greene, Alexandra Howson. London: Routledge, 2008.
Günal, Asena. "Health and Citizenship in Republican Turkey: An Analysis of the Socialization of Health Services in Republican Historical Context." Ph.D. diss., Boğaziçi University, 2008.
Güneş, Cengiz. *The Kurdish National Movement in Turkey: From Protest to Resistance*. New York: Routledge, 2012.
Hakan, Tolga. "Bir Aile Planlaması Program Denemesi Hakkari İli İçin." MA thesis, Hacettepe Üniversitesi, 1976.
Hakkari Valiliği (Governorship of Hakkari). *Cumhuriyetin 50. Yılında Hakkari: 1973 İl Yıllığı*. Istanbul: Pera Basımevi, 1974.
Hakkı, Naşit. *Derebeyi ve Dersim*. Ankara: Hakimiyet-i Milliye Matbaası, 1939.
Hall, Mark, Elizabeth Dugan, Beiyao Zheng, and Aneil K Mishra. "Trust in Physicians and Medical Institutions: What Is It, Can It Be Measured, and Does It Matter?" *Milbank Quarterly* 79, no. 4 (2001): 613–39.
Hansen, Thomas Blom, and Finn Stepputat. "Introduction." In *Sovereign Bodies: Citizens, Migrants, and States in the Postcolonial World*, edited by Thomas Blom Hansen and Finn Stepputat. Princeton, NJ: Princeton University Press, 2005.
Harootunian, Harry D. *Overcome by Modernity: History, Culture, and Community in Interwar Japan*. Princeton, NJ: Princeton University Press, 2000.
Hechter, Michael. *Containing Nationalism*. Oxford and New York: Oxford University Press, 2000.
Heckathorn, Douglas D. "Collective Sanctions and the Creation of Prisoner's Dilemma Norms." *American Journal of Sociology* 94, no. 3 (1988): 535–62.
Heper, Metin. *The State and Kurds in Turkey: The Question of Assimilation*. Basingstoke and New York: Palgrave Macmillan, 2007.
Hirschon, Renee, ed. *Crossing the Aegean: An Appraisal of the 1923 Compulsory Population Exchange between Greece and Turkey*, vol. 12. New York: Berghahn Books, 2003.
Holloway, John. *Change the World without Taking Power*. London and Sterling, VA: Pluto Press, 2002.
Horowitz, Donald L. *Ethnic Groups in Conflict*. Berkeley: University of California Press, 1985.
Horvitz, Leslie Alan, and Christopher Catherwood. *Encyclopedia of War Crimes and Genocide*. Facts on File Library of World History. New York: Facts on File, 2006.
İstatistik Genel Direktörlüğü (General Directorate of Statistics). *Genel Nüfus Sayımı 1935*. Ankara: Mehmet İhsan Basımevi, 1937.
Jongerden, Joost. *The Settlement Issue in Turkey and the Kurds: An Analysis of Spatial Policies, Modernity and War*. Leiden and Boston: Brill, 2007.

Jongerden, Joost, and Cengiz Gunes. "A Democratic Nation: The Kurdistan Workers' Party (PKK) and the Idea of Nation beyond the State." In *Beyond Nationalism and the Nation-State: Radical Approaches to Nation*, edited by İlker Cörüt and Joost Jongerden. London: Routledge, 2021.

Karaman, İsmail. *Hakkari Raporu*. Ankara: DPT, 1978.

Karpat, Kemal H. *Ottoman Population, 1830–1914: Demographic and Social Characteristics*. Madison: University of Wisconsin Press, 1985.

Keating, Michael. "Nations without States: The Accommodation of Nationalism in the New State Order." In *Minority Nationalism and the Changing International Order*, edited by Michael Keating and John McGarry. Oxford and New York: Oxford University Press, 2001.

———. "Social Citizenship, Solidarity and Welfare in Regionalized and Plurinational States." *Citizenship Studies* 13, no. 5 (2009): 501–13.

Kedourie, Elie. *Nationalism*. London: Hutchinson, 1961.

Keller, Richard C. "Geographies of Power, Legacies of Mistrust: Colonial Medicine in the Global Present." *Historical Geography* 34 (2006): 26–48.

Kelman, Herbert C. "Violence without Moral Restraint: Reflections on the Dehumanization of Victims and Victimizers." *Journal of Social Issues* 29, no. 4 (1973): 25–61.

Keyder, Çağlar, and Nazan Üstündağ. "Doğu Ve Güneydoğu Anadolu'nun Kalkınmasında Sosyal Politikalar." In *Doğu Ve Güneydoğu Anadolu'da Sosyal Ve Ekonomik Öncelikler*. Istanbul: Tesev Yayınları, 2006.

Kleinman, Arthur. *The Illness Narratives: Suffering, Healing, and the Human Condition*. New York: Basic Books, 1988.

Koca, Hüseyin. *Yakın Tarihten Günümüze Hükümetlerin Doğu-Güneydoğu Anadolu Politikaları*. Konya: Mikro Basım-Yayım-Dağıtım, 1998.

Koçak, Cemil. *Umumi Müfettişlikler, 1927–1952*. İstanbul: İletişim, 2003.

KOM Department. *Turkish Report of Anti-Smuggling and Organized Crime 2011*. Ankara: KOM Publication, 2012.

Konda. *Kürt Meselesi'nde Algı Ve Beklentiler*. İstanbul: İletişim, 2011.

Koonings, Kees, and Dirk Krujit. *Societies of Fear: The Legacy of Civil War, Violence and Terror in Latin America*. London and New York: Zed Books, 1999.

Kurban, Dilek, Yükseker Deniz, Ayşe Betül Çelik, Ünalan Turgay, and A. Tamer Aker. *Coming to Terms with Forced Migration: Post-Displacement Restitution of Citizenship Rights in Turkey*. Istanbul: TESEV, 2007.

Kutbay, Cemil. *Kalkınmada Öncelikli İllerde Sanayii Tesisleri*. Ankara: Başbakanlık Devlet Planlama Teşkilatı, Kalkınmada Öncelikli Yöreler Dairesi, 1993.

———. *Kamu Yatırımlarının Kalkınmada Öncelikli Yöreler ve Diğer İller İtibariyle Dağılımı: 1963–1981*. Ankara: Devlet Planlama Teşkilatı, 1982.

Küçük, Bülent, and Ceren Özselçuk. "'Mesafeli' Devletten 'Hizmetkâr' Devlete: AKP'nin Kısmi Tanıma Siyaseti." *Toplum ve Bilim* 132 (2015): 162–90.

Laclau, Ernesto. *Emancipation(S)*. New York: Verso, 1996.

Larner, Wendy. "Neo-liberalism: Policy, Ideology, Governmentality." *Studies in Political Economy* 63, no. 1 (2016): 5–25.

Latham, Alan. "Powers of Engagement: On Being Engaged, Being Indifferent; and Urban Life." *Area* 31, no. 2 (1999): 161–68.

Lecca, Pedro J., Ivan Quervalu, Joao V. Nunes, and Hector F. Gonzales. *Cultural Competency in Health, Social & Human Services: Directions for the 21st Century.* Florence, KY: Routledge, 2014.

Lechner, Norbert. "Some People Die of Fear: Fear as a Political Problem." In *Fear at the Edge: State Terror and Resistance in Latin America*, edited by Juan E. Corradi, Patricia Weiss Fagen, and Manuel A. Garretâon Merino. Berkeley: University of California Press, 1992.

Lecours, André. "Sub-State Nationalism in the Western World: Explaining Continued Appeal." *Ethnopolitics* 11, no. 3 (2012): 268–86.

Lefebvre, Henri. *The Production of Space.* Oxford and Cambridge, MA: Blackwell, 1991.

Lefort, Claude. *The Political Forms of Modern Society: Bureaucracy, Democracy, Totalitarianism.* Cambridge: Polity Press, 1986.

Mann, Michael. "The Autonomous Power of the State: Its Origins, Mechanisms and Results." *European Journal of Sociology/ Archives Européennes de Sociologie* 25, no. 2 (1984): 185–213.

———. *The Dark Side of Democracy: Explaining Ethnic Cleansing.* New York: Cambridge University Press, 2005.

Marcus, Aliza. *Kan ve İnanç: PKK ve Kürt Hareketi.* Translated by Ayten Alkan. Istanbul: İletişim Yayınları, 2009.

Marshall, Thomas Humphrey, and Tom Bottomore. *Citizenship and Social Class.* London: Pluto Press, 1992.

Massey, Doreen B. *For Space.* London and Thousand Oaks, CA: SAGE, 2005.

Mbembé, Achille. *On the Postcolony.* Berkeley: University of California Press, 2001.

McEwen, Nicola. *Nationalism and the State: Welfare and Identity in Scotland and Quebec.* Brussels: Peter Lang, 2005.

McEwen, Nicola, and Luis Moreno. "Exploring the Territorial Politics of Welfare." In *The Territorial Politics of Welfare*, edited by Nicola McEwen and Luis Moreno. London and New York: Routledge, 2005.

McLeod, John. *Beginning Postcolonialism.* Manchester and New York: Manchester University Press, 2000.

Mechanic, David, and Sharon Meyer. "Concepts of Trust among Patients with Serious Illness." *Social Science & Medicine* 51, no. 5 (2000): 657–68.

Merrifield, Andy. *Henri Lefebvre: A Critical Introduction.* New York: Routledge, 2006.

Mutlu, Servet. *Doğu Sorununun Kökenleri: Ekonomik Açıdan.* İstanbul: Ötüken, 2002.

———. "Economic Bases of Ethnic Separatism in Turkey: An Evaluation of Claims and Counterclaims." *Middle Eastern Studies* 37, no. 4 (2001): 101–35.

———. "The Economic Cost of Civil Conflict in Turkey." *Middle Eastern Studies* 47, no. 1 (2011): 63–80.

———. "Ethnic Kurds in Turkey: A Demographic Study." *International Journal of Middle East Studies* 28, no. 4 (1996): 517–41.

Nairn, Tom. *The Break-up of Britain: Crisis and Neo-Nationalism.* London: NLB, 1977.

Negri, Antonio. *Time for Revolution.* New York and London: Continuum, 2003.

Nielsen, Gritt B. "Peopling Policy: On Conflicting Subjectivities of Fee-Paying Students." In *Policy Worlds: Anthropology and the Analysis of Contemporary Power*, edited by Cris Shore, Susan Wright and Davide Però. New York: Berghahn Books, 2011.

O'Malley, Pat, Lorna Weir, and Clifford Shearing. "Governmentality, Criticism, Politics." *Economy and Society* 26, no. 4 (1997): 501–17.

O'Neil, John D. "The Cultural and Political Context of Patient Dissatisfaction in Cross-Cultural Clinical Encounters: A Canadian Inuit Study." *Medical Anthropology Quarterly* 3, no. 4 (1989): 325–44.

Oran, Baskın. "The Minority Concept and Rights in Turkey: The Lausanne Peace Treaty and Current Issues." In *Human Rights in Turkey*, edited by Zehra F. Kabasakal Arat. Philadelphia: University of Pennsylvania Press, 2007.

Öcalan, Abdullah. *War and Peace in Kurdistan*. Cologne: International Initiative Freedom for Öcalan-Peace in Kurdistan, 2008.

Öniş, Ziya. "The Triumph of Conservative Globalism: The Political Economy of the AKP Era." *Turkish Studies* 13, no. 2 (2012): 135–52.

Özbek, Nadir. *Cumhuriyet Türkiyesi'nde Sosyal Güvenlik ve Sosyal Politikalar*. İstanbul: Emeklilik Gözetim Merkezi: Tarih Vakfı, 2006.

Özbudun, Ergun. "AKP at the Crossroads: Erdoğan's Majoritarian Drift." *South European Society and Politics* 19, no. 2 (2014): 155–67.

———. "From Political Islam to Conservative Democracy: The Case of the Justice and Development Party in Turkey." *South European Society and Politics* 11, no. 3–4 (2006): 543–57.

Özcan, Ahmet. *"Ama Eşkiyalık Çağı Kapandı!": Modern Türkiye'de Son Kürt Eşkiyalık Çağı (1950–1970)*. Istanbul: İletişim, 2018.

Özdağ, Ümit. *Türk Ordusu PKK'yı Nasıl Yendi?: Türkiye PKK'ya Nasıl Teslim Oluyor*. Ankara: Kripto, 2010.

Özdemir, Rahmi, and Emine Kayataş. "Hakkari İlinde Tifo Salgını-Mart 2007: Etkilenen Pediatrik Olguların Değerlendirilmesi." *Journal of Dr. Behcet Uz Children's Hospital* 2, no. 3 (2012):137–40.

Özkahraman, Enver, and Nasrullah Müezzinoğlu. *Hakkari '94*. Ankara: Erk Yayincilik, 1996.

Özmert, Elif N. "Dünya'da ve Türkiye'de aşılama takvimindeki gelişmeler." *Çocuk Sağlığı ve Hastalıkları Dergisi* 51, no. 3 (2008): 168–75.

Pamuk, Şevket. *The Ottoman Empire and European Capitalism, 1820–1913: Trade, Investment, and Production*. Cambridge and New York: Cambridge University Press, 1987.

———. *Türkiye'nin 200 Yıllık İktisadi Tarihi*. Istanbul: Türkiye İş Bankası Kültür Yayınları, 2014.

———. *Uneven Centuries: Economic Development of Turkey since 1820*. Princeton, NJ: Princeton University Press, 2018.

Pamukoğlu, Osman. *Unutulanlar Dışında Yeni Bir Şey Yok: Hakkari ve Kuzey Irak Dağlarındaki Askerler*. İstanbul: Harmoni, 2004.

Payton, Robert L., and Michael P. Moody. *Understanding Philanthropy: Its Meaning and Mission*. Bloomington: Indiana University Press, 2008.

Peukert, D. J. K. *Inside Nazi Germany: Conformity Opposition and Racism in Everyday Life*. London: Batsford, 1987.

PKK. *Partiya Karkerên Kurdistan PKK Yeniden İnşa Kongre Belgeleri*. Istanbul: Çetin Yayınları, 2005.

Poulantzas, Nicos. "The Nation." In *State/Space: A Reader*, edited by Neil Brenner, Bob Jessop, Martin Jones and Gordon Macleod. Malden, MA: Blackwell Pub., 2003.

Pratt, Mary Louise. *Imperial Eyes: Travel Writing and Transculturation*. London and New York: Routledge, 2008.
Reid, Steve. "Community Service for Health Professionals: Human Resources." *South African Health Review*, no. 1 (2002): 135–60.
Republic of Turkey Prime Ministry Undersecretariat of Public Order and Security. *The Silent Revolution: Turkey's Democratic Change and Transformation Inventory 2002–2012*. Ankara: Undersecreteriat of Public Order and Security Publications, 2013.
Roseberry, William. "Hegemony and the Language of Contention." In *Everyday Forms of State Formation: Revolution and the Negotiation of Rule in Modern Mexico*, edited by Gilbert M. Joseph and Daniel Nugent. Durham and London: Duke University Press, 1994.
Rubel, Arthur J. "Compulsory Medical Service and Primary Health Care: A Mexican Case Study." In *Anthropology and Primary Health Care*, edited by Jeannine Coreil and J. Dennis Mull. Boulder: Westview Press, 1990.
Sağlık Bakanlığı (Ministry of Health). *Yataklı Tedavi Kurumları İstatistik Yıllığı 1995*. Ankara: Sağlık Bakanlığı Tedavi Hizmetleri Genel Müdürlüğü, 2001.
———. *Sağlık İstatistikleri 1996*. Ankara: Sağlık Bakanlığı Araştırma, Planlama ve Koordinasyon Kurulu Başkanlığı, 1997.
———. *Sağlık İstatistikleri 2002*. Ankara: Sağlık Bakanlığı Araştırma, Planlama ve Koordinasyon Kurulu Başkanlığı, 2003.
———. *Yataklı Tedavi Kurumları İstatistik Yıllığı 2003*. Ankara: Sağlık Bakanlığı Tedavi Hizmetleri Genel Müdürlüğü, 2004.
———. *Yataklı Tedavi Kurumları İstatistik Yıllığı 2006*. Ankara: Sağlık Bakanlığı Tedavi Hizmetleri Genel Müdürlüğü, 2007.
Sağlık ve Sosyal Yardım Bakanlığı (Ministry of Health and Social Assistance). *Sağlık İstatistik Yıllığı 1964–67*. Ankara: Güneş Matbaacılık, 1971.
Sakalys, Jurate A. "Restoring the Patient's Voice the Therapeutics of Illness Narratives." *Journal of Holistic Nursing* 21, no. 3 (2003): 228–41.
Sanford, Victoria. "Contesting Displacement in Colombia: Citizenship and State Sovereignty at the Margins." In *Anthropology in the Margins of the State*, edited by Veena Das and Deborah Poole. Santa Fe, NM: School of American Research Press, 2004.
Saraçoğlu, Cenk. "İslami-Muhafazakar Milliyetçiliğin Millet Tasarımı: AKP Döneminde Kürt Politikası." *Praksis* 26 (2011): 45–47.
———. "Türkiye Sağı, Akp Ve Kürt Meselesi." In *Türk Sağı: Mitler, Fetişler, Düşman İmgeleri*, edited by İnci Özkan Kerestecioğlu and Güven Gürkan Öztan. Cağaloğlu, İstanbul: İletişim, 2012.
Sarızeybek, Erdal. *Şemdinli'de Sınırı Aşmak*. Istanbul: Pozitif, 2011.
Scheper-Hughes, Nancy. *Death without Weeping: The Violence of Everyday Life in Brazil*. Berkeley: University of California Press, 1992.
———. "The Primacy of the Ethical: Propositions for a Militant Anthropology." *Current Anthropology* 36, no. 3 (1995): 409–40.
Schepher-Hughes, Nancy, and M. M Lock. "The Mindful Body: A Prolegomenon to Future Work in Medical Anthropology." *Medical Anthropology Quarterly* 1, no. 1 (1987): 6–41.

Schmitt, Carl. *Political Theology: Four Chapters on the Concept of Sovereignty.* Chicago: University of Chicago Press, 2005.

Scott, Joan W. "The Evidence of Experience." *Critical Inquiry* 17, no. 4 (1991): 773–97.

Shillony, Ben-Ami. "The Flourishing Demon: Japan in the Role of the Jews." In *Demonizing the Other: Antisemitism, Racism and Xenophobia*, edited by Robert S. Wistrich. Amsterdam: Harwood Academic, 1999.

Shore, Cris, and Susan Wright. "Policy: A New Field of Anthropology." In *Anthropology of Policy: Critical Perspectives on Governance and Power*, edited by Cris Shore and Susan Wright. London and New York: Routledge, 1997.

Silverman, David. *Communication and Medical Practice: Social Relations in the Clinic.* London: Sage, 1987.

Smith, Anthony D. *Nationalism: Theory, Ideology, History.* Cambridge: Polity Press, 2010.

Sohn-Rethel, Alfred. *Intellectual and Manual Labour: A Critique of Epistemology.* Atlantic Highlands, NJ: Humanities Press, 1978.

Steinmetz, George. "Introduction: Culture and the State." In *State/Culture: State-Formation after the Cultural Turn*, edited by George Steinmetz. Ithaca: Cornell University Press, 1999.

Straus, Scott. *The Order of Genocide: Race, Power, and War in Rwanda.* Ithaca: Cornell University Press, 2006.

Surbone, Antonella. "Telling the Truth to Patients with Cancer: What is the Truth?" *The Lancet Oncology* 7, no. 11 (2006): 944–50.

Şimşek, Selahattin. *Hakkâri Dedikleri.* Istanbul: Martı Yayınları, 1990.

Tang, Sannie Y., and Annette J. Browne. "'Race' matters: racialization and egalitarian discourses involving aboriginal people in the Canadian health care context." *Ethnicity and Health* 13, no. 2 (2008): 109–27.

Tanık, Bülent, ed. *Umumi Müfettişler Toplantı Tutanakları-1936.* Ankara: Dipnot Yayınları, 2010.

Taşkın, M. Fayik, ed. *Sağlık Kurultayı Belgeleri (3-4-5 Aralık 2010, Diyarbakır).* Diyarbakır: Aram Yayınları, 2012.

Taylor, Charles. "The Politics of Recognition." In *Multiculturalism: Examining the Politics of Recognition*, edited by Amy Gutmann. Princeton: Princeton University Press, 1994.

Tekeli, İlhan. *Türkiye'de Bölgesel Eşitsizlik ve Bölge Planlama Yazıları.* İstanbul: Tarih Vakfı, 2008.

The Gracious Quran: A Modern-Phrased Interpretation in English. Translated by Ahmad Zaki Hammad. Lisle, IL: Lucent Interpretations, 2009.

Tuğal, Cihan. *Passive Revolution: Absorbing the Islamic Challenge to Capitalism.* Stanford, CA: Stanford University Press, 2009.

Turan, Ömer. "Kudretli Devlet, Manevi Kalkınma, Ağır Sanayii: Türk Sağı Ve Kalkınma." In *Türk Sağı: Mitler, Fetişler, Düşman İmgeleri*, edited by İnci Özkan Kerestecioğlu and Güven Gürkan Öztan. Istanbul: İletişim, 2012.

TÜİK Türkiye İstatistik Kurumu (Turkish Statistical Institute). *Genel Sanayi ve İşyerleri Sayımı, 2002.* Ankara: TÜİK, 2006.

———. *Bölgesel Göstergeler 2009: TRB 2 Van, Muş, Bitlis, Hakkari.* Ankara: TÜİK, 2010.

———. *Seçilmiş Göstergelerle Hakkari 2012.* Ankara: TÜİK, 2013.

———. *Seçilmiş Göstergelerle Hakkari 2013.* Ankara: TÜİK, 2014.

———. *Yaşam Memnuniyeti Araştırması 2013.* Ankara: TÜİK, 2014

Üner, Ragıp, and Nusret Fişek. *Sağlık Hizmetlerinin Sosyalleştirilmesi ve Uygulama Planı Üzerinde Çalışmalar*. Ankara: SSYB, 1961.

Üsküll, Zafer. *Siyaset Ve Asker: Cumhuriyet Döneminde Sıkıyönetim Uygulamaları*. Ankara: İmge Kitapevi, 1997.

Wallerstein, Immanuel Maurice. *The Modern World System 1: Capitalist Agriculture and the Origins of the European World-Economy in the Sixteenth Century*. Berkeley, CA and London: University of California Press, 2011.

Weber, Max. *Economy and Society: An Outline of Interpretive Sociology*. 2 vols. Edited by Guenther Roth and Claus Wittich. Berkeley: University of California Press, 1978.

White, Jenny. *Muslim Nationalism and the New Turks*. Princeton, NJ: Princeton University Press, 2013.

Wibulpolprasert, Suwit, and Paichit Pengpaibon. "Integrated Strategies to Tackle the Inequitable Distribution of Doctors in Thailand: Four Decades of Experience." *Human Resources for Health* 1, no. 12 (2003): 1–17.

Williams, Robert R. *Hegel's Ethics of Recognition*. Berkeley: University of California Press, 1997.

Wilson, Fiona. "In the Name of the State? Schools and Teachers in an Andean Province." In *States of Imagination: Ethnographic Explorations of the Post-Colonial State*, edited by Thomas Blom Hansen and Finn Stepputat. Durham, NC: Duke University Press, 2001.

Winnicott, Donald Woods. *Playing and Reality*. New York: Basic Books, 1971.

Yadırgı, Veli. *The Political Economy of the Kurds of Turkey: From the Ottoman Empire to the Turkish Republic*. Cambridge: Cambridge University Press, 2017.

Yalçın-Heckmann, Lale. *Tribe and Kinship among the Kurds*. Frankfurt am Main: P. Lang, 1991.

Yavuz, Hakan. *Nostalgia for the Empire: The Politics of Neo-Ottomanism*. New York: Oxford University Press, 2020.

Yeğen, Mesut. *Müstakbel Türk'ten Sözde Vatandaşa: Cumhuriyet Ve Kürtler*. Istanbul: İletişim, 2006.

———. Introduction to *Kürtler'e Vurulan Kelepçe: Şark Islahat Planı*, 11–18, by Mehmet Bayrak. Beysukent, Ankara: Öz-Ge, 2009.

———. "The Kurdish Peace Process in Turkey: Genesis, Evolution and Prospects." In *Global Turkey in Europe III*, edited by Senem Aydın-Düzgit, Daniela Huber, Meltem Müftüler-Baç, E. Fuat Keyman, Michael Schwarz and Nathalie Tocci. Istanbul: Stiftung Mercator, 2015.

Yeşiltuna, Serap, ed. *Atatürk ve Kürtler: Resmi Kanun, Kararname, Rapor ve Tutanaklarla*. Istanbul: İleri Yayınları, 2007.

Yörük, Erdem. "The Politics of the Turkish Welfare System Transformation in the Neoliberal Era: Welfare as Mobilization and Containment." Ph.D. diss., The Johns Hopkins University, 2012.

———. "Welfare Provision as Political Containment the Politics of Social Assistance and the Kurdish Conflict in Turkey." *Politics & Society* 40, no. 4 (2012): 517–47.

Yörük, Erdem, and Murat Yüksel. "Class and Politics in Turkey's Gezi Protests." *New Left Review* 89, no. 1 (2014): 103–23.

Yurt Ansiklopedisi: Türkiye, il il. Istanbul: Anadolu Yayıncılık, 1982.

Zeydanlıoğlu, Welat. "The White Turkish Man's Burden: Orientalism, Kemalism and the Kurds in Turkey." In *Neo-Colonial Mentalities in Contemporary Europe? Language and the Discourse in the Construction of Identities*, edited by Guido Rings and Anne Ife. Newcastle upon Tyne: Cambridge Scholars Publishing, 2008.

Žižek, Slavoj. "The Spectre of Ideology." In *Mapping Ideology*, edited by Slavoj Žižek. London and New York: Verso, 1994.

———. *The Sublime Object of Ideology*. London and New York: Verso, 1989.

Zurn, Pascal, Mario R. Dal Poz, Barbara Stilwell, and Orvill Adams. "Imbalance in the Health Workforce." *Human Resources for Health* 2, no. 1 (2004).

Zürcher, Erik Jan. *Turkey: A Modern History*. London and New York: I.B. Tauris, 1993.

Index

Adalet ve Kalkınma Partisi (AKP) xv, xvi, xvii, xviii, xix, xx, 1, 2, 4, 6, 20, 29, 30, 43, 77, 84, 88, 90, 92, 94, 106, 119, 124, 131–136, 139–141, 144, 149, 168, 187, 203, 210, 212, 219, 221, 234, 238, 254, 283, 288, 290
   Hakkâri 38n10, 154, 160, 164, 166, 191, 199, 220, 281
   health reforms 3, 155, 180, 232, 236
   Kurdish strategy *see* Kurdish policy
   nationalism 5, 36, 37, 137, 142–148, 151, 160, 163, 167, 170n34 209, 223, 230, 279, 280, 284, 285
Animal Husbandry 18, 24, 46, 62, 65, 72, 89
Assyrians 20, 21, 89, 147

Bare Life 14, 16, 58, 60, 138, 238, 244, 282, 283
Biopolitics 2, 17, 87, 90, 138, 141, 142, 150, 167, 210
   biopolitical aspect of nationalism 16, 47
   biopolitical perspective 137, 140, 203

Border 3, 7, 15, 99, 104, 105, 116, 117, 135, 245, 247

cross-border trade *see* smuggling
Capitalism xvii, 90, 136
Citizenship 5, 30, 45, 97, 216, 218, 221–223, 227n46, 284–285, 288–291
   citizenly dissatisfaction 211–212, 221–222, 280
   equal citizenship 183, 210, 213–214, 219, 221, 223, 273
Collective Punishment 36, 43, 53–60, 65–68, 70–73, 77
Colonialism xix, 89, 187, 202, 210, 235, 236, 255
Compulsory Service 25, 30, 31, 37, 96, 176, 184, 229–231, 240, 242, 263, 269, 273, 274–275n19
   law 3, 99, 101–103, 105–106, 151, 154, 216, 232, 233, 236–238, 244
Contract System 105–106
Counter-Insurgency xv, xvii, 4, 18, 21, 54, 67, 89, 136, 150

Counter-Terror Strategy 69
Cumhuriyet Halk Partisi (CHP) 45, 59, 64, 73, 138
Çukurca 18, 20, 21, 23, 26, 32, 33, 66, 68, 69, 73, 81n77, 98, 104, 124, 199, 247, 257, 281
  health posts 26, 245

Dehumanization 55–57, 176, 210
Democratic Opening xvi, 140, 148
Demokrat Parti (DP) 59, 64, 126n28, 128n66
Development 4, 16, 27, 31, 37, 86, 88–90, 94, 107, 125, 138, 140, 167, 237, 253, 281
  narratives 13, 176, 213, 214, 284
  performance 47, 141
  uneven development 13, 285
Disciplinary Normalization 15, 16
Discrimination 37, 92, 146, 205, 207, 230, 257, 258, 260, 262, 280
  positive 93, 219, 220
Distribution of Doctors 230–232, 236
Doctor-Patient Encounter 175, 188, 202–203, 241, 257–258, 260, 263, 268

Eastern Reform Plan 46, 53, 61
Economy 17, 18, 23–24, 59, 61, 62, 64, 72, 86, 88, 89, 124, 132, 140, 174
Elections xv, 6, 45, 132, 133, 147, 232
Emergency Rule 4, 46, 55, 60, 66, 69, 70, 72, 76, 81n81
Erdoğan, Recep Tayyip 132, 134, 137, 138, 141, 142, 143, 145, 146, 149, 164, 170n36, 232, 281, 282, 283, 284
Ethnicity 3, 8, 20, 45, 46, 56, 77n4, 94, 143, 174
Ethnopolitical Challenges 6, 286, 289, 290, 291

ir/rationality 285, 287

Family Health Centers 25, 159, 160, 177, 178, 179, 196, 199, 269, 276n42, 281

Gendarmerie 18, 19, 50, 53, 54, 60, 62, 63, 65, 69, 73, 81n81, 116
  oppression 59, 66, 74–76
General Health Insurance Scheme 152, 180, 181, 215
General Inspectorate 4, 59–61, 64, 74, 76
General Practitioners (GP) 1, 3, 25, 26, 35, 37, 95–99, 101, 103, 104, 106, 107, 109, 122, 151, 152, 156, 157, 200, 229, 236, 238, 239, 240, 242, 243, 245, 247, 252, 256, 257, 269, 276n42
Green Card 115, 152, 157, 179–181

Hakkâri
  Hakkâri health centers 109, 110
  Hakkâri public hospital xvii, 84, 99, 102, 104, 105, 109, 110, 111, 112, 113, 115, 153, 154, 155, 177, 182, 183, 185, 186, 188, 189, 190, 191, 192, 193, 194, 195, 196, 197, 198, 199, 202, 204, 205, 241, 244, 252, 253, 256, 262, 264, 265, 266, 267, 268, 298
  University of Hakkâri 26, 34, 38n10, 161, 184, 200, 204, 205, 213, 214, 246, 261, 281
Halkların Demokratik Partisi (HDP) xvii, xx, 138, 139
Health Clerks 27, 95, 96, 98, 106, 269, 297
Health Personnel 17, 98, 101, 230, 232
Health Posts xvii, 25, 97–102, 104, 106, 107, 114, 115, 122, 128n70, 156, 157, 159, 207, 208, 239, 243,

245, 252, 258, 261, 262, 269–272, 277, 297
Health Professionals 1, 18, 27, 35, 99, 269, 271
Health Services 28, 30, 31, 97, 111, 116, 117, 120–123, 126n27, 154–158, 173, 174, 179, 180, 185, 187, 191, 199, 204, 205, 209, 210, 211, 212, 218, 221, 222, 223, 231, 232, 236, 265
Health Workforce 1, 95–97, 101–104, 106, 107, 167, 173, 176, 183, 194, 195, 230
Healthcare Providers 1, 107, 131, 174, 175, 177, 186
Healthcare Provision xvii, xix, 1, 3, 5, 28, 36, 37, 83, 85, 94, 96, 97, 101, 102, 107, 120, 124, 131, 132, 151, 152, 164, 166, 167, 173, 174, 175, 176, 177, 182, 183, 184, 185, 190, 191, 199, 200, 211, 212, 213, 214, 215, 216, 217, 218, 220, 221, 222, 232, 250, 264, 280, 281, 287, 288, 289, 290
Hegemony xvii, xix, 7, 45, 132, 135, 167, 173, 187, 223, 284, 289–291
Homo Sacer 15–16, 282

Identification 3, 5, 234, 235, 260, 269, 289
Identity 2, 4, 47, 56, 57, 136, 138, 141, 143, 146, 150, 167, 175, 220, 231, 232, 251, 275n30, 282, 283, 292n4
 Kurdish identity xx, 142, 148, 200, 202, 203, 205, 219, 285
 national identity 10, 15, 46, 47, 137, 210
 Turkish identity 48, 94
Immunization 115, 120, 123, 157–159, 173
Indirect State Racism 36, 49, 83–90, 92–94, 107, 117, 121, 175, 176, 185, 187, 206, 209, 210

Infant and Child Mortalities 117, 119–120
Iran 3, 18, 20, 21, 41, 46, 52, 59, 61, 62, 74, 80n52, 89, 104–105, 109, 116
Iraq xvi, 18, 21, 46, 59, 61–63, 81n77, 89, 98, 104, 108, 109, 162

Kemalism 138, 143, 146
Kemalist Turkey xv, xvii, 36, 43, 77, 84, 85, 88, 93, 95, 117, 136, 187, 223
Koma Civakên Kurdistan (KCK) 4, 149–151, 160–163, 167, 251, 282, 288
Kurds xv–xx, 4–6, 18, 20, 35, 37, 41n60, 44–47, 69, 73, 76, 77, 86, 90, 92, 93, 94, 132, 135, 136, 137, 139, 141, 142, 146, 148, 150, 151, 160, 165–168, 173, 200, 203, 205, 207, 210, 219, 231, 245, 246, 255, 258, 281, 284, 286, 290
 assimilation 2, 14–17, 25, 46, 51–53, 58–59, 77, 93, 135, 146, 209, 230, 234, 280, 282
 official discourse 1, 6, 9, 36, 55–57, 131, 141, 143, 147, 257, 282
Kurdish Issue *see* Kurdish Question
Kurdish Opening *see* Democratic Opening
Kurdish Question xv–xx, 2, 3, 6, 36, 43, 126n29, 131, 135–137, 140–142, 146–148, 187, 199, 220, 221, 227n47, 230, 242, 243, 290
Kurdish Policy xv–xx, 1–2, 6, 135–137, 142, 144, 148, 199, 219
Kurdish Strategy xviii, 131, 187
Kurdish Studies xviii, 6, 7, 9, 279
Kurdishness xviii, 37, 56–58, 77, 88, 93, 131, 132, 137, 141, 142, 144, 146, 167, 199, 200, 202–207, 242, 283, 284
 self-valorization 210–211

320 | Index

Kurdistan xvi, 4, 46, 89, 149, 162, 210, 219, 226, 258

Maternal and Infant/Child Health Services 121, 123, 156, 158, 178, 179
Medical Equipment 3, 97, 100, 103, 107, 109, 111, 113, 114, 151, 152, 154, 213, 215, 265
Milliyetçi Hareket Partisi (MHP) 68, 138, 143
Ministry of Health (MoH) 30, 96, 99, 113, 115, 118, 121, 123, 129n101, 180, 185, 214
Ministry of Health and Social Assistance (MHSA) *see* Ministry of Health
Modernity

Nation xvi, xx, 8, 9, 14–16, 37, 44, 45, 56, 86, 88, 131, 134–138, 140, 142–146, 148, 167, 170n29, 286
  becoming of nation 10–14, 223, 233
  being of nation 10–13, 232
Nationalism
  everyday nationalism 7–10
  sub-state nationalism 5, 289
Nation-Building 5, 8, 9, 14, 16, 20, 21, 138
Nation-State xvii, 2, 7, 9–10, 14–15, 20, 21, 44, 55, 59, 68, 89, 90, 94, 132, 136, 141, 160, 167, 213, 222, 223, 231
Negotiations xvi, xix–xx, 2, 29, 134, 136, 144, 147
Nursing and Midwifery Professionals 1, 27, 95, 97, 98, 99, 105, 106, 114, 118, 119, 123, 176, 198, 261, 262, 269–273, 277n56, 297

Ottoman Empire 20, 43–45, 61, 62, 88, 89, 90, 129n95, 134, 143

heritage 137, 144, 145, 146
Öcalan, Abdullah xvi, xx, 20, 136, 149, 210

Passive Revolution xvii, 148, 150
Patients xix, 3, 18, 27, 28, 96, 97, 98, 99, 100, 102, 103, 104, 105, 106, 107, 108, 109, 110, 111, 112, 113, 114, 153–156, 160, 191–198, 200–205, 207, 209, 213–215, 217, 231, 236, 240, 241, 257, 258, 260, 261, 262, 264–268, 270, 281, 283, 298
Patient Rights Unit 26, 191, 201, 218, 219, 268
Patient Satisfaction 26, 174, 177, 182, 185–188, 190, 199, 225n17, 263
  dissatisfaction xvii, xviii, 168, 173–177, 187, 199, 210–212, 222, 230, 273, 280, 290
  distrust 117, 121–123, 175, 183, 184, 188, 190, 195, 208–209, 221
  questionnaires 187
Partiya Karkerên Kurdistanê (PKK) xvi–xvii, xix–xx, 1, 2, 4, 32, 36, 39n10, 49, 50, 51, 58, 69, 70, 77, 81n77, 89, 134, 137, 141, 147, 149, 157, 162, 205, 211, 219, 242, 249, 251, 255, 258, 260, 262, 270
  guerilla 19, 21, 47, 48, 54–55, 62, 67–68, 71–72, 76, 135, 148, 160, 161, 164, 165, 166, 210, 247, 261
  insurgency 20, 47, 60, 67, 135
Politics of Identity 2, 136–138, 141–143, 220, 232, 282–283
Politics of Service 2, 3, 4, 136, 137–138, 141, 142, 150, 167, 220, 232, 282–283
Pre-AKP Period xvi, 36, 43, 77, 84, 88, 92–94, 119, 124, 135, 154, 164, 212, 221
Preventive Medicine 1, 98, 109, 121, 128, 156–158

Production of Space 37, 233, 234
  endurance 230, 235–238, 240, 243, 244, 248, 249, 252, 253, 256, 257, 258, 260, 262–265, 268, 269, 271, 273, 276n39, 281
  instrumentalism 235, 238, 242–244, 251, 253, 257, 260, 263–265, 269, 270, 273, 276n49
  national space 230, 232, 233
Public Health 106, 107, 108, 115, 117, 120, 122–123, 128n70, 297
Public Investment xviii, 17, 88, 90–93, 131, 132, 136, 138, 139, 141, 151, 152

Recognition xviii, xx, 17, 55, 56, 58, 132, 137, 141, 148, 218, 229, 248, 283–284, 288, 292n4
Resistance xvi, xviii, 1, 7, 10, 13, 31, 32, 54, 75, 122, 123, 133, 158, 207, 210, 262, 270, 272
Rights-Bearing Citizens 217
Rotation System 99–101, 103–104
Rural Areas 52, 73, 89, 101, 231, 266

Shortage of Doctors 98, 101, 105, 231, 236
Smuggling 18, 21, 54, 59, 61–63, 64–66, 74, 76, 80n52, 116
Social Assistance xviii, 133, 137, 139, 140, 156, 171n47, 219, 267
Social Policy xvii–xviii, 1–2, 4–6, 17, 38, 131, 132, 136, 220, 222, 231
  decentralization 287–289
Sovereignty xv, 2, 16, 36, 40n49, 43, 46, 48, 52, 53, 59, 75–76, 86, 148–150, 286, 289, 290
  sovereign violence 36, 46, 55, 58, 73, 77, 117, 131, 136, 149, 160, 164–165, 167, 175, 176, 185, 206, 209– 210, 282
  Turkish sovereignty 4, 73, 77, 146, 161

(Medical) Specialists 1, 3, 25, 26, 35, 37, 84, 95–107, 110, 111, 114, 151, 154–155, 171n46, 176, 179, 187, 191, 193–197, 198, 200, 202, 206, 207, 208, 209, 216, 229, 231, 236, 237, 240–244, 247, 248, 252–256, 258, 262–267, 269, 273, 275n21
State-Citizen Relations xix, 36, 37, 43, 84, 174, 175, 185–186, 188, 221
Stereotypes 35, 245, 246, 248, 254, 255, 259, 263
Stigmatization 32, 35, 88, 245, 246, 248, 254, 259, 262, 272
Şemdinli 17, 18, 20, 25, 51, 63, 68, 71, 82n81, 102, 106, 124, 243, 280
  Şemdinli health posts 156, 157, 297
  Şemdinli public hospital 104, 114, 156, 193, 200, 243, 253

Terror 4, 69, 70, 147, 150, 161, 258, 282
Turks 2, 27, 35, 44, 45, 46, 56, 58, 77n4, 93, 94, 142, 204, 205, 207, 245, 246, 251
Turkish Nationalism 7, 44, 47, 56–58, 93–94, 131–132, 134, 137, 140, 142–148, 151, 160, 163, 167, 187, 209, 210, 248, 259, 269, 284, 285
  state-nationalism 2, 5, 9–10, 32, 36, 37, 131, 138, 148, 151, 167, 279, 284
Turkish Studies 6
Turkishness 2, 35, 43, 45, 46, 56, 58, 61, 93, 137, 142–148, 170n34, 221, 223, 242

Underdevelopment 31, 36, 94
Unitary Theory of Space 233
Urban Areas 17, 18, 20, 22, 24, 25, 27, 47, 90, 97, 99, 118, 119, 120, 121, 124, 150, 177, 230, 231, 238
Vaccination 3, 116–117, 120, 122–123, 152, 156–157, 160, 207, 272

Villages 34, 47, 48–49, 50, 55, 59, 62, 63, 65, 69, 72, 74–75, 96, 97, 102, 104, 117, 118, 119, 123, 205, 208, 212, 214, 236, 237, 251, 253, 254, 255, 265, 272
  evacuation xvii, 4, 17, 18, 21–24, 33, 54, 60, 67–68, 77, 89, 124, 150, 271, 280, 295
  evacuees 32, 178, 196, 206
  guards 32, 70, 71, 76, 81n77

Yüksekova 3, 4, 17, 18, 20, 21, 22, 23, 25, 26, 27, 41n68, 63, 68, 73, 74, 76, 102, 106, 107, 115, 123, 124, 144, 151, 157, 176, 193, 207, 219, 227n48, 254, 258, 280, 281
  Yüksekova health posts 207, 258, 262, 270, 271, 277n56, 297
  Yüksekova public hospital 104, 114, 192, 194, 198, 203, 217, 218, 256, 261

Culture, Society and Political Economy in Turkey

Isabel David and Kumru Toktamiş
General Editors

The series provides a publishing platform for pioneering research on understudied aspects of culture, society, and political economy in Turkey, including minorities, local politics, social movements, gender, popular culture, political parties, religion, and related fields. This series captures critical perspectives in response to the authoritarian context that may pose obstacles to rigorous research. As such, the series welcomes work on the methodological challenges of studying Turkey as the country is going through a process of accelerated societal, political, and economic change, generating clashes between competing interests and projects. The series aims to fully address these contentions by expanding knowledge on these areas. Both established and emerging scholars are invited to publish their research, either as monographs or as edited volumes. With such an approach, the ultimate purpose of the series is to decisively shape the field of studies on Turkey and became a reference for scholars working in the field.

To receive more information, please contact:

editorial@peterlang.com

To order books, please contact our Customer Service Department:

peterlang@presswarehouse.com (within the U.S.)
orders@peterlang.com (outside the U.S.)

Visit our website at www.peterlang.com.

www.ingramcontent.com/pod-product-compliance
Ingram Content Group UK Ltd.
Pitfield, Milton Keynes, MK11 3LW, UK
UKHW022151230426
12049UKWH00003BA/37